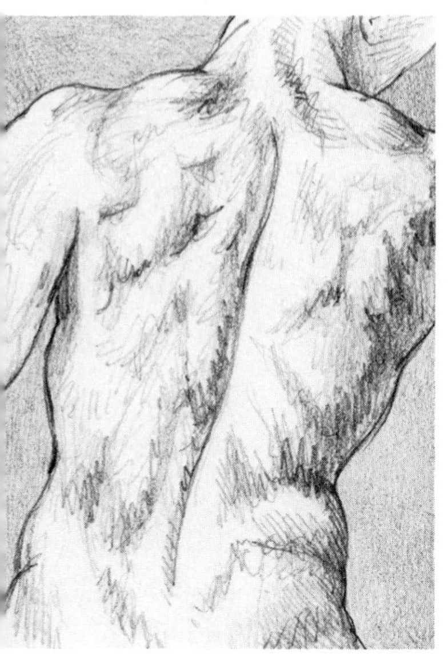

the spine in sports

Edited By

Stephen H. Hochschuler, M.D.

Co-Founder, Texas Back Institute
Plano, Texas

HANLEY & BELFUS, INC./Philadelphia
MOSBY—YEAR BOOK/St Louis • Baltimore • Boston • Chicago • London
Philadelphia • Sydney • Toronto

Publisher: HANLEY & BELFUS, INC.
210 South 13th Street
Philadelphia, PA 19107
(215)546-7293

North American and worldwide sales and distribution:

MOSBY—YEAR BOOK, INC.
11830 Westline Industrial Drive
St. Louis, MO 63146

In Canada: THE C.V. MOSBY COMPANY, LTD.
5240 Finch Avenue East
Unit 1
Scarborough, Ontario M1S 4P2
Canada

THE SPINE IN SPORTS ISBN 1-56053-005-7

Library of Congress catalog card number 90-82772

Last digit is the print number: 9 8 7 6 5 4 3 2 1

CONTENTS

Chapter **Page**

CONTRIBUTORS

Stephen L. Aronoff, M.D.
Endocrine Associates of Dallas; Clinical Assistant Professor, University of Texas Southwestern Medical Center, Dallas, Texas

F. Alan Barber, M.D., FACS
Staff, Plano Orthopedic and Sports Medicine Center, Plano, Texas; Clinical Assistant Professor of Orthopedic Surgery, University of Texas Southwestern Medical Center, Dallas, Texas

Bradley T. Britt, M.D.
Staff, Plano Orthopedic and Sports Medicine Center, Plano, Texas

Charles V. Burton, M.D.
Medical Director, Institute for Low Back Care, Minneapolis, Minnesota

William H. Dillin, M.D.
Staff, Kerlan-Jobe Orthopaedic Clinic, Inglewood, California

Steven G. Dorfman, M.D.
Endocrine Associates of Dallas; Clinical Associate Professor, University of Texas Southwestern Medical Center, Dallas, Texas

David F. Fardon, M.D.
Assistant Clinical Professor of Orthopedic Surgery, University of Tennessee, Knoxville; Knoxville Orthopedic Clinic, St. Mary's Medical Center, Knoxville, Tennessee

Larry Charles Feeler, P.T.
President, Odessa Physical Therapy, P.C.; Guest Lecturer, Texas Tech Health Science Center, Lubbock, Texas

Stanley Feld, M.D.
Endocrine Associates of Dallas; Clinical Associate Professor of Internal Medicine, University of Texas Southwestern Medical Center, Dallas, Texas

Jeffrey E. Flemming, M.D.
Clinical Instructor, Orthopedics, Oregon Health Sciences University, Portland, Oregon

John W. Frymoyer, M.D.
Professor of Orthopedic Surgery and Director, McClure Musculoskeletal Research Center, Department of Orthopaedics and Rehabilitation, University of Vermont, Burlington, Vermont

Robert W. Gaines, Jr., M.D., FACS
Professor of Orthopaedic Surgery, University of Missouri Health Sciences Center, Columbia, Missouri

Billy Glisan, M.S.
Director of Training, Back WeRCs, Texas Back Institute, Plano, Texas

Serge Gracovetsky, Ph.D.
Associate Professor, Concordia University, Montreal, Quebec, Canada

Richard D. Guyer, M.D.
Medical Director of Research, Texas Back Institute Research Foundation, Plano, Texas; Associate Clinical Professor, Division of Orthopaedic Surgery, University of Texas Southwestern Medical School, Dallas, Texas

David T. Hanks, Ph.D.
Consulting Clinical Psychologist, Texas Back Institute, Plano, Texas

John A. Herring, M.D.
Department of Orthopaedic Surgery, Texas Scottish Rite Hospital, Dallas, Texas

Stephen H. Hochschuler, M.D.
Co-founder of the Texas Back Institute, Plano, Texas; Clinical Instructor, Division of Orthopaedic Surgery, University of Texas Southwestern Medical School, Dallas, Texas

Thomas Edgar Hyde, D.C., CCSP
Postgraduate Faculty; Logan College of Chiropractic, Chesterfield, Missouri; Staff, North Miami Chiropractic Center, North Miami, Florida

James R. Kasser, M.D.
Assistant Professor, Harvard Medical School; Staff, Boston Children's Hospital, Boston, Massachusetts

Thomas A. Lorren, P.T.
Director of Rehabilitation, Texas Back Institute, Plano, Texas

Clinton Maxwell, M.D.
Staff, Texas Back Institute, Plano Texas

James Maxwell, M.D.
Staff, Kerlan-Jobe Orthopaedic Clinic, Inglewood, California

Mary Lynn Mayfield, R.N., B.S.N.
Educational Coordinator, Back WeRCs, Texas Back Institute, Plano, Texas

Lyle J. Micheli, M.D.
Director, Division of Sports Medicine, Children's Hospital Medical Center; Assistant Clinical Professor of Orthopaedic Surgery, Harvard Medical School, Boston, Massachusetts

S. James Montgomery, M.B., B.Ch., FFARCS(I)
Physician to The Dallas Cowboys; former Assistant Professor, University of Texas Southwestern Medical Center, Dallas, Texas

Donna D. Ohnmeiss, M.S.
Research Coordinator, Texas Back Institute Research Foundation, Plano, Texas

Stanley V. Paris, Ph.D., P.T.
Professor and Chairman, Institute of Graduate Physical Therapy; Clinical Professor, Medical College of Georgia; Director, Flagler Physical Therapy Associates, St. Augustine, Florida

John H. Peloza, M.D.
Staff, Dallas Spine Group, Dallas, Texas

Ralph F. Rashbaum, M.D.
Co-founder of the Texas Back Institute, Plano, Texas; Clinical Instructor, Division of Orthopaedic Surgery, University of Texas Southwestern Medical School, Dallas, Texas

John J. Regan, M.D.
Staff, Texas Back Institute; Clinical Instructor, Division of Orthopaedic Surgery, University of Texas Southwestern Medical School, Dallas, Texas

Jose E. Rodriguez, M.D.
Spine Surgery Fellow, Texas Back Institute, Plano, Texas

Jeffrey A. Saal, M.D.
Director, Research and Education, San Francisco Spine Institute, Daly City, California

Barton L. Sachs, M.D.
Staff, Concord Hospital; Concord Orthopaedics, Concord, New Hampshire

Richard Sachson, M.D.
Endocrine Associates of Dallas; Clinical Associate Professor, University of Texas Southwestern Medical Center, Dallas, Texas

David K. Selby, M.D.
Clinical Professor of Orthopaedic Surgery, University of Texas Southwestern Medical School; Staff, Dallas Spine Group, Dallas, Texas

Philip R. Shalen, M.D.
Neuroradiologist and Diagnostic Radiologist, Radiology Consultants of North Dallas and Medical City Dallas Humana Hospital, Dallas, Texas

Chris G. Sheets, B.S.
Assistant Manager, Back WeRCs, Texas Back Institute, Plano, Texas

Alexis P. Shelokov, M.D.
Staff, Texas Back Institute, Plano, Texas

Amy Spiegel, B.A.
Staff, Texas Back Institute, Plano, Texas

J. Richard Steadman, M.D.
Staff, Dallas Spine Group, Dallas, Texas

William J. Stith, Ph.D.
Director, Texas Back Institute Research Foundation, Plano, Texas; Assistant Clinical Professor, Division of Orthopaedic Surgery, University of Texas Southwestern Medical School, Dallas, Texas

John J. Triano, M.A., D.C.
Professor and Chief of Clinics Staff; Director, Spinal Ergonomics Lab; The National College of Chiropractic, Lombard, Illinois

Valerie VanderLaan, P.A.-C.
Physician Assistant, Texas Back Institute, Plano, Texas

Robert G. Watkins, M.D.
Staff, Kerlan-Jobe Orthopaedic Clinic, Inglewood, California

Arthur H. White, M.D.
Medical Director, San Francisco Spine Institute, Daly City, California

Leon L. Wiltse, M.D.
Orthopaedic Staff, Memorial Medical Center of Long Beach, Long Beach, California

PREFACE

The Spine in Sports is a much-expanded version of a recent issue of SPINE: State of the Art Reviews, a review series on the spine from the same publisher. This freestanding book contains several chapters not in the SPINE:STARs issue plus a series of case reports by authorities on the care of the spine-injured athlete. The intent is to make this valuable information available to a wider audience of orthopedic surgeons, neurosurgeons, sports medicine physicians, other team physicians, and athletic trainers—to any health care provider whose responsibilities include caring for athletes at risk for spinal injury or other spinal disorders.

An attempt is made to give an overview of current information regarding basic science, prevention, diagnosis, treatment, rehabilitation, and return-to-sporting activities for athletes with spinal injuries and other spine-related disorders. In recent years, the fitness craze has helped establish the importance of conditioning. Whether the individual is young or middle-aged, proper nutrition, flexibility, strength, and endurance are key ingredients both for preconditioning and rehabilitation.

At the time of injury it becomes important to understand the role of modified, limited, and monitored activity in trying to avoid deconditioning. Prior to engaging (or re-engaging) in sports, a thorough evaluation of the musculoskeletal system is indicated. This should include a careful history and physical examination, a discussion as to the nature of the sport in which the individual wishes to participate, and the general, as well as specific, potential problems associated with that sport.

It has become commonly accepted that for the middle-aged individual who wishes to return to sporting activities from an otherwise sedentary lifestyle, a cardiovascular analysis is in order. In addition, it is quite important to test flexibility, strength, muscle imbalance, leg-length inequality, and nutritional requirements, and to educate the individual with regard to warm-up procedures, proper equipment, and what to do in case of injury.

The majority of injuries to the spine are self-limiting. Most athletes are well motivated, and it is estimated that only approximately 10% of injuries associated with sports are related to the spine. However, no sport is immune from spinal injury, and this is readily understood when one considers Dr. James A. Nicholas's linkage concept. This doctrine basically relates that the spine acts as the link between the upper and lower extremities and absorbs as well as transmits forces while providing support and balance. Injuries to the limbs affect the spine and injuries to the spine affect the limbs.

The sports medicine approach for the prevention and care of spinal disorders is not only quite appealing but also logical. Complete rest has a significant physical and psychological impact on the athlete. Most authors in this book would agree that continued (although modified and limited) activity, within an essentially nonpainful range, is indicated when spinal injury does occur.

This compendium of papers brings together a broad spectrum of health care professionals, including exercise physiologists, physical therapists, and psychologists, as well as physicians, to address issues concerning medical and surgical management of spinal injuries in sports. The book is divided into four sections, including general considerations, spinal problems in specific sports, evaluation and treatment of spinal injuries associated with sports, and a final section of case reports concerning the management of difficult spinal problems in accomplished athletes. We are not aware of any other book that provides the overall approach to spinal problems in sports contained herein and hope it offers useful guidance for physicians and other health professionals faced with the often difficult challenge of the spine-injured athlete.

I would like to take this opportunity to thank all the contributors and make special mention of gratitude to Donna Ohnmeiss, Research Coordinator for the Texas Back Institute Research Foundation, for her diligent efforts in coordinating this project.

STEPHEN H. HOCHSCHULER, M.D.

PART I

THE SPINE AND SPORTS
GENERAL CONSIDERATIONS

Chapter 1

EXERCISE AND THE INTERVERTEBRAL DISC

William J. Stith, PhD

The intervertebral disc plays a crucial role in the flexibility and stability of the spinal column and must survive very high loads during various physical activities.[3,40,41] The disc itself appears to be the major load-carrying component of the spine, absorbing and distributing forces applied to the vertebral column.[24,33] At relatively small loads, force is taken up by the disc, but with increasing load, energy is transferred to the vertebral body, which can ultimately result in fracture of the vertebral endplates.[56] Sports such as weight lifting have been shown to result in tremendous loads on the lumbar spine.[20] The importance of the mechanical and structural properties of the intervertebral disc are of considerable interest in the relationship of injury to various sports activities. The following article addresses the biochemistry of the intervertebral disc and how it is affected by exercise.

DISC COMPOSITION

The intervertebral disc consists of three distinct tissues: (1) the nucleus pulposus, (2) the annulus fibrosus, and (3) the vertebral endplates, which are primarily hyaline cartilage. The nucleus and the annulus blur into one another, so it is best to think of them as a gradient of tissue rather than distinct entities. Collagen of the annulus fibrosis merges into the hyaline cartilage of the endplates.[3,11,12,15]

The annulus fibrosus consists of concentric lamella of collagen fibers arranged in parallel arrays at an angle of 60° to the spinal axis. The anterior

90 concentric layers of helicoid laminated fibers are present in the annulus, with adjacent bands oriented in opposing directions.[4]

The central feature of all collagen is the very stiff helical structure that makes it insoluble and imparts great tensile strength to the molecule. The helix consists of three protein chains, each containing approximately 1,055 amino acids, with a high concentration of proline and hydroxyproline. These amino acids force the polypeptide chains into a left-handed helix, greatly limiting motion and therefore stabilizing the triple helix.[18] The collagen of the outer rim of the anterior annulus is principally type I collagen, which forms the larger diameter (50–60 mm) fibers in the disc, serving to impart structure to the disc and to resist tension.[11,69] In contrast to the regular arrangement of dense collagen fibers in the annulus, the nucleus pulposus is a loose collagen fibril network contained within an extensive gelatinous matrix. The collagen of the nucleus pulposus is primarily type II collagen, which has smaller diameter (30 mm) fibrils.[11,14] Type II collagen of the nucleus pulposus readily adheres to the proteoglycans, which are the primary constituents of the nucleus pulposus. While proteoglycans contribute a minor proportion of the dry weight of the structure, they bind large quantities of water and convert the matrix into a highly structured gel.

In contrast to collagens, which are principally protein in composition, proteoglycans are composed of 5% protein and 95% glycosaminoglycan. The proteoglycan molecule consists of a core of protein with distinct regions for binding of glycosaminoglycan molecules of hyaluronic acid, keratin sulfate, and chondroitin sulfate. These glycosaminoglycans are negatively charged linear polysaccharide chains of repeating disaccharide units. One of the disaccharides is always an amino sugar (glycose amino) along with large carbohydrate polymers known as glycans. These molecules have high negative charges from sugars containing carboxylate and sulfate groups.[18]

One hundred to 500 proteoglycan subunits will attach to the hyaluronic acid at intervals of about 300 angstroms. The binding of these glycosaminoglycans to the core protein is stabilized by small (40,000–60,000 mw) link proteins. The hyaluronic acid chain is anchored in turn to collagen fibers scattered throughout the matrix. The proteoglycan subunits vary in core protein length, in glycosaminoglycan proportions as well as the degree of sulfation.[18]

In the extracellular matrix of the nucleus, proteoglycans are found as aggregates, with the size of the aggregate determined by the length of hyaluronic acid. These aggregates are extremely large (greater than 100 million daltons) with a highly negative-charged density that allows the aggregate to fill the maximum possible volume.[18] These aggregates trap or organize water into a shell of hydration within the aggregate, much as a sponge entraps water.[18]

The proteoglycans act to impart function to the intervertebral disc by allowing compression to squeeze fluid out and absorb some of the load. The interactive negative forces resist load by strongly repelling each other and resisting further deformation. After removal of the compressive force, the aggregate quickly expands and reabsorbs the water lost.[62,65] Studies in the rabbit intervertebral disc have shown that the swelling pressure is highest in the nucleus pulposus and lowest in the anterior annulus.[23]

DISC FUNCTION

The intervertebral disc functions to provide flexibility, resist compressive forces and shock, and transfer forces between adjacent vertebrae.[4] In flexion, extension, and lateral bending, fibers on the convex side of the bend resist deflection by tension, whereas annular fibers on the concave side bulge outward. In torsion, half of the annular fibers are loaded in tension.[4] In flexion or extension the nucleus pulposus may change position,[59,60] but, if so, it appears to return quickly back once the opposing movement is initiated.[66] Discs with normal morphology appear to show more consistent changes in position than do discs with abnormal morphology.[59]

In compressive loading, the nucleus pulposus acts hydrostatically to increase intradiscal pressure to approximately 1.5 times the applied load.[44] This phenomena is interpreted as the nucleus acting to transform compression loads into radially directed tensile forces in the annulus, causing hoop stress where the value can be 3.5 times the applied pressure.[3,36] As the nucleus solidifies with age, its efficiency in distributing stresses uniformly to the annulus decreases. The annulus then sustains most of the vertical load and little tangential load.[42] Increases in type II collagen in the annulus at the expense of type I may lower the tensile strength of the annulus, making possible rupture of the thinner, more parallel posterior fibers of the annulus where loads may be six to seven times as great as the applied load. This has been observed in studies when the disc was tilted backward.[43]

Imposed loads on the lumbar spine as high as 18.8 to 36.4 kilonewtons have been found in world championship power lifters.[20] This externally applied load produces stresses and strains of both the vertebral body and disc. The vertebral body is composed of a more stiff material and has a greater elastic modulus than does the disc. Therefore, strains can be produced more easily in the disc, which in turn must distribute the resultant forces.[33,69] Stresses in the disc resulting from these extreme loads or degeneration from mechanical trauma, such as from dynamic loading, may result in tearing of the tissue, including cracks and crevices that progressively weaken the disc, making annular rupture possible.[7,58]

Release of components from the disc may result in the production of back pain.[12] An inflammatory response has been obtained from homogenized autogenous nucleus pulposus injected into the lumbar epidural space of dogs. This material was shown to irritate dura and nerve roots.[39]

A high incidence of spondylolysis and Schmorl's nodes has been found in both weight lifters and track and field athletes who have been doing weight training exercises for more than four years.[2] It is thought that Schmorl's nodes may be healed microscopic endplate fractures.[51,67] If true, then disc degeneration could result from repair processes, including endplate calcification.[16,53,55] The structure that fails first in axial compression is the vertebral endplates.[7,16,41,53,56]

Low back injuries are the dominating complaint among weight lifters.[5,35] A recent study has examined the incidence of low back pain among retired wrestlers and heavy weight lifters.[21] The lifetime incidence and prevalence of back pain were greatest among wrestlers and may have resulted from damage to posterior elements, which is frequent during wrestling and often overlooked. Such damage could be from torsional forces, which would be more readily evident with wrestlers than weight lifters. The peripheral surface structures of the disc are subjected to the greatest stresses and subsequently develop the greatest strains, depending on the distance from the peripheral annulus to the axis of rotation. This stress is maximal at the posterolateral region of the annulus, which has fewer fibers and whose fibers are thinner than those present anteriorly.[16,17,31–33,69] Combinations of movements such as twisting, bending, and bending with rotation will result in increased stresses and strains on a disc, especially with a superimposed load, and are the most likely to result in disk injury.[16,33,42] Combined loading is the most likely to result in disc failure with back pain.[4]

DISC DEGENERATION

Disc degeneration has been associated with changes in the composition of the annulus, nucleus pulposus, and the endplates. There may be an increase in type II collagen in the annulus, since the nucleus is already predominantly type II.[13] The ratio of keratin sulfate to chondroitin sulfate also increases, with the greatest increase in keratin sulfate occurring in the nucleus.[1] As the aging or degeneration process progresses, the nucleus loses water (from 85–90% at birth to 70% by the seventh decade),[10,46] becoming firm and white rather than soft and translucent. The infantile type of nucleus pulposus, with cells from the notochord surrounded by firm fibrous tissue, is replaced with an adult type of cell, with a firmer structure composed of fibrocartilage and dense fibrous tissue at the first half of the second decade. The cell number decreases in the central portion of the nucleus, and a cell population is observed only in the region near the cartilaginous endplates.[47] In the elderly, the nucleus appears as a solid plate of cartilage surrounded by an outer lamella of annulus fibrosis. Associated with the decreased water is a concomitant decrease in hexosamine content with a loss of sulfated glycosaminoglycans.[12,50,65] Oxidation of lipid can also occur in the disc, leading to an accumulation of brown deposits. This oxidation of lipid forms dialdehydes, which can react to crosslink further the collagen fibers, altering their mechanical properties as well as blocking their already slow turnover. Therefore, changes in diet and metabolism that deposit lipid in the disc may alter its mechanical properties and accelerate degeneration.[11]

With aging, there is a progressive increase in vertebral endplate concavity associated with decreased bone density. In the cancellous bone of vertebral bodies, a decrease in the number of support structures for the endplates has also been observed.[63] A recent study evaluated the biomechanics and structural properties of the endplate. Decreases in proteoglycan concentration and an increase in microscopic anomalies thought to be early Schmorl's nodes were observed. These anomalies had a random collagen orientation rather than the regular parallel arrangement of fibers seen in younger specimens, which should be more effective in withstanding nuclear pressure.[55] Strength of the endplate has been shown to decrease with age.[44,51] The endplate breaking point for those over 40 is, on the average, approximately 50% of that for those under 40.[51] MRI was used successfully to diagnose traumatic Schmorl's node formation in a patient following forced lumbar flexion which resulted in an injury.[34]

Increased disc degeneration has been shown by means of MRI analysis, whereby gross morphology and decreased proteoglycan concentration could be correlated with a grading system for T-2 weighted images from MRI scans. MRI was found to more closely reflect proteoglycan concentration than did gross morphology. The decrease in proteoglycans was correlated with a decrease in hydration, which could be visualized with T-2 weighted spin-echo sequences.[12] Actual determination of water content is difficult, since MRI is only sensitive to mobile proton centers. Thus, protein and tightly bound water give solid-like signals that go undetected in MRI.[49]

A significant effect of the aging process is the loss of blood vessels in the disc. By age 12, the disc is largely avascular.[22] Nutrient transport in and out of the disc is primarily by passive diffusion, with sulfate and other negatively charged anions diffusing mostly from the periphery of the annulus; small uncharged solutes such as glucose and oxygen diffusing through the endplates and annulus; and small cations primarily through the endplates.[38,64] Overall, about 40% of the bone-disc interface is permeable.[38] With increasing age there is an increase in calcification of the endplates. These changes may be intensified through mechanical loading or trauma.[12] Calcification of the endplate can lead to obliteration of the disc space.[47]

Within the disc itself, the pH is already low, presumably from lactic acid buildup from glycolysis taking place in the low oxygen tension of the disc.[9,25,38,45] Calcification of the endplates can result in a decreased solute interchange, which can further compound the problem by lowering pH. Lysosomal enzymes such as glycosidases, proteases, and sulfases are stimulated by an acid environment, with pH5 being optimum.[18] Stimulation of the lysosomal enzymes may hasten the degradation or aging process inside the disc.[52] Exercise has been shown to have an ameliorative effect on disc degeneration by increasing the flow of nutrients into the disc and waste products out. Exercise results in increased aerobic metabolism in the outer annulus and the central portion of the nucleus pulposus, bringing about reduction of lactate concentration.[27] A decrease in activity has just the opposite effect.[26] In addition, physical and chemical factors such as vibration and smoking have been shown to decrease sulfate transport to the disc as well as to lower the intradiscal oxygen tension,[28,29] which could result in an increased accumulation of lactate.

Diffusion into degenerative discs and peridiscal scar tissue has been observed through the use of gadolinium-diethylene triamine penta-acetic acid (Gd-DPTA).[30,57] Gadolinium-DPTA is a small molecule (mol. wt. 938) that does not cross intact cell membranes and can thus be used as a leak detector in damaged or degenerative vertebral endplates. Since enhancement does not appear to occur in normal discs, Gd-DPTA may serve as a means of studying nutritional pathways, inflammatory changes, and the effects of therapeutic agents.[12]

The disc appears to have a limited ability to resynthesize and repair its matrix. Chymopapain injected into the discs of 9-month-old beagles resulted in a rapid decrease in disc height of 30–60%, depending on the dose administered. Some dogs showed defects at the higher doses. By 24 months, disc height was not significantly different from noninjected controls.[19] The action of the enzyme appears to be primarily on proteoglycans with little action on collagen.[68] A similar replacement of disc cellular tissue with fibrous scar has also been seen after laser discectomy.[61]

In human discs, proteoglycans are reported to have a total life of 2 years, with that of collagen being significantly less.[38] The enzymes involved in collagen synthesis require ferrous iron, molecular oxygen, and vitamin C.[18] It is not known whether the repairs are of sufficient quality to produce long-term functional restoration of the disc.[12]

Repair remodeling of the components within the disc may follow Wolff's law, whereby structure may be dictated in response to stress, as has been shown in patients with scoliosis.[6] Type I collagen content of the annulus is increased on the concave side of the curve and decreased on the convex side, most noticeably in the outer annulus. Collagen content is also increased in the nucleus, particularly in vertebrae located at apices of the curve.[8] There is also significantly higher levels of aggregate and larger nonaggregating monomers, similar to that seen in cerebral palsy patients.[48] In a patient with a tear of the posterior annulus, there appeared to be loss of collagen and an increase of proteoglycan and water, which occurred around the tear and which were not apparent in the remainder of the disc.[54] These findings appeared to be similar to results in rabbits with surgically induced ventral disc herniation. After injury there was metaplasia into fibrocartilage, originally from cells along the margins of the annular wound, with proliferation of cells changing almost the entire disc space into fibrocartilage. Water content initially fell and then rose rapidly again before showing a gradual loss over an extended period. Proteoglycan levels paralleled changes in water content. Hyaluronic acid content decreased rapidly after herniation, but there was no change in the size of proteoglycan monomers.[37]

CONCLUSION

The components of the intervertebral disc, nucleus pulposus, annulus, and vertebral endplates all act in concert to stabilize the spine and absorb load while allowing the spine to flex or extend. The nucleus plays a crucial role in shock absorption by deforming in response to load and by transferring vertical forces into ones that are radially directed to the annulus. To adequately perform their function, the cells of the nucleus must receive adequate nutrition, which comes from passive diffusion primarily through the endplates. Flow of nutrients into the disc and waste products out is aided by exercise. Excessive static loading or repetitive dynamic loading can result in fracture of the endplates with subsequent calcification and decreased transport. Increasing age and/or duration of activity may intensify these effects. Endplate damage appears to be present in weight lifters and track and field athletes who have engaged in weight-lifting activities for more than 4 years. Impairment in the nucleus' functional ability can result in nonuniform forces being transferred to the annulus with possible rupture in the posterolateral section, where the fibers are thinner and fewer in number. Failure of disc components has been associated with back pain as well as with accelerated degeneration of adjacent structures such as the facet joints, which may also be involved in the production of pain.

REFERENCES

1. Adams P, Muir H: Quantitative changes with age of proteoglycans of human lumbar discs. Ann Rheum Dis 35:289–296, 1976.
2. Aggrawal ND, Kaur R, Kumar S, Mathur DN: A study of changes in the spine in weight lifters and other athletes. Br J Sports Med 13:58–61, 1979.
3. Akeson WH, Woo SLY, Taylor TKF, et al: Biomechanics and biochemistry of the intervertebral disks: The need for correlation studies. Clin Orthop 129:133–140, 1977.
4. Ashman RB: Disc anatomy and biomechanics. Spine: State of the Art Reviews 3(1):13–26, 1989.
5. Brady TA, Cahill BR, Bodnar LM: Weight training-related injuries in the high school athlete. Am J Sports Med 10:1–5, 1982.
6. Brickley-Parsons D, Glimcher MJ: Is the chemistry of collagen in intervertebral discs an expression of Wolff's law? Spine 9:148–163, 1984.
7. Brown T, Hansen RJ, Yorra AJ: Some mechanical tests on the lumbosacral spine with particular reference to the intervertebral discs: A preliminary report. J Bone Joint Surg 39A:1135–1164, 1957.
8. Bushell GR, Ghosh P, Taylor TKF, Sutherland JM: The collagen of the intervertebral disc in adolescent idiopathic scoliosis. J Bone Joint Surg 61B:501–508, 1979.
9. Diamant B, Karlsson J, Nachemson A: Correlation between lactate levels and pH in discs of patients with lumbar rhizopathies. Experientia 24:1195–1196, 1968.
10. Durning RP, Murphy ML: Lumbar disk disease: Clinical presentation, diagnosis, and treatment. Postgrad Med 79:54–74, 1986.
11. Eyre DR: Biochemistry of the intervertebral disc. In Hall DA, Jackson DS (eds): International Review of Connective Tissue Research. New York, Academic Press, 1979, pp 227–290.

12. Eyre DR, et al: Intervertebral disc. In Frymoyer JW, Gorden SL (eds): New Perspectives on Low Back Pain. Park Ridge, IL, American Academy of Orthopedic Surgeons, 1988, pp 131–214.
13. Eyre DR, Muir H: Types I and II collagens in intervertebral disc: Interchanging radial distributions in annulus fibrosis. Biochem J 157:267–270, 1976.
14. Eyre DR, Muir H: Quantitative analysis of types I and II collagens in human intervertebral discs at various ages. Biochim Biophys Acta 492:29–42, 1977.
15. Eyring EJ: The biochemistry and physiology of the intervertebral disc. Clin Orthop 67:16–28, 1969.
16. Farfan HF: Mechanical disorders of the low back. Philadelphia, Lea & Febiger, 1973.
17. Farfan HF, Cossette JW, Robertson GH, et al: The effects of torsion on the lumbar intervertebral joints: The role of torsion in the production of disc degeneration. J Bone Joint Surg 52A:468–497, 1970.
18. Gamble JG: The musculoskeletal system. New York, Raven Press, 1988.
19. Garvin PJ, Jennings RB: Long term effects of chymopapain on intervertebral discs of dogs. Clin Orthop 92:281–295, 1973.
20. Granhed H, Jonson R, Hansson T: The loads on the lumbar spine during extreme weight lifting. Spine 12:146–1449, 1987.
21. Granhed H, Morelli B: Low back pain among retired wrestlers and weight lifters. Am J Sports Med 16:530–533, 1988.
22. Hassler O: The human intervertebral disc: A micro-angiographical study on its vascular supply at various stages. Acta Orthop Scand 40:765–772, 1970.
23. Hirano N, Tsuji H, Ohshima H, et al: Analysis of rabbit intervertebral disc physiology based on water metabolism: I. Factors influencing metabolism of the normal intervertebral discs. Spine 13:1291–1302, 1988.
24. Hirsh C, Nachemson A: New observations on the mechanical behavior of lumbar discs. Acta Orthop Scand 23:254–283, 1954.
25. Holm S, Maroudas A, Urban JPG, et al: Nutrition of the intervertebral disc: Solute transport and metabolism. Connective Tissue Research 8:101–119, 1981.
26. Holm S, Nachemson A: Nutritional changes in the canine intervertebral disc after spinal fusion. Clin Orthop 169:243–258, 1982.
27. Holm S, Nachemson A: Variations in the nutrition of the canine intervertebral disc induced by motion. Spine 8:866–874, 1983.
28. Holm S, Nachemson A: Nutrition of the intervertebral disc: Effects induced by vibration. Orthop Trans 9:451, 1985.
29. Holm S, Nachemson A: Nutrition of the intervertebral disc: Acute effects of cigarette smoking. An experimental animal study. Ups J Med Sci 93:91–99, 1988.
30. Hueftle MG, Modic MT, Ross JS, et al: Lumbar spine: Postoperative MR imaging with Gd-DPTA. Radiology 167:817–824, 1988.
31. Jackson DW: Low back pain in young athletes: Evaluation of stress reaction and discogenic problems. Am J Sports Med 7:364–366, 1979.
32. Jayson M, Barks JS: Structural changes in intervertebral discs. Ann Rheum Dis 32:10–15, 1973.
33. Jensen GM: Biomechanics of the lumbar intervertebral disk: A review. Phys Therapy 60:765–773, 1980.
34. Kornberg M: MRI diagnosis of traumatic Schmorl's node. Spine 13:934–935, 1988.
35. Kotani T, Ichikava N, Wakabeyashi W: Studies of spondylolysis found among weight lifters. Br J Sports Med 6:4–8, 1971.
36. Kulak RF, Belytschko TB, Schultz AB, Galante JO: Nonlinear behavior of the human intervertebral disc under axial load. J Biomech 9:377–386, 1976.
37. Lipson SJ, Muir H: Proteoglycans in experimental intervertebral disc degeneration. Spine 6:194–210, 1981.
38. Maroudas A: Nutrition and metabolism of the intervertebral disc. In White AA, Gordon SL (eds): Symposium on Idiopathic Low Back Pain. St Louis, CV Mosby, 1982, pp 370–390.
39. McCarron RF, Wimpee MW, Hudkins PG, Laros GS: The inflammatory effect of nucleus pulposus: A possible element in the pathogenesis of low-back pain. Spine 12:760–764, 1987.
40. Morris JM: Biomechanics of the spine. Arch Surg 107:418–423, 1973.
41. Morris JM, Lucas DB, Bresler B: Role of the trunk in stability of the spine. J Bone Joint Surg 43A:327–351, 1961.
42. Nachemson A: Some mechanical properties of the lumbar intervertebral discs. Bulletin Hospital Joint Diseases 23:130–143, 1962.
43. Nachemson A: The influence of spinal movements on the lumbar intradiscal pressure and on the tensile stresses in the annulus fibrosis. Acta Orthop Scand 33:183–207, 1963.

44. Nachemson A: The load on lumbar discs in different positions of the body. Clin Orthop 45:107–122, 1966.
45. Nachemson A: Intradiscal measurements of pH in patients with lumbar rhizopathies. Acta Orthop Scand 40:23–42, 1969.
46. Naylor A, Happey F, MacRae T: Changes in the human intervertebral disc with age: A biophysical study. J Am Geriatr Soc 3:964–973, 1955.
47. Oda J, Tanaka H, Tsuzuki N: Intervertebral disc changes with aging of human cervical vertebra: From the neonate to the eighties. Spine 13:1205–1211, 1988.
48. Oegema TR, Bradford DS, Cooper KM, Hunter RE: Comparison of the biochemistry of proteoglycans isolated from normal, idiopathic scoliotic and cerebral palsy spines. Spine 8:378–384, 1983.
49. Panagiotacopulos ND, Pope MH, Krag MH, Bloch R: Water content in human intervertebral discs: Part I. Measurement by magnetic resonance imaging. Spine 12:912–917, 1987.
50. Pearce RH, Grimmer BJ, Adams ME: Degeneration and the chemical composition of the human lumbar intervertebral disc. J Orthop Res 5:198–205, 1987.
51. Perey O: Fracture of the vertebral end-plate in the lumbar spine: An experimental biomechanical investigation. Acta Orthop Scand 25(suppl):1957.
52. Pope M, Wilder D, Booth J: The biomechanics of low back pain. In White AA, Gordon SL (eds): Symposium on Idiopathic Low Back Pain. St Louis, CV Mosby, 1982, pp 252–295.
53. Roaf R: A study of the mechanics of spinal injuries. J Bone Joint Surgery 42B:810–823, 1960.
54. Roberts S, Beard HK, O'Brien JP: Biochemical changes of intervertebral discs in patients with spondylolisthesis or with tears of the posterior annulus fibrosis. Ann Rheum Dis 41:78–85, 1982.
55. Roberts S, Menage J, Urban JPG: Biochemical and structural properties of the cartilage end-plate and its relation to the intervertebral disc. Spine 14:166–174, 1989.
56. Rolander SD: Motion of the lumbar spine with special reference to the stabilizing effect of posterior fusion. Acta Orthop Scand 90(suppl):1966.
57. Ross JS, Delamarter R, Heuftle MG, et al: Gadolinium-DTPA-enhanced MR imaging of the postoperative lumbar spine: Time course and mechanism of enhancement. AJR 152:825–834, 1989.
58. Sandover J: Dynamic loading as a possible source of low back disorders. Spine 8:652–658, 1983.
59. Schnebel BE, Simmons JW, Chowning J, Davidson R: A new digitizing technique for the study of movement of intradiscal dye in response to flexion and extension of the lumbar spine. Spine 13:309–312, 1988.
60. Shah JS, Hampson WGJ, Jayson MIV: The distribution of surface strain in the cadaveric lumbar spine. J Bone Joint Surg 60B:246–251, 1978.
61. Sherk HH, Rhodes A: Laser discectomy. In Sherk HH (ed): Lasers in Orthopedics. Philadelphia, J.B. Lippincott, 1990.
62. Stevens RL, Ryvan R, Robertson WR, et al: Biological changes in the annulus fibrosis in patients with low back pain. Spine 7:223–233, 1982.
63. Twomey LT, Taylor JR: Age changes in lumbar vertebrae and intervertebral discs. Clin Orthop 224:97–104, 1987.
64. Urban JPG, Holm S, Maroudas A, Nachemson A: Nutrition of the intervertebral disc: Effect of fluid flow on solute transport. Clin Orthop 170:296–302, 1982.
65. Urban JPG, McMullin JF: Swelling pressure of the lumbar intervertebral discs: Influence of age, spinal level, composition, and degeneration. Spine 13:179–187, 1988.
66. Vanharanta A, Ohnmeiss DD, Stith WJ, et al: Effect of repeated trunk extension and flexion movement as seen by CT/discography. Presented at Federation of Spine Associations, Las Vegas, Nevada, Feb. 1989.
67. Vernon-Roberts B, Pirie CJ: Healing trabecular microfractures in the bodies of the lumbar vertebrae. Ann Rheum Dis 32:406–412, 1973.
68. Watts C, Knighton R, Roulhac G: Chymopapain treatment of intervertebral disc disease. J Neurosurg 42:374–383, 1975.
69. White AA, Panjabi MM: Clinical Biomechanics of the Spine. Philadelphia, J.B. Lippincott, 1978.

Chapter 2

THE SPINE AS A MOTOR IN SPORTS: APPLICATION TO RUNNING AND LIFTING

Serge Gracovetsky, PhD

It is generally believed that the spine is essentially a supporting column linking pelvis to shoulders. Physical activities appear to involve mainly the upper and lower limbs. For instance, as an individual walks or runs, his trunk is believed to be carried passively by this legs. However, this simple and attractive idea leads to numerous contradictions. For example, why is the spine curved in the form of an 'S' instead of being straight, when it would appear that a straight column would support compressive loads better than a curved one? If that were the case, the spine, which is impacted at each heel strike, would be at a disadvantage. The argument that spinal lordosis is a transient condition that will be eliminated as a matter of evolutionary improvement contradicts the fact that monkeys already have a straight spine and, as far as can be observed, are quadrupeds. The uniqueness of human bipedalism suggests that the features of the human spine may be related in a fundamental way to our locomotor process, and indeed perhaps to all physical activities.

In the search for an answer, consider the 20-year-old male subject in Figure 1. He has reduced arms and no legs. The drawing of his pelvis clearly demonstrates the absence of lower extremities. Therefore, this young man is standing on his ischium.

The problem is this: If it is true that legs are necessary for human locomotion, then a person with the anatomy depicted in Figure 1 would not be able to walk. This perspective of human locomotion is so ingrained in our culture that, to date,

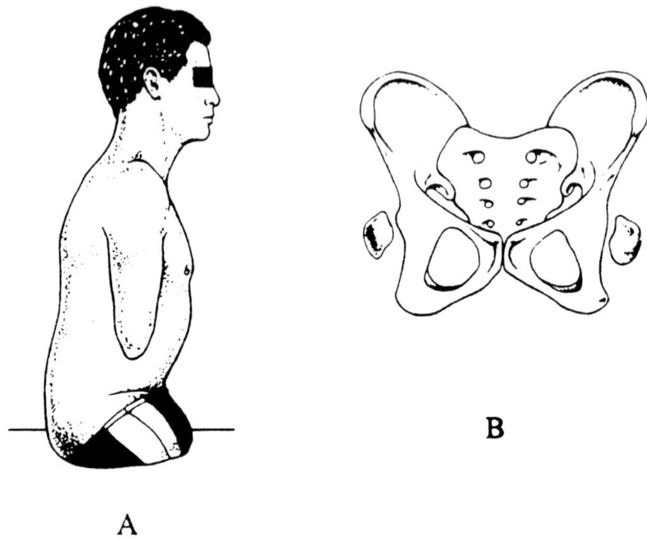

FIGURE 1. *A,* Lateral view of a subject with no legs and reduced upper extremities. *B,* Anteroposterior (AP) view of the pelvis showing clearly the absence of lower extremities.

the study of human gait has been principally an exercise in analyzing the motion of the legs. The rhythmic, alternating trunk motions are considered the result of jostling by the legs[10] likewise, the associated muscular contractions are assumed to be part of the effort required to keep from falling over—an aspect of the widely held view that locomotion is a precarious process.[12] The graceful, flowing stride of the Olympic runner has even been described as "essentially a series of collisions with the ground."[7] However, there are substantial mathematical and clinical arguments to reject this rather crude representation of human gait.

In most studies, the head, arm, and trunk masses are lumped together and not assigned any function essential to the dynamics of walking. Numerous objections to such a representation have been raised: the motion of the shoulders cannot be hampered without disturbing the locomotion process; people with fused spines exhibit gait modifications; 77% of patients with failed fusions are nonetheless satisfied with the results[11]; and if the torso is in a brace or cast, "walking at moderate or higher speeds becomes awkward and the energy requirements as measured by oxygen consumption rise sharply."[5] Also, the fact of the vertical displacement of the body's center of gravity during locomotion becomes incomprehensible—why do we not flex the knees more in order to clear the ground rather than lift the entire trunk? Indeed, Newton's first law encourages the straightest possible trajectory for the center of gravity; yet it is impossible to walk while maintaining the center of gravity in the horizontal plane. Clearly, there must be an evolutionary advantage to our body's close interaction with the gravitational field.

This is not a philosophical argument. Living organisms do exploit their environment, either as a source of energy or for other important purposes. Pigeons assess the direction of the earth's gravitational field as a support for their navigation. The earth's gravitational field is remarkably constant, and it seems unrealistic not to exploit it in some important way.

Furthermore, from an evolutionary point of view it is difficult to think of the trunk, arms, and head as passive (i.e., nonfunctional) elements in the locomotor process. It would be a waste of muscular mass not to use them in some essential way, instead of just dragging them about while walking and running.

The fact is that legs are not necessary for human locomotion. The subject shown in Figure 1A walks using the same spinal pelvic motion as an individual with legs, albeit with a greater amplitude of pelvic axial rotation.[3,4] The lack of detectable difference in locomotive patterns between a person with legs and our subject without legs raises some serious issues of consistency. Quite clearly, the representation of the spine as a passive structure totally reliant on the motion of the legs to carry it cannot be maintained. A radical change in our perception of the role of the spine must be made. To resolve this and other contradictions, it was proposed in 1985 that the spine be considered as a sort of engine driving the pelvis.[3]

The basic problem of human bipedal locomotion is that the pelvis must be rotated axially using a muscular system that is more or less parallel to the spine. There are small pelvic muscles that could conceivably contribute to the axial rotation of the pelvis. However, the anatomical arrangement of these muscles does not provide for efficient axial pelvic rotation.

The theory of the spinal engine is an attempt to explain how the spine participates in our locomotive efforts in conjunction with our natural environment, i.e., the earth's gravitational field. According to this theory, the mechanism by which the spine drives the pelvis is the following (Fig. 2):

1. The hip extensors contract and the body is lifted in the gravitational field. This can be clearly seen as the runner's feet leave the ground.

2. During the flight phase, the unloaded spine fires its erectors to rearrange its posture by bending to one side. This requires a relatively small amount of muscular power that can be easily supplied by the trunk muscles.

3. The coupled motion of the spine transforms this lateral bend into an axial torque as the legs prepare for landing.

4. Upon heel strike, a substantial pulse propagates through the leg and is shaped by the mechanical response of knee, hip, and sacroiliac joints. This compressive pulse applied to the intervertebral joint has the effect of enhancing the latter's ability to resist axial torque.

5. At the same time, the descending thorax, arrested by the impact of the heel striking the ground, converts its potential energy into kinetic form. The net

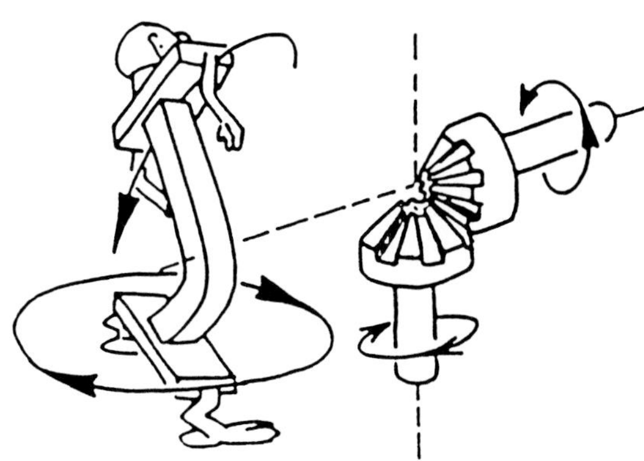

FIGURE 2. The primitive lateral bend of the spine inherited from our fish ancestors is converted by the lordosis into an axial torque. This property of the spine is in fact common to any rod, as realized in 1903 by Lowett.

effect is to enhance the lateral pull on the spine initiated by the erectors during flight. Through this elaborate sequence of energy transformation, which requires the existence of the earth's gravitational field, the hip extensors flex the spine laterally. In that sense, the hip extensors become lateral spine flexors. As shown elsewhere, the hip extensors are also spine extensors in the sagittal plane via the strong lumbodorsal fascia. Hence, the hip extensors represent the primary source of "economical" power, which the spinal engine transforms in the execution of physical activities. The associated trunk muscles "control" the flow of power to and from the extremities, using the gravitational field as temporary storage whenever required.

6. Here again, the coupled motion of the spine transforms this lateral bend into the axial torque needed to rotate the pelvis axially. The power delivered by this torque is enhanced by two factors: (1) by the lordosis and (2) by the joint stiffness that is increased by the compression pulse propagated through the spine at heel strike. Hence, it could also be argued that the hip extensors end up being the primary axial rotators of the spine.

7. From this point on, the legs follow the pelvic motion to enhance the stride.

This theory neatly explains the need for a runner to use shoes that do not unduly absorb shocks; indeed the shape of the compressive pulse returned to the spine must be very specific in order to permit the chemical energy liberated by the hip extensors to be transformed into pelvic motion. An incorrect pulse shape, as is produced when walking on sand, forces the trunk musculature to directly generate the energy needed by the spine to drive the pelvis. This source of energy is inefficient and the body tires rapidly. Athletic excellence requires an understanding of proper body mechanics so that the output power of the spine can be maximized without exceeding safety limits.

THE IMPORTANCE OF LORDOSIS

The coupled motion of the spine is crucial to the locomotor process because it converts the primitive lateral bend of our fish ancestors into an axial torque. This conversion is possible only because the spine is not straight, that is, it has a curvature, or lordosis. The coupled motion of the spine was first demonstrated by Lowett in 1903.[6] The theory of the spinal engine suggests that the control of lordosis is perhaps the most important feature that makes locomotion possible. Hence, in the event of spinal injury, control of lordosis must be restored; this is achieved through a variety of exercises. Pelvic tilt exercises are one example. Other methods achieve the same result indirectly: for instance, asking a golfer to bend his knees also results in pelvic tilt.

IMPLICATION IN THE UNDERSTANDING OF SPINAL INJURIES

The influence of the theory of the spinal engine on the appreciation of the mechanical etiology of spinal disorders is significant. If, for example, the spine is envisioned as some kind of passive structure carried by the legs, then the signs and symptoms of an injured patient will be interpreted as manifestations of weaknesses in that passive column (Fig. 3). The corresponding diagnoses and rehabilitation procedures may then be targeted to reinforcing the strength of that passive column through such steps as fusion, bracing, or installing plates and screws.

FIGURE 3. A passive trunk is carried away by the legs.

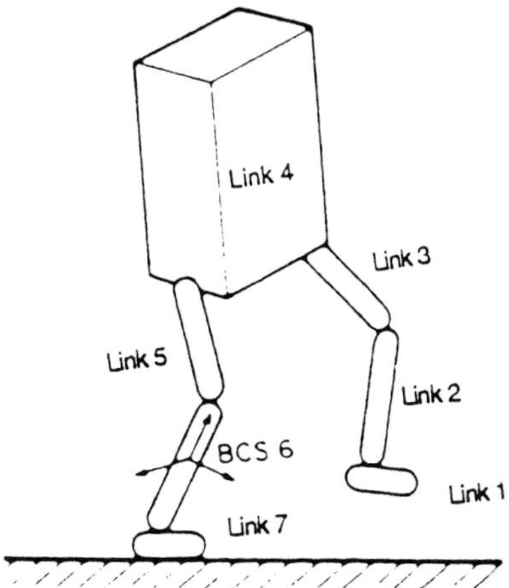

If, however, the spine were an engine, namely the primary engine inherited from our fish ancestors, then it might be necessary to review the interpretation of signs and symptoms leading to diagnosis, as well as the corresponding protocol for the rehabilitation of injured spines. Obviously, repairing an active engine cannot possibly be the same as repairing a passive column.

The theory of the spinal engine affects our perceptions of numerous human activities. Here, we will examine how this theory is likely to modify the way we evaluate and measure the function of the spine.

THE HIGHLY VARIABLE RELATIONSHIP BETWEEN ANATOMY AND SPINAL FUNCTION

The evaluation of spinal function often involves the use of radiography. Radiography, however, is essentially a quasi-static way to qualitatively assess the anatomical condition of a joint. The problem is that anatomical imperfections are not always associated with a corresponding loss in spinal function, which is what the athlete is interested in. Indeed, the relationship between anatomy and spinal function is highly variable: an injury to the disc may be compensated for by a rearrangement of the geometry of the facets so that overall spinal function is maintained in spite of the injury. In this way injured athletes may recover near normal function despite anatomical damage to the spine.

DIFFICULTIES IN SPINAL FUNCTION ASSESSMENT

The difficulties involved in objectively assessing spinal functioning are rather formidable. Besides the fact that the spine consists of 24 individual intervertebral joints (all of which are mobile, and any one of which can be the site of an injury), the whole assembly is mounted on the pelvis, which itself moves. The strong connective tissues that attach the vertebrae directly to the ilium ensure that the motions of the spine and pelvis are inextricably linked (Fig. 4). This is why all the various isokinetic, isotonic, isoinertial, and related machines intended to measure muscular trunk strength do not do justice to the biomechanical complexity of the spine (Fig. 5). By attempting to mechanically isolate the spine from the pelvis using harnesses and belts, and allowing its movement around a fixed axis of rotation, these machines interfere substantially with the normal functioning of

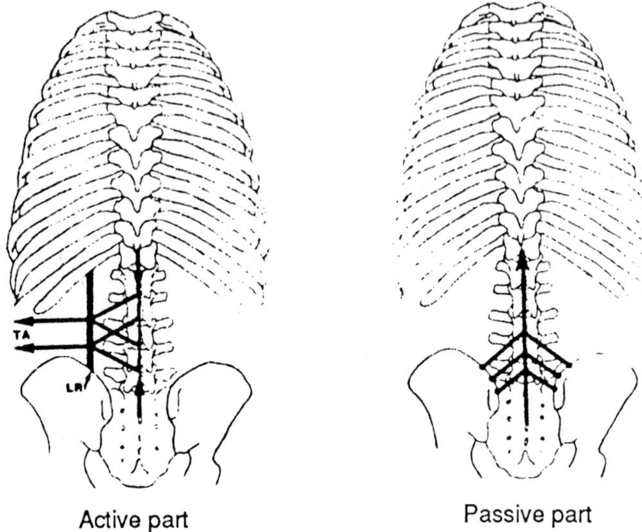

FIGURE 4. The lumbodorsal fascia is made of a thick network of collagen fibers connecting the pelvis to the spinous processes.

the spine. What they measure is in fact the disturbance of the spine's function by the machine. While this disturbance may be repeatable, it is not necessarily relevant. After all, most workplace tasks are not performed with the worker's pelvis restrained by a belt, nor are they performed isokinetically, isoinertially, or in any other such artificial way. The evaluation of spinal function must be done dynamically as the spine moves freely.

Spine function can be approximated by a machine called the Spinoscope (Fig. 6). The Spinoscope obtains geometric data from the patient using a dual camera system, while the activity of the musculus multifidus is recorded using skin surface EMG electrodes. Through mathematical analysis, detailed information about the coordination among spine, pelvis, and muscles can be deduced. For a normal individual, this coordination is task-specific and can be used as a

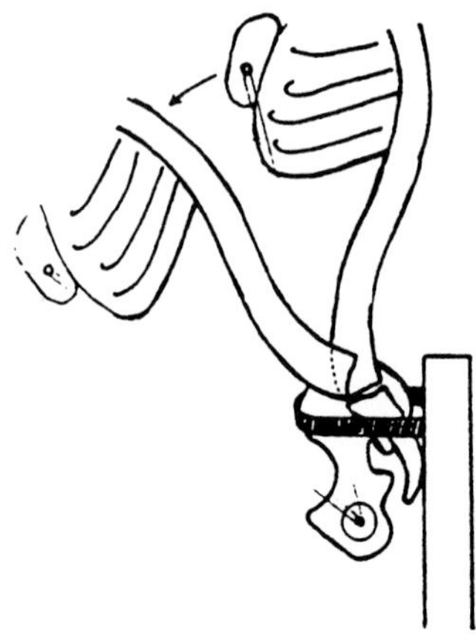

FIGURE 5. Harnessing the pelvis to isolate the spine is part of a common evaluation procedure. Unfortunately, spinal function is inextricably linked to that of the pelvis.

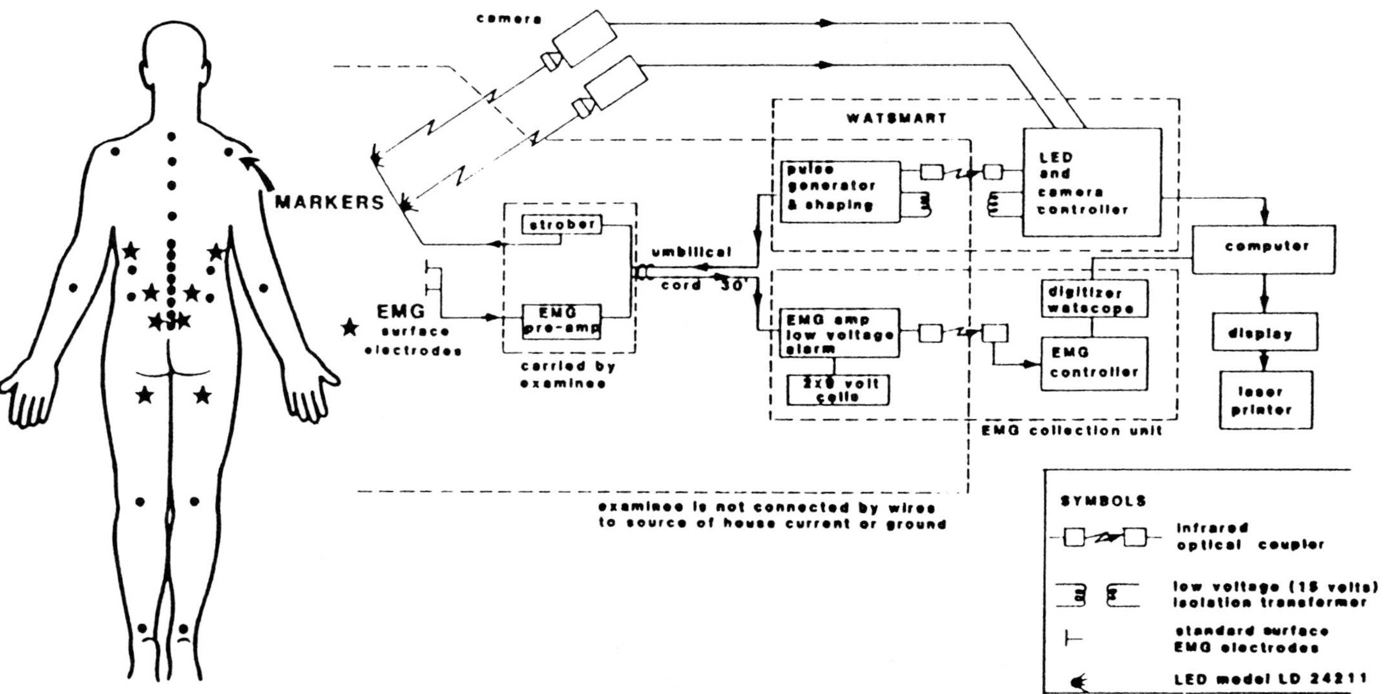

FIGURE 6. Overview of the Spinoscope.

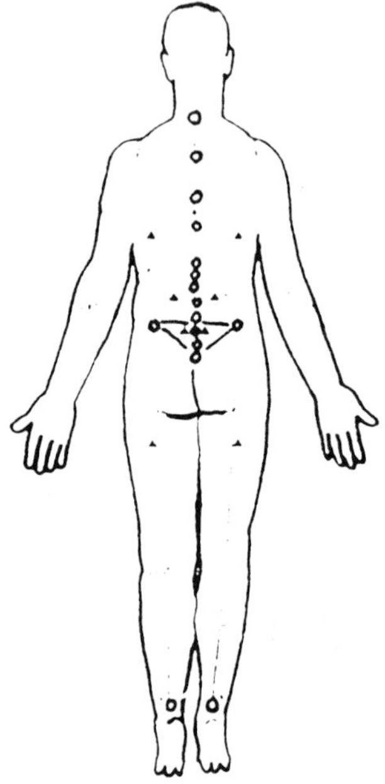

FIGURE 7. Twelve markers are placed above the midline of the spine, while two more are placed above the iliac crest and two above the Achilles tendons.

reference. When a patient with an unknown condition is tested, his spinal and pelvic coordination can be compared with the reference obtained from the normal individual. Any discrepancy between them is interpreted as a loss of spinal function.

The kinematics of the spine are extracted by tracking the motion of markers placed on the skin with adhesive tape (Fig. 7). These markers are small light-emitting diodes. Twelve of them are distributed along the spine. Only two of these markers need to be located with precision. The first one must be above the spinous process of C7, and the ninth below must be above L4. With this accomplished, the other markers can be placed approximately, because their relation to the underlying vertebrae can be calculated using anthropomorphic tables. In addition, two more markers are placed above the iliac crest, and two more on the achilles tendon. The EMG electrodes are placed above the multifidus at L5. In this region, the multifidus stands alone and the electrical signal is not disturbed by the activities of the iliocostalis and the longissimus.

During data collection, each marker emits a short pulse of infrared light. The infrared light is invisible to the naked eye, but the markers flashing in slow motion can be seen through a special viewer. At full speed, each marker flashes about 5,000 times per second. This allows the reconstruction of spinal motion at a rate of 180 images per second. The reconstructed motion can be played back for detailed analysis of the kinematics of the spine. Figure 8 illustrates the basic three-dimensional data used for spinal evaluation.

When the patient bends forward, the motion of the markers in the sagittal plane contains information on the intersegmental mobility and lordosis reduction (Fig. 9). This information, however, is corrupted by skin motion, which introduces an error into the measurement process. Despite this error, useful data can be obtained from these measurements. This can be demonstrated by an experiment that compares the motion of markers placed on the skin with the corresponding motion of the vertebrae (Fig. 10).

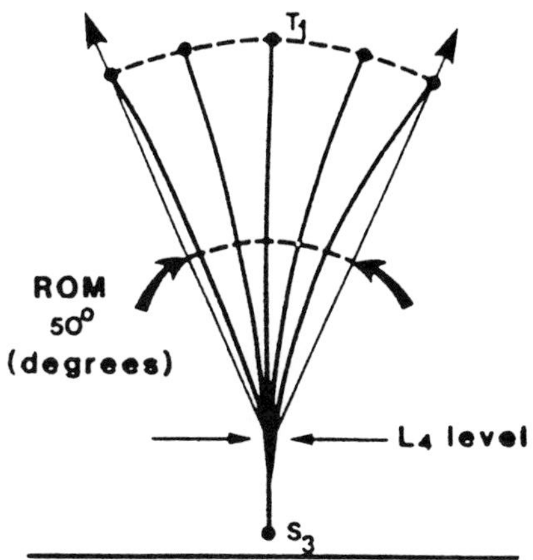

FIGURE 8. Subject bending laterally with the corresponding markers' positions tracked by the camera.

The correlation between the motion of skin markers and vertebrae can be determined by using radiography (Fig. 10A). A string of steel balls is taped onto the skin, and radiographs are taken while the patient bends forward and laterally. The radiographs give the position of the markers with respect to the vertebrae. It is therefore possible to relate the variations in position of the markers with the motion of each individual vertebra. For example, we can measure the variation in distance between two markers placed above L5 and T12 and compare this with the displacement of the spinous processes of L5 and T12 (Fig. 10B). The cumulative data on 7 patients shown in the figure demonstrate a good correlation.

The accuracy of the other measurements can also be assessed using this method (Fig. 11). For example, lordosis is an important parameter that can be

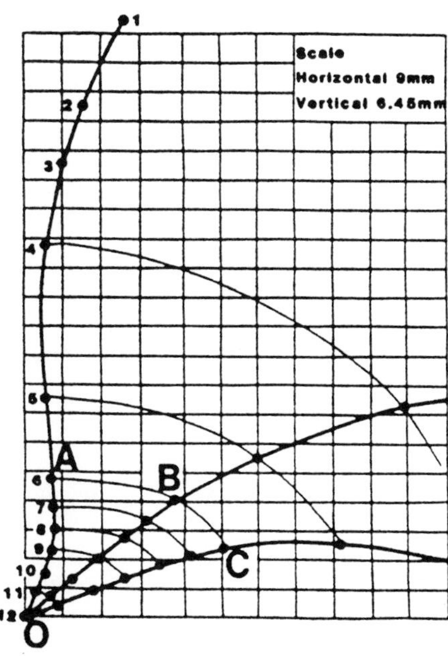

FIGURE 9. Subject in flexion with the reconstructed motion of the markers in the sagittal plane.

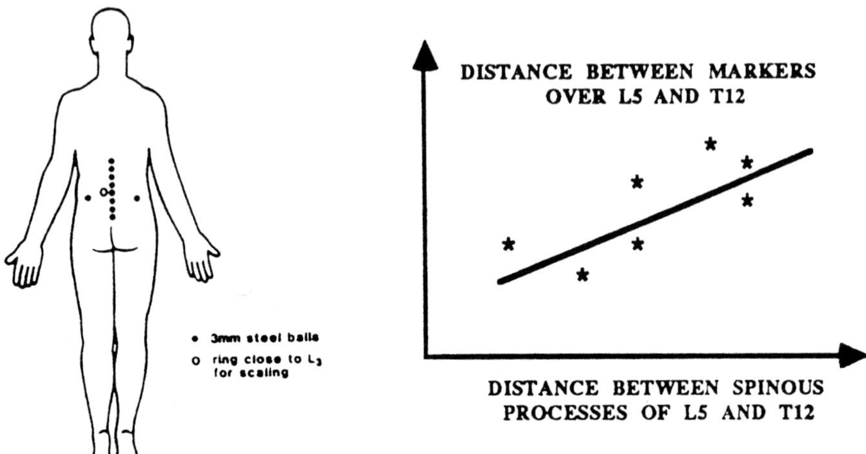

FIGURE 10. *A,* AP view of the spine with a string of steel balls placed on the skin. *B,* Cumulative data on seven individuals showing the correlation between the variation in the distance between the L5 and T12 vertebrae and the variation in distance between markers placed above the spinous processes of L5 and T12.

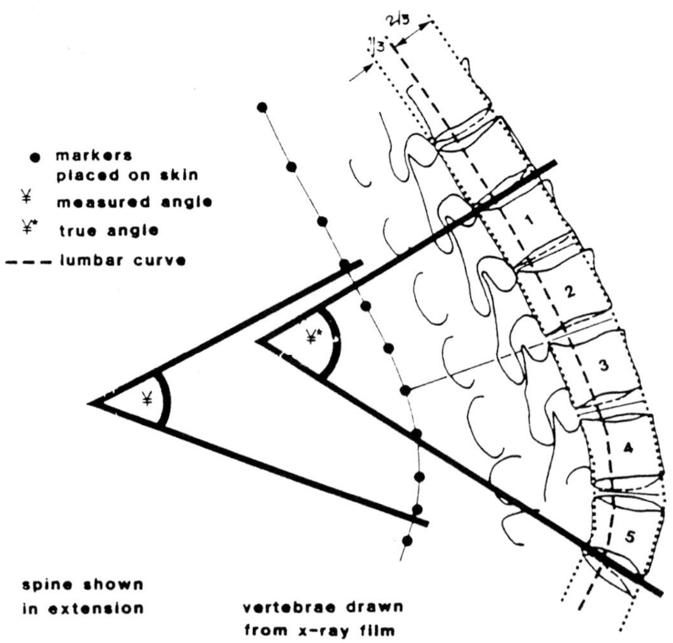

FIGURE 11. Lateral view showing the relative position of vertebrae and steel balls. These define the lumbosacral angle Ψ^* as the angle between L5/1 and T12/L1, and the angle Ψ as the estimate of Ψ^* calculated from the positions of the steel balls.

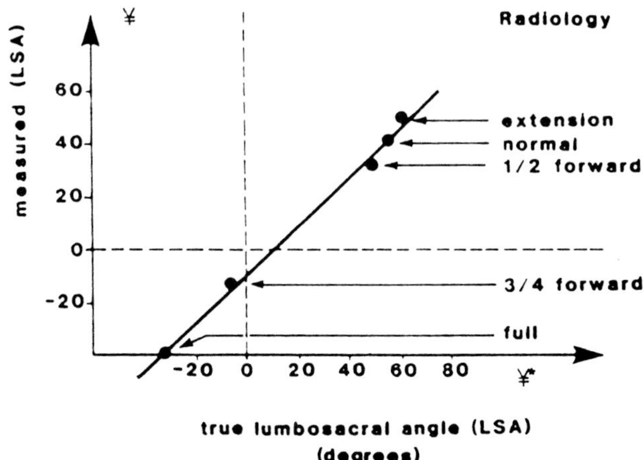

FIGURE 12. The correlation between Ψ^* and Ψ is fairly linear, indicating that the motion of external markers placed on the skin does contain information relevant to the estimation of the true lumbosacral angle.

characterized by the lumbosacral angle, which is defined to be the angle Ψ^*. This true lumbosacral angle can be approximated by the angle Ψ, obtained from the position of the steel balls placed on the skin.

While the lumbosacral angle derived from the position of the skin markers is plotted as the vertical axis, the lumbosacral angle derived from the true position of the vertebrae is shown on the horizontal axis (Fig. 12). The relationship, as determined from five lateral radiographs of the same patient moving from full flexion to full extension, is fairly linear.

NEAR-NORMAL RESPONSE OF HEALTHY INDIVIDUALS

The question of normality is important, because it suggests a mechanism for ranking a given patient vis-à-vis a reference. Ideally, the clinician would like to have a machine with two lights: a green one if the patient is normal, and red one if abnormal. The difficulty in the low back pain (LBP) is that over the course of a lifetime, the spine is exposed to considerable wear and tear and hence the probability of finding an undamaged spine (which we would presumably like to call a healthy or "normal" spine) becomes very small indeed. This is why the numerous attempts to define a normal patient are bound to be arbitrary. For example, it has been suggested that a normal patient would not have had an episode of LBP for one year. Here, a normal patient is defined to be asymptomatic during a specific period of time. Is an asymptomatic patient a normal one? Probably not. Being asymptomatic is a necessary condition of good health but not the only one.

Clinical evaluation of normality usually includes some degree of radiological investigation, although it has become clear that these anatomical data have a poor correlation with function. This brings us back to square one: what conditions need to be present for a healthy spine? It seems that this simple question has yet to be answered in the literature. In the meantime there exists no consensus as to what a normal reference would be.

However, the situation is not hopeless. The definition of normality must be rooted in the identification of some kind of desirable property that a normal spine must have. For example, we may want to recognize that survival implies the maintenance of the mechanical integrity of the spine, and therefore a normal spine should execute tasks in such a way that the stresses within it are as low and as equalized as possible to prevent injury. To do that requires a very specific coordination among spine, pelvis, and musculature.

It is possible to calculate what this coordination ought to be[4] and to design in vivo experiments to verify whether the calculations are consistent with the clinical observations. So far, the data do not contradict the view that a normal spine attempts to minimize and equalize the stress it has to support during the execution of a task. This finding gives us a clinical method for the evaluation of normality. The reasoning goes as follows: if all intervertebral joints are normal, then the central nervous system will see that all joints contribute to the transfer of forces. This, in turn, will result in the stresses being distributed evenly throughout the spine, thus minimizing the possibilities of injury. The resulting coordination can then be said to be normal.

This definition of normality is useful in clinical practice. Consider a normal volunteer (i.e., young, no history of back pain, otherwise in fine health). This volunteer is asked to lift a series of weights ranging from zero to 100 kilograms. The style of lifting is free. As the load lifted increases, the general appearance of the trunk suggests that the volunteer adopts a "flat back" posture. A flat back posture is generally believed to imply a lordotic spine. Thus, it is concluded that the posterior ligamentous system is slack and therefore that the lift must result from the activity of the erectors. Unfortunately, this is erroneous; the pelvic rotation has flexed the spine to a point where the posterior ligaments are so tight that the erectors relax. This phenomenon was noted as early as 1955 by Floyd and Sylver.[2] Subsequently, the anatomical descriptions of Bogduk[1] demonstrated that it is biomechanically impossible for the relatively small erector spinae to generate the moments necessary to sustain any load but the most trivial. Let us now have a closer look at how the lift is performed.

APPLICATION TO THE ANALYSIS OF A COMMON SPORT ACTIVITY: THE SAGITTAL DEADLIFT

The sagittal deadlift (Fig. 13) comprises two distinct phases:

1. From a relaxed upright stance, the subject bends forward to pick up a weight (a barbell). The knees may or may not be locked, depending upon the person's choice.

2. The barbell is then lifted. The subject returns to the upright posture, keeping the barbell at arm's length in such a way that the arms always hang down from the shoulders.

Data are collected on the position of 12 markers placed along the spine, with two more on the iliac crests together with the integrated electromyogram (IEMG) of the multifidus (L5), longissimus, and iliocostalis (L3) taken bilaterally.

Phase One

The basic problem of lifting is transferring the loads from the shoulders to the ground. This transfer is made possible by the continuity in the anatomical arrangement of soft tissues as shown in Figure 14. This arrangement is not obvious because different names are assigned to different sections of the fibers

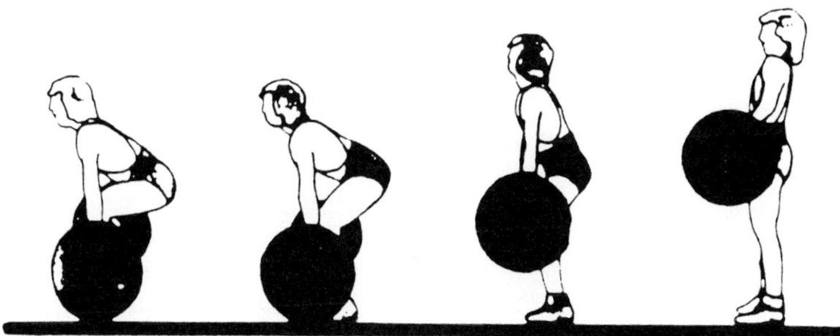

FIGURE 13. Sagittal deadlift. The subject bends forward to pick up a barbell (phase 1) and returns to the erect stance with the barbell against his hips (phase 2).

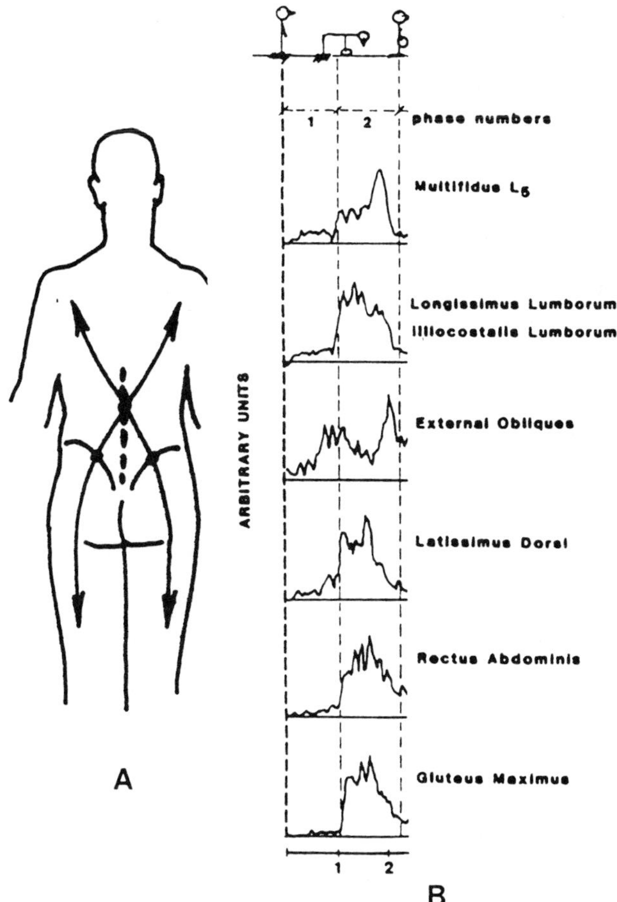

FIGURE 14. *A,* Path of forces from the arm to the ground. *B,* IEMG of several muscles recorded during the four phases of the lift. The raw EMG spinal is band filtered (5 Hz to 300 Hz), digitized at 1 kHz, rectified, averaged, and plotted. On this graph, the signal from the right and left electrode of each muscle has been added.

transmitting the forces; as they pass over the ilium, the muscle fibers of the hip extensors become the deep layer of the lumbodorsal fascia; then, once they cross the midline, they become the tendinous part of latissimus dorsi, which then turn into the latissimus dorsi itself, which inserts into the humerus. These different names obscure the unity of this anatomy, which can be imagined as a cable. It is clear, however, that forces will be transmitted properly by that cable only if each portion is taut. The cable is made of two distinct components: a muscular component, which can easily be conceived of as being contracted; and a ligament component, which must also be taut. Ligaments are passive structures and, thus, to be tightened they require geometrical changes such as lordosis reduction. This is the key to understanding proper lifting techniques.

As the subject bends forward to pick up the 20 kg barbell, the multifidus, longissimus, and iliocostalis lumborum are essentialy silent. Control of the descent depends entirely on the proper positioning of the body in the earth's gravitational field, so that minimum muscular activity is required. The fascia fibers are attached to the ilium, whose position is controlled by the hip extensors. Restraining the pelvis tightens the lumbodorsal fascia. The forces are now directly transmitted to the shoulders and the erectors can relax. The IEMG data of selected muscles are shown in Figure 14B. From the motion of the markers, several quantities can be analyzed and correlated with the IEMG of muscle of the trunk.

The Angle of Forward Flexion of the Trunk. This is the angle between an imaginary line passing through markers 1 and 12 (Fig. 15A) and the plumb line, and is denoted α. The variation of α is shown (Fig. 15B) as the subject executes the four phases of the lift. Since the total motion characterized by the angle α is due to the combined motion of both spine and hip, the spinal motion can be deduced by measuring the motion of the hip and subtracting it from the motion of the trunk. To relate the geometrical changes of the trunk to the muscular activity, the activity of the multifidus is shown in both 15A and 14B.

The Hip Motion. The hip motion is derived by tracking the motion of the plane defined by markers 12, 17, and 18, i.e., the markers placed above S_3 and both crests of the ilium (Fig. 15A). The intersection of this plane with the sagittal plane yields a straight line. The angle between this line and the vertical characterizes the motion of the hip and is plotted in Fig. 15B.

Notice the peculiarity of the hip angle variation. During the first phase, as the subject bends to pick up the barbell, the hips rotate forward by 30 degrees, then backwards by about 15 degrees. This backward motion is due to the flexion of the knee as the subject squats to reach for the barbell. Nonetheless, the total trunk motion still increases.

Indeed, the spinal motion, as defined by the difference between the total trunk motion and hip motion, continues to increase even as the pelvis is restrained by the bending of the knees. This increase in spinal flexion is responsible for setting the posterior lumbar spine (PLS) under tension, thus allowing the erectors to shut down. This muscle relaxation phenomenon is confirmed by the IEMG of the multifidus, iliocostalis, and longissimus lumborum depicted in Figure 14B.

The tightening of the PLS due to reduction in lumbar lordosis is further confirmed by the variation in lumbosacral angle or its equivalent Ψ, as shown in Figure 16. The decrease in Ψ demonstrates a significant reduction in lumbar lordosis as the spine straightens out.

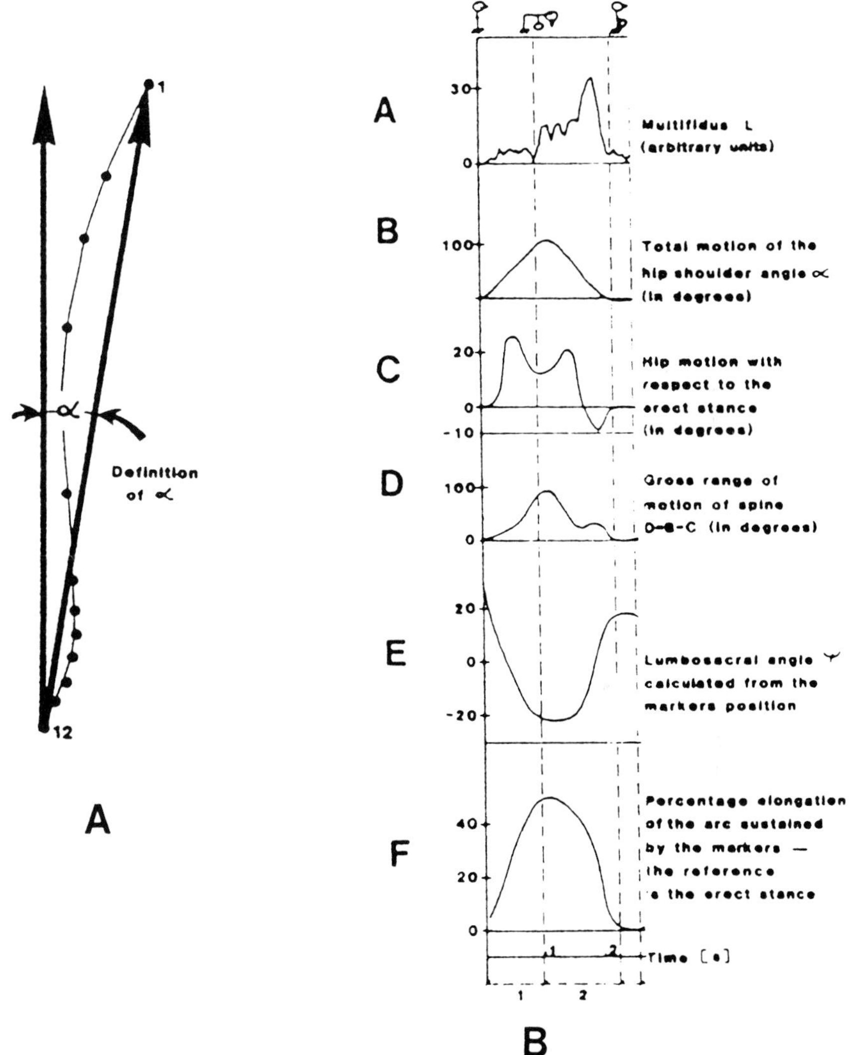

FIGURE 15. *A,* Definition of the angle α, which is the angle of the trunk with the plumb line. Definition of the pelvic angle, which characterizes the motion of the pelvis. The contribution of the spine is deduced by subtracting the pelvic angle from the trunk angle. *B,* Geometric data on the trunk, spine, and hip motion derived from the position of the external markers.

Lordosis. The effect of the reduction in lumbar lordosis on the rotation of the intervertebral joint is illustrated in Figure 15A. In this example, the distance between markers 12 (point zero) and 6 (point A) is 113 mm when the subject adopts an erect, relaxed stance. This distance increases to 153 mm (point B) and eventually extends to 170 mm (point C) when the subject is fully bent and is touching the barbell.

From the percentage increase plotted in Figure 16, it is evident that this increase mirrors the variation in the lumbosacral angle Ψ. It should be noted that

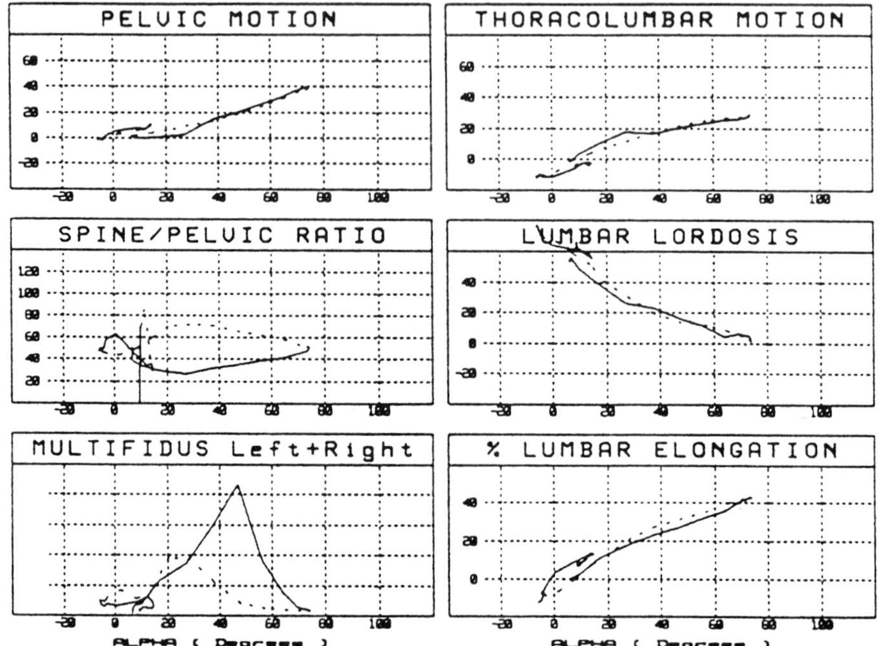

FIGURE 16. This is a rerarrangement of the data given in Figure 15. Instead of plotting the various parameters versus time, they are now plotted versus α. The figure A was derived by scaling and superimposing the IEMG of the multifidus with the calculated moment at L5. The muscle relaxation phenomenon is obvious. Note the sharp drop in muscle contribution at the very instant it is needed most, according to the proposition that back muscles do the lifting. The muscle relaxation phenomenon clearly demonstrates that this aspect of spine mechanics should be reviewed.

the 50% increase in the distance OA is quite significant, as it allows the PLS to be stretched. That this subject is able to rotate all his intervertebral joints during forward flexion is also evidence that they are likely to be in good condition. The subject lifted 60 kg with similar results, thus indicating that his lifting capacity exceeds 60 kg.

Phase Two

The subject now grips the barbell and lifts it while returning to the erect stance. The moment required to execute this movement is generated by the hip extensors, as evidenced by the sharp rise in activity of gluteus maximus (Fig. 14B). The action of the arm sustaining the barbell is demonstrated by latissimus dorsi. The longissimus and iliocostalis lumborum fire immediately in order to stabilize the spine laterally. Their contribution to the lift, however, is not very efficient because their attachment to the transverse process gives them a much shorter lever arm than the PLS.

Note again that the multifidus exhibits the characteristic response called "muscle relaxation." At the instant of lift-off when maximum effort is needed, the multifidus does not contribute very much. Interestingly, it is only when the subject attains an almost erect stance, at about a 25-degree angle of forward flexion, that the maximum EMG signal from the multifidus is recorded.

A direct measure of the distribution of tasks between muscles and ligaments cannot be made, because there is no existing experimental procedure capable of measuring the tension in the various collagen fibers of the PLS. Nonetheless, it is possible to correlate an estimation of the total moment at L, that must be balanced during the lift with the measured EMG activity of the multifidus.

The total moment calculated by using a previously published mathematical model of the spine[44] for a similar 20-kg lift may be plotted against the total angle of flexion of the trunk α. The IEMG scale was chosen to fit the calculated muscular response, a choice that would be fully justified if the relation between IEMG and the corresponding force produced by the muscle were linear. In fact, it is known that for the erectors, the relationship between IEMG and force is monotonic and nearly linear for small loads.[8,9] Hence, the appropriateness of this scaling procedure may be challenged.

As the subject begins to pull up on the barbell, the load on his spine increases along with the moments to be balanced at each intervertebral joint. The pelvis rotates (Fig. 15) to flex the spine until the PLS develops enough tension to transmit the forces generated by the hip extensors to the upper extremities. The barbell only begins to rise from the ground after phase 2 has started. At that time, the contribution of the ligaments is maximum. As the barbell clears the subject's knees while he returns to an erect posture, the moment to be balanced drops off rapidly as the lordosis (characterized by the lumbosacral angle Ψ) increases. The increase in lordosis results in the rapid slackening of the PLS, which is associated with a rapid rise in the activity of the multifidus. Indeed, as the forces generated by the hip extensors can no longer be transmitted through the slackening PLS, they must use a different channel. The only anatomical solution to this problem is the path offered by the contracting erectors. Hence there is a switchover from a ligament-predominant transmission to muscle-predominant transmission. The sudden rise in muscular activity occurs for a range of α between 35 and 50 degrees; it is the reverse of the muscle relaxation phenomenon.

Because the lordotic change is due primarily to the motion of the hips, the gross motion of the spine remains fairly constant during this transition. After the switchover, the motion of the subject's spine is controlled by the erectors.

It is difficult to compare these data to those available in the literature, since no equivalent studies have been published. Although various theoretically possible muscular combinations have been observed and reported, the work described either does not assign any particular role to lordosis or else entirely neglects the PLS. Therefore, we suggest that the interpretation of the data in the available literature is not straightforward.

SPINAL RESPONSE AS THE LOAD LIFTED INCREASES

It is instructive to compare the responses of a volunteer as he lifts a series of increasingly heavier loads. This is shown in Figure 17, which contains the overlayered responses from lifts of 0, 20, 40, 60, 80, and 100 kilograms. These responses are virtually identical. Note the absence of significant changes in lordosis as the load to be lifted increases; these data demonstrate that lordosis variation is essentially independent of the load lifted, provided it is accompanied by a corresponding change in trunk velocity (Fig. 17). Indeed, since the erectors are incapable of lifting anything above 20 kg, the tightening of the lumbodorsal fascia must increase with the load, so that the forces generated by the powerful hip extensors may be transmitted all the way to the upper

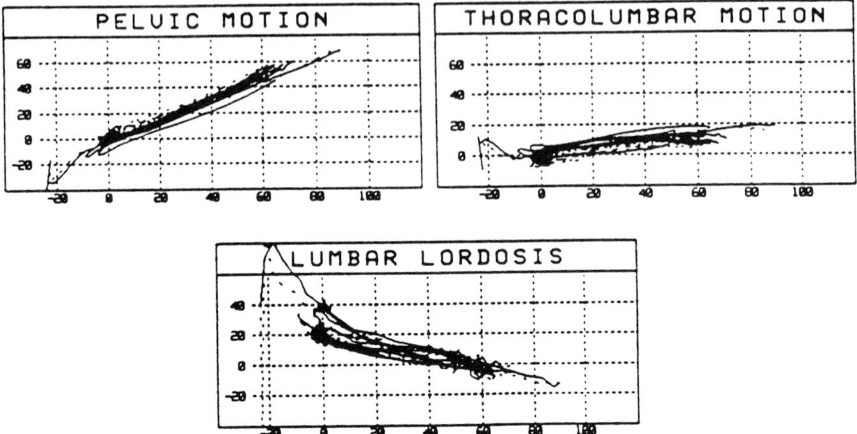

FIGURE 17. The data from several lifts of increasing loads are overlayed. Notice the similarity of the responses. The data suggest that the coordination chosen by the volunteer is independent of the load to be lifted, as long as the task can be executed (see Fig. 18).

extremities. It is well known that the ability of collagen to transmit force is a function of the rate of elongation, i.e., trunk speed. The higher the speed, the stiffer the collagen.

There is a limit as to what collagen can transmit. As the load exceeds a comfortable limit, the trunk velocity begins to decrease. To maintain its ability to transmit an increasingly higher level of forces, the collagen must stretch more; this cannot be done arbitrarily, since the soft tissues of the spine may be damaged. At this point, the lifter rapidly approaches his physiological limits. This observation suggests a measure for estimating the safety of a load. It is proposed that the load is safe as long as the trunk velocity increases. The value of the load at which the velocity begins to decrease would indicate the asymptomatic maximum for safe loading.

The general trend of the responses discussed above is respected even in the presence of an injury. And similarly, the safe limit of an injured patient can be evaluated. In Figure 19, the trunk velocity profile as the load increases suggests that this patient has a safe load of 9 kg.

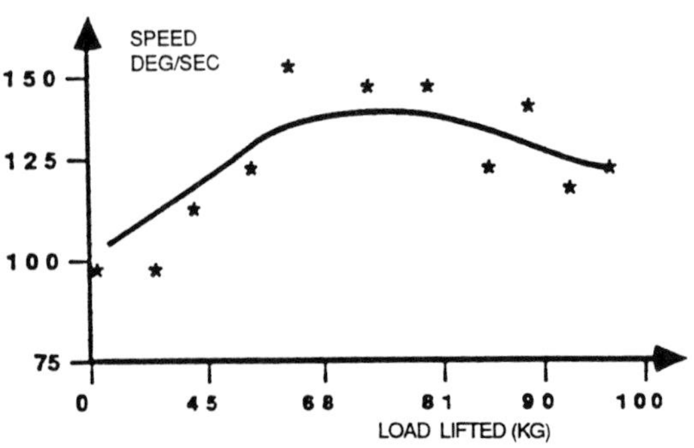

FIGURE 18. For each load lifted, the trunk velocity changes. The velocity peaks for a certain angle of forward flexion. Note that the maximum velocity first increases when the load to be lifted increases, then begins to decrease. It is suggested that the point at which this velocity begins to decrease reflects the limit of ligaments stretching and as such represents a reasonable index of safe load for the lift.

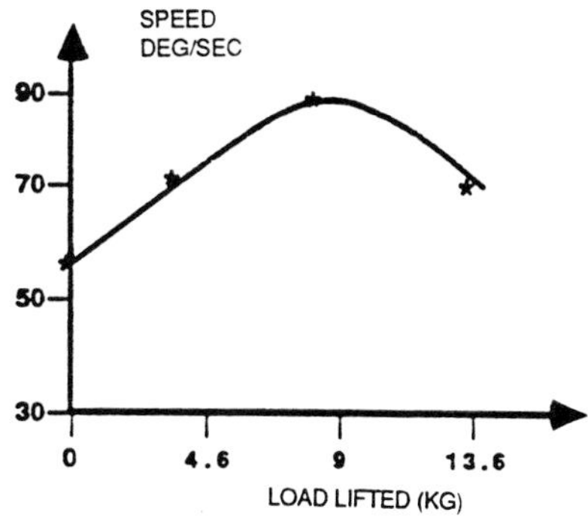

FIGURE 19. This patient had a fusion of L4/5/S1. There is little change in discomfort as the load lifted increases to 14 kg. Yet the analysis of trunk velocity indicates a slow-down when the load exceeds 9 kg.

RESPONSES OF THE SPINE UNDER FATIGUE CAUSED BY REPETITIVE LIFTS

Another interesting element is the variation in response as the patient becomes tired by repeated loading. In the experiment depicted in Figure 20, the patient is requested to lift a load equal to a quarter of his previously determined maximum safe load. This lift must be repeated up to 75 times, at a rate of one lift every two seconds or so. Data are collected every 15 lifts. Note the lack of significant changes in the response during this exercise. This suggests that this patient can safely execute this task.

RANGE OF MOTION VERSUS COORDINATION OF MOTION

There is an important distinction to be made between range of motion and coordination. Range of motion is under voluntary control and can be easily altered. Coordination is harder to change because it is largely out of conscious control. For example, it is not easy to rotate L4 over L5. Individual joints cannot be rotated at will. The coordination between joints in the execution of a motion task appears to be a characteristic of a healthy spine and represents a desirable signature that should be measured.

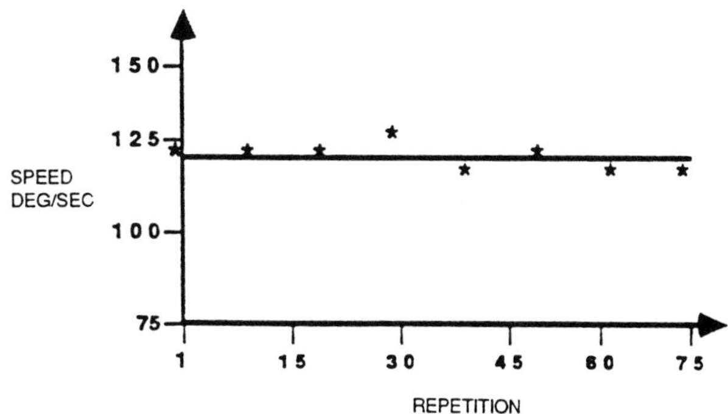

FIGURE 20. The patient lifts a load equal to a quarter of the maximum safe load determined above. The lift is repeated 75 times at 2-second intervals. The overlayed data of lift numbers 1, 15, 30, 45, 60, and 75 show no significant changes, thereby suggesting that such a repetitive effort is well within this patient's limits.

There are no objections to measuring the lifting capacity of an asymptomatic spine by monitoring the coordination between spine and pelvis as the load increases. The theory predicts that the coordination between spine and pelvis is independent of the weight of the load lifted, as long as the spine can safely support it (Fig. 17). As the spine approaches its limit, the spine-pelvis coordination breaks down. The consistency of spine-pelvis coordination throughout the range of acceptable loads is surprising in view of the external appearances of the various styles of lifting.

CONCLUSION

The theory of the spinal engine predicts that the coordination between spine and pelvis is determined by the need to minimize the level of stress on the spine, regardless of the task to be executed. This unique optimum coordination will be affected by injury, and the resulting changes can be readily detected. The avoidance of injury requires strict adherence to this optimum coordination. It is hoped that during the training of athletes, coaches will teach training and performance techniques that do not interfere with the body's natural optimum coordination.

REFERENCES

1. Bogduk N, Twoney LT: Clinical Anatomy of the Lumbar Spine. New York, Churchill Livingstone, 1987.
2. Floyd WF, Sylver PHS: The function of the erector spinae muscles in certain movements and postures in man. J Physiol (Lond) 129:184–203, 1955.
3. Gracovetsky S: A hypothesis for the role of the spine in human locomotion: A challenge to current thinking. J Biomed Eng 7:205–216, 1985.
4. Gracovetsky S: The Spinal Engine. New York, Springer Verlag, 505 pp, 1988.
5. Inman TI, Ralston JH, Todd F: Human Walking. Baltimore, Williams & Wilkins, 154 pp, 1981.
6. Lowett AW: A contribution to the study of the mechanics of the spine. Am J Anat 2:457–462, 1903.
7. McMahon TA, Greene P: Reflex stiffness of man's anti-gravity muscles during kneebends while carrying extra weights. J Biomechanics 12:881–891, 1979.
8. Ortengren R, Andersson GB, Nachemson AL: Studies of relationship between lumbar disk pressure, myoelectric back muscle activity, and intra-abdominal pressure. Spine 6(1):98–103, 1981.
9. Schultz AB, Andersson GB, Ortengren R, et al: Analysis and quantitative measurements of loads on the lumbar spine when holding weights in standing postures. Spine 7(4):390–397, 1982.
10. Thurston, AJ, Harris JD: Normal kinematics of the lumbar spine and pelvis. Spine 8:199–205, 1983.
11. White AA, Panjabi MM: Clinical Biomechanics of the Spine. Philadelphia, JB Lippincott, 534 pp, 1978.
12. Winter DA: Biomechanical motor patterns in normal walking. J Motor Behavior 15(4):302–330, 1983.

Chapter 3

GENERAL FITNESS IN THE TREATMENT AND PREVENTION OF ATHLETIC LOW BACK INJURIES

Billy Glisan, MS, and Stephen H. Hochschuler, MD

Since the 1970s, the number of Americans involved in recreational sports has increased exponentially. Hundreds of thousands of youths and adults are now involved in recreational sports activities such as basketball, softball, soccer, or flag football. Others prefer racquet sports such as racquetball, squash, or tennis. A great proportion of joggers from the past decade have merged with a new group of "fitness enthusiasts" involved in some type of routine physical fitness activity, such as cycling, weight training, and/or aerobics. In preparation for personal challenges, highly competitive endurance athletes have channeled their almost fanatic behavior into conditioning programs designed to achieve peak physical performance.

The rapid growth in the pursuit of physical fitness has resulted in a remarkable increase in the incidence of orthopedic injuries, many related to the spine. This drastic increase in the reported number of injuries, especially in contact sports such as football or basketball, is in part unavoidable because of the physical demands placed on the spine. However, others are more likely related to an insufficient conditioning program.

Individuals involved in endurance events at near-professional levels understand the importance of regular conditioning in preparation to obtain their ultimate performance. Others, however, do not dedicate adequate time to condition their bodies for the demands of their particular sports. In fact, a large proportion of those involved with many sports such as softball and flag football use weekend activities to actually "get in shape" entirely, ignoring conditioning and flexibility training. Most of us know this individual as the classic "Weekend Warrior"!

The purpose of this chapter is to emphasize the need to develop a preliminary level of overall conditioning and fitness. This not only increases one's level of general health and energy, but also helps develop specific physiological adaptations necessary to reach a maximal level of performance and perhaps more importantly to reduce the risk of injury. These principles are also critical to the rehabilitation of spine-injured individuals.

CARDIOVASCULAR FITNESS

Cardiovascular fitness is synonymous with cardiovascular endurance, aerobic capacity, and functional capacity. These terms relate to the ability of the heart, lungs, and blood vessels to acquire, transport, and deliver oxygen to muscles. Oxygen is mandatory to release the energy from fat, carbohydrate, and protein at the cellular level. This energy, in the form of adenosine triphosphate (ATP), is used to perform muscular work.[16] ATP can be produced in muscles in either an aerobic or anaerobic process. The aerobic system uses oxygen to release the stored energy from the organic fuels with drastically improved efficiency.

Anaerobic metabolism can form ATP without the use of oxygen, primarily from the breakdown of carbohydrates. The catabolism of fat and protein requires sufficient oxygen to release their stored energy; thus they are not utilized as fuels in substantial quantities during anaerobic exercise.

Our bodies are constantly employing both energy systems to produce ATP. At rest, the delivery of oxygen is adequate to meet the body's energy demands, and the aerobic energy system is primarily engaged. As the body's need for energy increases to perform muscular work (the energy requirement increasing with increasing exercise intensities), the need for greater oxygen delivery to the exercising muscles occurs. There is a direct relationship between exercise intensity and oxygen demand. All individuals reach a point during exercise when the demand for oxygen exceeds the supply. This point, referred to as the anaerobic threshold, occurs when one is primarily limited to the breakdown of carbohydrates as the predominant fuel supply for ATP production. Concurrently, lactic acid, a by-product of anaerobic metabolism, accumulates in working muscle cells. This increased acidity results in a lower pH at the cellular level, which in turn inhibits ATP production resulting in muscle fatigue and exhaustion.

Maximum oxygen uptake (VO_2max) represents the maximal volume of oxygen transported to the exercising muscles.[3] VO_2max is the objective measurement of aerobic capacity or cardiovascular fitness. The greater this value, the greater an individual's level of cardiovascular fitness and potential exercise performance.

Studies that compare aerobic capacity with the incidence of back injury are few. Results from these studies do not clearly indicate the benefits of a cardiovascular fitness program to diminish back insults. One prospective study estimated VO_2max by treadmill testing. No significant correlation between VO_2max and the occurrence of back injuries was demonstrated.[5] This study, however, included a large number of subjects who smoked, which may have biased the results.

In a series of studies involving various cardiovascular measures, one investigator initially demonstrated a preventive value from increasing levels of physical fitness.[9] In a follow-up study, the same investigator demonstrated a 25% decrease in workers' compensation costs (possibly reflecting a reduced incidence of compensation claims), which appeared to be directly related to improvements in cardiovascular fitness and the initiation of a policy allowing for more rapid return to work. This occurred while flexibility and muscular strength parameters did not significantly change.[10]

There is no conclusive evidence that cardiovascullar fitness decreases the risk for back injury. Further research is warranted in this area. It is difficult to separate aerobic capacity from muscular endurance, strength, and other measures of general physical fitness, due to their complex interrelationships. The end result may well be that increasing levels of all components of physical fitness (aerobic capacity, muscular strength and endurance, flexibility, and body composition) may be equally important in both decreasing the incidence of back injuries and assisting in the expeditious rehabilitation of an injury.

The American College of Sports Medicine (ACSM) has made the following recommendations pertaining to the quality and quantity of exercise.[2] Five factors must be successfully structured to obtain optimal gains in cardiovascular fitness. These include:

1. Type/mode of activity
2. Intensity
3. Duration
4. Frequency
5. Rate of progression

TYPE OF ACTIVITY

To attain maximal gains in cardiovascular fitness, an activity must incorporate large muscle mass and must be performed for a prolonged period of time in a continuous, rhythmic fashion. Exercises such as walking, swimming, jogging/running, cycling, and cross-country skiing usually meet the established criteria. Other activities such as hiking, figure skating, dancing, etc. can also significantly improve aerobic capacity if structured appropriately. Although less tedious than cycling or treadmill walking, these activities do not provide as great a control of exercise intensity and therefore should be employed cautiously with novices or rehabilitation participants until a base level of conditioning is developed.

The injured athlete must maintain cardiovascular fitness to avoid deconditioning often associated with increased pain and depression. Specifically designed exercise protocols consistent with the patient's working diagnosis must be adhered to. In the case of a herniated disc, flexion exercises should be avoided. Bicycling in the upright position or swimming should be considered. In spondylolisthesis, extension exercises beyond neutral should be avoided and appropriate abdominal strenghtening and dynamic stabilization instituted.

Rotation often exacerbates symptoms in the spine-injured patient. Rotational exercises should first be accomplished in an unloaded or slightly loaded position prior to more aggressive endeavors. Exercising on specific types of equipment such as the Schwinn Air-Dyne, the UBE, or on a standard treadmill are all cardiovascular exercises that have inherent rotational components and consequently should be employed cautiously.

Jogging and running warrant special attention. These activities transmit impact-loading to the spine. These forces can be as much as three to four times the person's body weight. Jogging causes more vertical load than running and consequently may be more damaging to the spine. Hence, running might well be a better choice than jogging. Either may not be tolerated and hence should be prescribed cautiously. Lower impact cardiovascular activities such as bicycling, swimming, walking, and stair climbing may indeed prove less hazardous and a better choice than jogging or running.

EXERCISE INTENSITY

To maximize gains in aerobic capacity, exercise intensity should correspond to 65 to 90% of an individual's maximal heart rate or 50 to 85% of his functional capacity (VO_2max). This value varies depending on the patient's initial level of cardiovascular fitness. The greater an individual's aerobic capacity, the greater his exercise intensity must be in order to achieve significant improvements in VO_2max.

Provided the total energy expenditure is the same, individuals may be able to exercise at lower intensities for a longer duration and obtain similar improvements in VO_2max as they would exercising for a shorter time but at a greater intensity.[15,32,40] Exercise adherence is improved when subjects exercise at lower training intensities.[36] In addition, high-intensity training programs have been associated with a greater incidence of musculoskeletal injuries[26,30] and cardiovascular symptoms.[14,21,33] Therefore, it appears advantageous to have patients exercise at lower intensities for longer durations. Exercise intensity may be monitored by a variety of techniques. The heart rate method will be discussed.

Generally, unless disturbed by environmental conditions, disease, or psychological stimuli, a direct relationship exists between heart rate and exercise intensity.[46] Therefore, when exercising to increase aerobic capacity, heart rate can be effectively utilized to prescribe and monitor exercise intensity.

Training heart rate can be accurately assessed during an exercise stress test on a bicycle or treadmill ergometer. When access or costs restrict performing these objective measures, a less sophisticated estimate may be calculated as follows:

> 220 − age = maximal predicted heart rate (HRmax); subtract the resting heart rate* multiplied by % of maximal heart rate (ranges from 0.65 to 0.90); add the resting heart rate. This final quantity is the Target Heart Rate

It is difficult to maintain the heart rate at exactly a specified value, hence a range of approximately ± 5 bpm is established, which is the target heart rate zone. The goal is to exercise at a workload that allows the patient's heart rate to plateau and remain within this range for the duration of the session, excluding warm-up and cool-down.

DURATION OF EXERCISE

To obtain maximal improvements in functional capacity, the duration of the exercise session, excluding the warm-up and cool-down, can vary in length from 15–60 minutes. In general, the longer the duration of the exercise session, the greater the magnitude of improvements in VO_2max.[1,18,21,28,29,43] Significant improvements in aerobic capacity have been demonstrated with high-intensity (greater than 90% max), short-duration (5–10 minutes) sessions. However, high-intensity sessions are associated with a greater risk for orthopedic injury and cardiovascular problems. Hence, for sedentary individuals lower intensity (40 to 70% of functional capacity), moderate-duration (20–30 minutes) exercise sessions are recommended. An individual should not experience undue fatigue an hour

---

* Resting heart rate should be determined upon waking in the morning or while lying supine. Heart rate should be taken for 3–5 minutes and then averaged to determine beats per minute (bpm).

after an exercise session.[2] Lower intensity exercises can be sustained for a longer duration with less fatigue. A low- to moderate-intensity and longer-duration exercise session is recommended for nonathletic adults, when the goal is to improve aerobic capacity and not athletic performance.

A patient recovering from an orthopedic injury may not be able to tolerate even low-intensity and moderate-duration exercises. Repeated brief bouts of low-intensity exercise ranging from 15–20 seconds to 2–3 minutes may be appropriate initially until a base level of exercise tolerance is developed.

FREQUENCY OF EXERCISE

The ACSM's general recommendation for training frequency is 3 to 5 days per week.[2] The greater the initial fitness level, the more frequently exercises can be performed. Frequency can vary from numerous daily exercise sessions of low-intensity and short-duration, to three to seven single daily sessions per week. Training more frequently than 5 days per week is possible; however, 95% of the potential improvement in aerobic capacity is obtained in a jog/run program of 4 to 5 days per week.[31] The risk for orthopedic injuries increases exponentially with jog/run-type exercises following increased training frequency and duration. When exercise frequency exceeds 4 days per week, the participant is encouraged to employ "cross-training" techniques to minimize the potential for an overuse syndrome as well as to decrease the possibility of boredom and staleness.

RATE OF EXERCISE PROGRESSION

Progression of aerobic exercise activities is highly dependent upon the health, age, functional capacity, and needs of the participant. Exercise progression is currently divided into three stages: initial, improvement, and maintenance.

Initial Conditioning Phase. A base level of conditioning is accomplished by initiating a low-level conditioning program that minimizes muscle soreness resulting from exercise. The length of time required to establish the base fitness level depends on an individual's adherence to the program. The initial conditioning phase consists of a 4 to 6 week period, but may extend to as much as 10 weeks.

The initial exercise duration is typically no more than 10–15 minutes per session; however, for some patients, it is not uncommon to have total exercise sessions lasting 5 minutes or less. Exercise duration may be limited by local muscle fatigue, breathlessness, symptoms of cardiac disease (angina), or increased pain. Exercise prescriptions must be individualized.

Improvement Conditioning Phase. This phase differs from the initial phase of conditioning in that individuals are progressed at a much quicker rate. The duration of exercise sessions is typically increased every 1 to 3 weeks. If the individual is not already exercising at an intensity that corresponds to 50–85% of his or her functional capacity, then this level should be accomplished within the improvement phase. Fitness level determines progression of exercise intensity and frequency. The duration of exercise should be increased to 20–30 minutes before increasing the exercise intensity. Older individuals may take longer to adapt to the stresses of exercise and hence may require a slower rate of progression.

Maintenance Conditioning Phase. Most individuals will obtain the greatest proportion of cardiovascular improvements within the first 6 months of a training program. The purpose of this phase is to maintain the improvements accomplished in the previous phases.

MUSCULAR STRENGTH

Muscular strength is defined as the maximal tension or force that can be generated by a muscle or group of muscles.[3] Maximal muscular strength is obtained from exercises of high-resistance and low-repetition. Muscular strength can be classified as static, dynamic, or explosive.

Static strength is the ability of a muscle to exert a maximal force for an extended period of time. A high level of static strength is required by a gymnast when performing movements such as the iron cross. Static strength requires isometric muscular contractions that generate muscle tension; however, there is little or no muscle shortening, lengthening, or joint movement. No external work is performed; however, internal muscular work is performed, which is reflected by the liberation of heat. Static strength may be assessed by a tensiometer or dynamometer.

Dynamic strength is the ability to repeatedly create forces to move or support a portion of the body weight for an extended period of time. This is exemplified by the repeated muscular contractions of the long-distance runner. Dynamic strength efforts utilize isotonic muscular contractions. The length of the muscles constantly varies from decreasing lengths (concentric contractions) to increasing lengths (eccentric contractions), both of which cause joint movement. Dynamic strength may be assessed by performing calisthenics, various forms of weight lifting, or with cable tensiometers or dynamometers. An isokinetic dynamometer may be utilized to objectively measure dynamic strength.

Finally, **explosive strength** is the ability to exert a maximal, short burst of force. This type of strength is demonstrated by the shot-putter, who combines the explosive strength capabilities of various muscle groups to propel the shot into space. Explosive strength is essentially the same as muscle power. Power is defined as the amount of external work performed divided by time.[1,38] Power is typically more important in athletic pursuits when the velocity of force production, joint movement, and external work completed are key to successful performance.

MUSCULAR ENDURANCE

Muscular endurance is defined as the ability of a muscle or group of muscles to work at a less than maximal level for an extended period of time.[38] Improvements in muscular endurance are demonstrated from a conditioning program that applies low-resistance, high-repetitions against the muscle(s). The development of adequate levels of muscular endurance affords an individual the ability to perform repeated muscular contractions or work tasks for an extended period of time without undue fatigue. As muscular endurance increases, normally lesser improvements are seen in muscle strength and vice versa.

The development of strength and endurance is very specific to the muscle group trained and the type of contractions (i.e., isometric, isotonic, concentric, eccentric, etc.) and positions (joint angles) in which the muscle is trained. Even though some transfer of strength is demonstrated via isokinetic or isometric testing methods, if an individual trains in an isotonic or isometric manner, then he or she should be tested isotonically or isometrically, respectively.

THE KINETIC CHAIN

The human body is a conceptual kinetic chain, consisting of many bones, joints, muscles, and connective tissues. A balance in the strength, endurance, and length of these tissues must be maintained to ensure proper motion, stability, and function. Often, if an imbalance of strength and/or length (tissue shortness, or hypomobility) exists on one side of a joint, there will exist weakness and/or excess muscle or connective tissue length (hypermobility) on the opposing side. When these conditions exist, the related joint is considered to be at risk for an injury.

Under normal conditions, the trunk muscles, including the back extensors, flexors, lateral flexors, and rotators, provide movement and stability to the trunk. When trauma has affected the musculotendinous unit or joint, changes in the muscle and/or connective tissue length, strength, or function associated with disuse and inhibition can occur. An accurate objective assessment of a patient's muscular strength compared to a normative data base is essential in rehabilitation. This information helps set goals.

Strength Ratios. Numerous investigators have attempted to identify the appropriate muscle agonist/antagonist strength ratios for the trunk.[7] There is great variation in the assessment of trunk muscle strength. This is coincident with the variety of testing methods available (i.e., isometric, concentric, eccentric, and isokinetic). Most studies indicate the peak torque ratios of the trunk muscles for healthy individuals (extensors to flexors) range from 1.0–2.0 to 1 (1–2:1). The most commonly cited ratio is 1.3:1, indicating the trunk extensors are 30% stronger than the flexors. In the low-back-pain patient population, ratios from 0.79 to 1.23 for extension/flexion have been reported.

Since the articulations of the back allow movement in multiple planes, it is important to look beyond just extension/flexion ratios and to identify the ideal ratios for lateral flexion and rotation. The generally accepted ratio for lateral flexion and rotation is 1:1. Further studies are warranted to analyze functional activities incorporating flexion/extension coupled with rotational and side-bending components.

Once muscle balance and strength have been assessed, the information must be integrated into a conditioning or rehabilitation plan that includes specific strengthening and stretching exercises to correct imbalances. The information that follows highlights pertinent relationships of the various muscle groups of the trunk and lower extremities to the pelvis.

Muscular Stability of the Vertebral Column

Stability of the trunk is provided by anterior, lateral, and posterior musculature. Anteriorly these include the rectus abdominis and internal and external oblique muscles. The combined forces of these muscles act to oppose hyperextension of the vertebral column.[24] The anterior musculature assists in the maintenance of an ideal standing posture. Weakness or paralysis of these muscles may lead to excessive lordosis of the lumbar spine, increasing the potential risk for spinal injuries.

Posteriorly, the erector spinae, quadratus lumborum, intertransversarii, interspinalis, transversospinalis, and levator muscles function together to provide posterior stability for the vertebral column, as well as opposing the forces of gravity. They also function as antagonists to the anterior musculature. These major muscle groups are assisted by multiple other muscle groups, including the neck, arm, buttock, and leg, to maintain an erect posture.[38] Therefore, appropriate leg-length strength of all these muscle groups is essential to maintain ideal posture.

Postural Alignment of the Lumbar Spine and Pelvis

The pelvis is the critical link joining the vertebral column to the lower extremities. During ambulation the mobile pelvis transmits the motion of gait to the vertebral column via strong ligamentous attachments to the lumbar spine.

The relationship of the pelvis to the spine is critical in the prevention and treatment of low back injuries. The pelvis may be tilted anteriorly or posteriorly in the sagittal plane. An extenuation of anterior pelvic tilt may result in hyperlordosis. This is caused from abdominal weakness and may be associated with contracture of the lumbodorsal fascia. A posterior tilt of the pelvis in the sagittal plane is often the result of lumbar or thoracic kyphosis and is associated with weakness of the paraspinal extensor muscles. Either of these sagittal plane abnormalities changes the normal transfer of motion from the pelvis to the lumbar spine. This can accelerate the degenerative process involving the lumbar discs and facets. Critical to any rehabilitation program is an attempt to normalize this biomechanical relationship by balancing the strength and length of the appropriate trunk muscles.

Anterior Pelvic Tilt

Hip flexors, abdominals, hamstrings, low-back extensors, and gluteal muscles may be responsible for anterior pelvic tilt. Hip flexors insert along the anterior portion of the lumbar vertebrae and exert a forward and downward pull on the vertebrae. Excessive shortening of the hip flexors may be responsible for exaggerated anterior pelvic tilt. Although this situation may be counteracted by strong abdominal muscles, frequently the abdominal musculature is weak and elongated, contributing to hyperlordosis.[25] The elongated hamstring and gluteal muscles cannot counteract the hip flexors, creating further pelvic tilt. Furthermore, adaptive contracture of the lumbodorsal fascia contributes to the problem. Treatment consists of a stretching program for the lumbodorsal fascia and hip flexors, as well as strengthening of abdominal, gluteus maximus, and hamstring muscles to reduce excessive lumbar lordosis.

Posterior Pelvic Tilt

Posterior pelvic tilt causes a reduction in the lordosis of the lumbar spine, commonly called flat back. Contracture of hamstrings and hip extensors with concomitant elongation of the hip flexors and back extensors predispose to this posture. A specific rehabilitation program consisting of hip flexor and back extensor strengthening along with hamstring, abdominal, and hip extensor stretching is recommended.

FLEXIBILITY

Empirical evidence suggests that generalized flexibility is essential for successful athletic performance.[6,17,19,20,35] Maintenance of flexibility is also apparently important in the prevention of injuries.[8,19,39] Consequently, most coaches include stretching exercises as part of their team's required workout routine.[41,42]

Although flexibility is considered synonymous with range of motion, it is more correctly considered a combined result of the function of different anatomic structures. Muscles, tendons, ligaments, cartilage, joint surfaces, and synovial fluid all play a crucial role in joint mobility under both normal and pathologial conditions.[38]

Flexibility may be classified as static or dynamic. Passive motion to an anatomic endpoint is referred to as the static flexibility of a joint.[25] Dynamic flexibility, on the other hand, is the active range of motion that results from muscular contracture. Dynamic flexibility usually occurs through the mid-range of motion and is not considered to be a reliable indicator of true joint motion. Dynamic flexibility is noted to increase athletic performance while decreasing risk of injury. For example, hamstring tightness places a runner at considerable disadvantage due to reduced knee extension, with a concomitant decrease in running speed. Static flexibility is also noted to be related to a decrease in musculotendinous injury during athletic activities.

When static or dynamic motion deficits are diagnosed, an effort to reestablish physiologic range of motion should be attempted. Hypermobility should be avoided. This is especially important in spinal fusion, in which an aggressive stretching program may cause hypermobility above or below the previously fused levels.

Neurophysiology

The muscle spindle and the Golgi tendon organ (found within the muscle tissue) are receptors that send vital sensory information regarding the position of joints and muscles, as well as the degree of stretch experienced by these structures to the central nervous system. This information allows the complex interaction between agonist and antagonist groups to be formulated into purposeful motion. These receptors send vital sensory information via neural afferent pathways to the central nervous system (CNS). The CNS processes the information and sends impulses via neural efferent[5] back to the agonist and antagonist muscles, providing them with information concerning agonist muscle. The muscle spindles and the Golgi organs are both sensitive to changes in muscle length. The muscle spindle is responsible for what is called the "stretch reflex."[19,35] The Golgi organ is also sensitive to changes in muscle tension. The interaction between these two receptors to control muscle length is quite complex. For example, when an agonist muscle (the hamstring) is stretched, the muscle spindles, because of their parallel arrangement to the muscle fibers, are also stretched, which causes them to send sensory information to the CNS that the muscle is being stretched. If the (hamstring) muscle and associated muscle spindles stretch too fast or too far, the agonist muscle (hamstring) will, through the stretch reflex (caused by the muscle spindles), stimulate the hamstring muscle to contract. The strength of this contraction will be proportionate to the degree and speed of the stretch. The greater the stretch and/or the faster the stretch, the greater the reflex contraction in the hamstring. This series of actions is executed as a safety mechanism designed to limit further stretching of the (hamstring) agonist muscles.[41,42] If the stretch is held for 6–10 seconds, the Golgi organs, being sensitive to the increase in muscle tension, will send their own impulses to the CNS, which will cause a reflex relaxation of the agonist (hamstring) muscle. This reflex reaction has been called the "inverse stretch reflex."[6] This protective mechanism allows the agonist muscle to be stretched in a relaxed fashion, so that its extensibility limits are not exceeded, which reduces the potential for trauma or damage to the muscle and related joint(s).

STRETCHING PROTOCOLS

There are different types of stretching exercises designed to increase flexibility. The oldest, termed the "ballistic stretch," uses repetitive bouncing movements to elongate soft tissues.[17,19] In contrast, the "passive stretch" often requires another person utilizing external forces to elongate the tissues.[6] "Static stretch" techniques are intended to elongate muscles and related tissues to a point of mild tension or mild discomfort. This position is then held for a specified time.[11,17,19] Finally, "proprioceptive neuromuscular facilitation" (PNF) utilizes alternating submaximal muscular contractions with static stretching exercises.[27,34,35]

Ballistic stretching has been abandoned due to the associated risk of joint and/or soft-tissue injury.[42] The rapid forceful movements utilized in this technique elicit a vigorous stretch reflex from the muscle spindles[6] and a concomitant muscle contraction, which may cause injury and should be discouraged. Correctly performed passive stretching, on the other hand, can be very effective in increasing range of motion. Care must be taken to minimize the risk of muscle or tendon injury due to too vigorous an external force. Static stretching that is performed in a gentle fashion generates the least amount of muscle tension. When correctly performed, the spindle's stretch reflex is avoided and the Golgi tendon organ is stimulated to cause muscle relaxation. This technique decreases the risk of soft-tissue injury and may be the safest of all.[6] Finally, PNF stretching techniques also use the Golgi organ's ability to override the muscle spindle's stretch reflex by eliciting the inverse stretch reflex mechanism and therefore are very successful in stretching contracted tissues.

Physiological Responses to Stretching. Although stretching programs are designed to increase the range of motion in specific muscles, often the connective tissue surrounding the joint is affected most significantly.[39] When a relaxed muscle is stretched, the most significant resistant to stretch is derived from the connective tissue in and around the muscle and not from stretching of the myofibrils.[4,23,37,45] Often following trauma or surgery, pathological changes occur in connective tissue in the form of scar formation, adhesions, and fibrotic contracture. Thus, stretching these contracted connective tissues may help achieve the goal of improved range of motion.

The success of stretching protocols also depends on the mechanical behavior of connective tissues under a tensile stress. Connective tissue responds to stretch with both plastic and elastic properties.[38] In response to a tensile stress, the tissues initially respond in an elastic fashion. Once the tensile stress is removed, the tissues return in spring-like fashion to their prestretched length. The results of this form of stretching are temporary. If the tensile stretch is increased, however, plastic deformation may occur in the target tissue. When tensile load is removed, the tissue does not return to its prestretched length, and a more permanent clinical result is obtained. Those tissues that contain plastic elements are said to have a viscous property. In fact, connective tissues have both plastic and elastic components within their physiological range. Therefore, connective tissues function as a viscoelastic material in which both elastic and plastic deformation occur, depending on the stretching technique and force used.[39,44]

Successful tissue stretching therefore requires appropriate force and duration. In connective tissue models (tendon), the amount of time required to obtain tissue stretching varies inversely with the force used.[39,44,45] It has been observed that methods using long duration and low force result in greater long-term elongation of connective tissues than those those protocols in which high force and short duration are used. Because permanent elongation of muscle-tendon units is the goal of a stretching program, exercises that preferentially alter the plastic rather than the elastic elements of tendons should be promoted.

Clinical Guidelines for Stretching Exercises. A well-designed stretching program should include exercises for all major muscle groups. Specialized exercises should be undertaken for specific areas where contracture has been demonstrated. These exercises should be conducted slowly and gently and elongation of the specific structure carried to the point of mild tension or mild discomfort and held for 30–60 seconds. These may be repeated in sets three to four times in an effort to obtain the maximum increase in range of motion.

SUMMARY

In this chapter we have attempted to review the preventative and therapeutic benefits of cardiovascular fitness, flexibility, muscle strength, and endurance. An incorporation of these findings into a daily exercise program can decrease athletic injury and may also favorably influence the incidence of occupational injury. When a back injury has occurred, these same techniques applied to rehabilitation can speed the recovery of a disabled individual and potentially decrease the chance of recurrent injury.

REFERENCES

1. American College of Sports Medicine. Position statement on the recommended quantity and quality of exercise for developing and maintaining fitness in healthy adults. Med Sci Sports 10:vii–x, 1975.
2. American College of Sports Medicine. Blair SN, et al (eds): Resource Manual for Guidelines for Exercise Testing and Prescription. Philadelphia, Lea & Febiger, 1986.
3. American College of Sports Medicine. Blair SN, et al (eds): Resource Material for Guidelines for Exercise Testing and Prescription. Philadelphia, Lea & Febiger, 1986.
4. Banus MG, Zetlin AM: The relation of isometric tension to length in skeletal muscle. J Cell Comp Physiol 12:4403–420, 1938.
5. Battie MC, Bigos SJ, Fisher LD, et al: A prospective study of the role of cardiovascular risk factors and fitness in industrial back pain complaints. Spine 14(2):141–147, 1989.
6. Beaulieu JE: Developing a stretching program. Phys Sportsmed 9(11):59–69, 1981.
7. Beimborn DS, Morrissey MC: A review of the literature related to trunk muscle performance. Spine 13(6):655–660, 1988.
8. Bobath B: The treatment of motor disorders of pyramidal and extrapyramidal origin by reflex inhibition and by facilitation of movement. Psychotherapy 41:146, 1955.
9. Cady LD, Bischoff DP, O'Connell ER, et al: Strength and fitness related to subsequent back injuries in firefighters. J Occ Med 21(4):269–272, 1979.
10. Cady LD, Thomas PC, Karwasky RJ: Program for increasing health and physical fitness of firefighters. J Occup Med 2:111–114, 1985.
11. Cornelius WL: Two effective flexibility methods. Athletic Training 16:23–25, 1981.
12. Cureton TK: Flexibility as an aspect of physical fitness. Res Q Am Assoc Health Phys Educ 12(suppl):382, 1941.
13. De Vries HA: Evaluation of static stretching procedures for improvement of flexibility. Res Q 33:222–228, 1962.
14. Firoelicher VF: Exercise testing and training: Clinical applications. J Am Coll Cardiol 1:114–125, 1983.
15. Gettman LR, Pollock ML, Durstine JL, et al: Physiological responses of men to 1, 3, and 5 day per week training programs. Res Q 47:638–646, 1976.
16. Glisan B, Stith WJ, Kiser S: Physiology of active exercise in rehabilitation of back injuries. Spine: State Art Rev 3(1):1989.
17. Harris ML: Flexibility: A review of the literature. Phys Ther 49:591–601, 1969.
18. Hartung GH, Smolensky MH, Harrist RB, Runge R: Effects of varied durations of training on improvements in cardiorespiratory endurance. J Hum Ergo 6:61–68, 1977.
19. Holland GJ: The physiology of flexibility: A review of the literature. Kinesiol Rev 00:49–62, 1968.
20. Hole LE, Travis TM, Okita T: Comparative study of three stretching techniques. Perceptual & Motor Skills 31:611–616, 1970.
21. Hossack KF, Hartwig R: Cardiac arrest associated with supervised cardiac rehabilitation. J Card Rehabil 2:402–408, 1982.
22. Jensen C, Fisher G: Scientific Basis of Athletic Conditioning. Philadelphia, Lea & Febiger, 1979.
23. Johns RJ, Wright V: Relative importance of various tissues in joint stiffness. J Appl Physiol 17:824–828, 1962.

24. Kareighbaum E, Barthelis KM: Biomechanics: A Qualitative Approach for the Study of Human Motion, 2nd ed. Edina, MN, Burgess Publishing Company, 1985.
25. Kendall FP, McCreary EK: Muscles: Testing and Function, 3rd ed. Baltimore, Williams & Wilkins, 1983.
26. Kilbom A, Hartley L, Saltin B, et al: Physical training in sedentary middle-aged and older men. Scand J Clin Lab Invest 24:315–322, 1969.
27. Knott M, Voss DE: Proprioceptive Neuromuscular Facilitation: Patterns and Techniques, New York, Harper & Row, 1968.
28. Liang MT, Alexander JF, Taylor HL, et al: Aerobic training threshold. Scand J Sports Sci 4:5–8, 1982.
29. Milesis CA, Pollock ML, Bah MD, et al: Effects of different durations of training on cardiorespiratory function, body composition and serum lipids. Res Q 47:716–725, 1976.
30. Oja P, Teraslinna P, Partaner T, Kapava R: Feasibility of an 18 month physical training program for middle-aged men and its effect on physical fitness. Am J Public Health 64:459–465, 1975.
31. Pollock ML: The quantification of endurance training programs. In Wilmore JM (ed): Exercise and Sport Sciences Reviews, Vol. 1. New York Academic Press, 1973, pp 155–158.
32. Pollock ML, Dimmick J, Miller HS, et al: Effects of mode of training on cardiovascular function and body composition of middle-aged men. Med Sci Sports 7:139–145, 1975.
33. Pollock ML, Miller H, Janeway R, et al: Effects of walking on body composition and cardiovascular function of middle-aged men. J Appl Physiol 30:126–130, 1971.
34. Prentice WE: An electromyographic analysis of the effectiveness of heat or cold and stretching for inducing relaxation in injured muscle. J Orthop Sports Phys Ther 3(3):133–140, 1982.
35. Prentice WE: A comparison of static stretching and PNF stretching for improving hip joint flexibility. Athletic Training 18:56–59, 1983.
36. Price C, Pollock ML, Gettman LR, Kent DA: Physical Fitness Programs for Law Enforcement Officers: A Manual for Police Administrators. Washington D.C., U.S. Government Printing Office, No. 027-000-00671-0, 1978.
37. Ramsey R, Street S: The isometric length-tension diagram of isolated skeletal muscle fibers of the frog. J Cell Comp Physiol 15:11–34, 1940.
38. Rasch PJ, Burke RK: Kinesiology and Applied Anatomy: The Science of Human Movement. 1978.
39. Sapega AA, Quedenfeld TC, Moyer RA, Butler RA: Biophysical factors in range-of-motion exercise. Phys Sportsmed 9(12):57–65, 1981.
40. Sharkey BJ: Intensity and duration of training and the development of cardiorespiratory endurance. Med Sci Sports 2:197–202, 1970.
41. Shellock FG: Physiological benefits of warm-up. Phys Sportsmed 11(10):134–139, 1983.
42. Shellock FG, Prentice WE: Warming-up and stretching for improved physical performance and prevention of sports-related injuries. Sports Med 2:267–278, 1985.
43. Terjung RL, Baldwin KM, Codesey J, et al: Cardiovascular adaptation to 12 minutes of mild daily exercise in middle-aged sedentary men. J Am Geriatr Soc 21:164–168, 1973.
44. Warren CG, Lehmann JF, Koblanski JN: Heat and stretch procedures: An evaluation using rat tail tendon. Arch Phys Med Rehabil 57:122–126, 1976.
45. Warren CG, Lehmann JF, Koblanski JN: Elongation of rat tail tendon: Effect of load and temperature. Arch Phys Med Rehabil 52:465–474, 1971.
46. Wasserman K, Hansen JE, Sue DY, Whipp BJ: Principles of Exercise Testing and Interpretation. 1987.

Chapter 4

ISOKINETIC TRUNK TESTING

Thomas A. Lorren, PT

Prior to the 1960s and 70s, any serious discussion of muscular performance measurement was limited to evaluating the performance of muscle or muscle complexes against two types of resistance: isometrics, a zero-speed static mode with no observable angular velocity (i.e., manual muscle or grip strength testing), and isotonics, a movement in which the resistance is fixed, but which may be performed at variable velocities. If we exclude the changes in lever arm and effects of inertia, an example would be using free weights or machine weight stacks. However, in 1968 Perrine developed the concept that totally revolutionized the way we look at objective muscle testing. This concept was called isokinetics and is one of the most commonly used methods of assessing muscular performance today.

DEFINITION

The term "isokinetics" was defined by Thistle et al.[22] and has had wide acceptance in the field of sports medicine. Isokinetics is essentially a movement in which the speed is fixed but the resistance is variable. Although there are many fine points separating the various aspects of isotonic and isokinetic concepts, for simplicity's sake it can be said that isotonic and isokinetic procedures are essentially the opposite with respect to velocity and resistance. Muscular force varies throughout the range of motion due to different biomechanics within the musculoskeletal system. With isokinetics, an application force throughout a range of motion will give a proportional resistance to that muscle group through the different joint angles, resulting in optimal dynamic loading.[3] This contrasts with isotonic loading, which allows loading only up to the weakest point on a muscle force curve before a full movement can no longer be achieved.

TRUNK TESTING

The use of isokinetics has been well documented in testing and treating the extremities, but has only been applied to the back since the late 1970s.[13] Prior to that time, testing for back strength was done isotonically by having a subject stabilized in the supine or prone position with weights for resistance attached to the trunk, and the number of flexion or extension movements that the individual could complete determined the flexor or extensor strength. Back strength was also measured isometrically (usually in a neutral upright position) in the flexion or extension direction against a strain gauge.

Early isokinetic trunk research was often performed using experimental devices. These were often single creations specific for the research design. Since the information obtained varies from device to device, the research data must be used with caution for direct application.

With the emergence of isokinetics in trunk testing, the primary niche for trunk dynamometry has been within the industrial research and occupational field. Although it has had wide acceptance, the use of spinal dynamometry has had little if any specific application to the field of sports medicine. The reasons for this are unclear but have resulted in a dearth of comparative data about the athletic population. It is our purpose here to review the literature and our personal experience to discuss the model of isokinetic athletic assessment used at the Texas Back Institute.

The need to objectively measure spine strength in athletics is fairly obvious. Both trunk and hip strength are important in sports to maintain balance, stability, and control. Since the trunk comprises greater than 50% of the body mass,[23] trunk muscles must maintain body equilibrium in the various motor tasks, as well as provide a central role in locomotion.[12]

Advantages. Isokinetic testing and treating, although expensive, does have several distinct advantages. It provides a testing procedure with minimal variables that allows the inclusion of virtually all individuals and further provides an accurate comparison of athletes to their representative groups. It permits training at higher speeds than would be possible with isotonics and still obtains objective data. It allows the measurement of consistency in patient performance based solely on the individual's previous contractions. In providing totally accommodating variable resistance, isokinetic testing is safe for testing and rehabilitation, but allows the maximum accommodation of force in resistance-training programs. It is also used to assess the affect of various treatment regimens.

Contraindications. As with any applied resistance, isokinetics, despite its inherent safety, may be contraindicated for certain individuals. For back testing, contraindications include individuals with sensory deficits, with acute or unstable fractures, with acute musculoskeletal injury, with hypertension, and anyone with moderate-to-severe pain exacerbated to an intolerable level by the activity or position of exercise. Patients with nerve root signs should also not be tested, especially those with signs or symptoms that are exacerbated by applied resistance. Although these are absolute contraindications, there are a few relative contraindications that should be addressed prior to discussion of spinal dynamometry. These include facet synovitis, spondylosis/spondylolisthesis, pars defect, Schmorl's nodes, scoliosis, and spinal stenosis. In individuals with these conditions it is possible to do a trunk isokinetic test safely. However, care must be taken to ensure that the process of testing does not exacerbate any unwanted signs or symptoms and that precautions are taken not to put the individual being tested at risk. This is usually done through specific patient positioning or administering the test in a modified manner.

Warm-up. As with any strenuous activity, it is imperative that the athlete be thoroughly warmed up before undergoing a maximal test. This can be achieved through 5 to 10 minutes of light stretching and active exercises, with particular attention to the muscles that will be used in the test. For trunk flexion these are the rectus abdominis, the internal and external obliques, and the iliopsoas. For trunk extension they are the hamstrings, gluteus maximus, and erector spinae. Since the lower extremities will be involved, they should be warmed up as part of the functional flexion and extension kinetic chain. Of prime importance in the pretest sequence is sustained static stretching, which should be held for 30 to 60 seconds to enhance muscle relaxation and avoid stimulating the Golgi tendon organs. This type of stretch has been shown to decrease muscle tension by half in comparison with ballistic stretching.[24]

TEST PROCEDURE

After making sure the patient is warmed up and stretched, the main keys to successful testing are giving clear consistent instructions and familiarizing the athlete with the examiner, the test, and the equipment. This includes making sure the athlete is wearing appropriate clothing and has removed all jewelry, especially earrings and chest/neck chains. The latter is of prime importance, since most trunk testing requires the application point for equipment resistance to be across the upper portion of the pectoral muscles and the sternum.

In addition to familiarizing the athlete with the test and equipment, a baseline blood pressure and pulse should be taken. This allows assessment of exertional recovery before progressing on to the next stage of the test. It is also a good idea to find out if the individual has a history of smoking and has eaten a meal within the last 3 to 4 hours. Although it is inadvisable to test a patient immediately after eating, this will not generally cause concern in the absence of other contraindications. However, occasionally problems such as fainting and nausea have been encountered, especially in young adult males. These are usually smokers who have had no breakfast and are tested late in the morning. Although it is impossible to say that these are specific contributing factors, in the absence of these factors and with repeated admonition not to hold their breath, these subjects seem to do quite well.

Positioning for Back Testing. The ability to test in multiple positions is of prime importance in back testing. The standing position gives information about the combination of the spine and hip action from a functional posture. Sitting posture helps to minimize the effective motion of the hips and the lower extremities. It is also believed that in sitting the pelvis is secure to the extent that the iliopsoas (a major contributor to spinal strength) is relaxed throughout the entire test. If this is the case, the primary results are obtained from the abdominal and paraspinal muscles.[15] Comparing the torque generated between seated and standing positions, involvement of the iliopsoas in the flexion movement increased the values by 100%.[15] In testing an individual with pathologic conditions (in the absence of absolute contraindications), the best results are usually obtained by making the patient comfortable. When working with individuals with known instabilities, testing in the seated position has been shown to be better tolerated than standing. This may be accounted for by the inherent "close-packed" position of the lower spine in the seated position. If there is a concern about exacerbating a previous disc problem, the individual may be tested standing and limited to 30 to 45 degrees of flexion movement. This provides good low-speed data without bringing on unwanted signs and symptoms.

Repetitions. In isokinetic trunk testing, various authors have described the optimal number of repetitions as being between two and six. We have elected to use five repetitions, since this number allows the maximum amount of consistent cycles before the onset of fatigue. In the case of individuals who are more symptomatic, a minimum of three repetitions may be used, since this is the lowest number that will allow a comparison of consistency.

Speeds. Testing speeds for isokinetic back testing are generally listed as 30, 60, 90, 120, 150, and 180 degrees per second. Although 30 degrees per second is an excellent speed for running sub-maximal tests, it is generally too slow for athletes. At 30 degrees per second, a tremendous amount of force can be generated, particularly in the standing position, and may actually lead to "false-positives." A false-positive is defined as discomfort generated with high forces and slow speeds that is not the result of any specific disorder. This is commonly seen in lower extremity testing and is attributed to a large increase in shearing forces. At high speeds (180 and above), we have found that even normal individuals tend to become inconsistent. In testing at high speeds, the large body mass and dynamometer arm take an increased amount of time to be accelerated and decelerated. In addition to causing increased errors in torque calculation due to inertia, many individuals, especially those of smaller size, only "catch" the testing speed for a very brief amount of time, rendering the data obtained minimally useful. Generally, test speeds for isokinetic testing are 60, 90, 120 and 150 degrees per second.

Screening for Isokinetic Testing. As with all high-exertion activity, athletes and nonathletes alike should be screened prior to generating maximum isokinetic values. This can be accomplished by having the athlete progressively push harder and faster in both directions of flexion and extension over ten repetitions. If the patient can produce maximum values without any undue discomfort or symptoms, he or she has then demonstrated an ability to undergo a maximum test. If the athlete is unable to reach a maximum effort due to the onset of unwanted signs and symptoms, then a decision needs to be made from a clinical standpoint whether to discontinue the process or to proceed with a submaximum test.

Sub-maximum Testing. A sub-maximum test is a method of obtaining data from an individual in an isokinetic mode that demonstrates maximum output before the onset of signs and symptoms prevents the individual from going further. Generally, isokinetic testing is considered to be a maximal effort phenomenon. However, at the Texas Back Institute, we have had success with delineating the maximum pain-free response even in our symptomatic patients. This is done by discussing with the athlete the specific signs and symptoms that are characteristic for him or her. Once the athlete has these firmly in mind, he is requested to slowly flex and extend within a comfortable range. If this does not produce symptoms, he is requested to progressively push harder and harder on both flexion and extension while verbally expressing the absence or onset of symptoms. At the onset of signs or symptoms, the athlete is requested to immediately stop. The highest values generated are then used in establishing a baseline for future measurement of clinical progress.

Importance of Lead-in Sequence. We have found that it is virtually impossible, even for athletes, to generate maximum isokinetic values on the first repetition. To increase the accuracy of testing and to give the subject a good lead-in, we have found that the following sequence provides optimum results. The athlete is given instructions to provide a repetition of 50% effort, followed by a repetition of 75% effort, and then 6 to 7 maximal repetitions. These are done as hard and as fast as possible in both directions. The test is started at the end of the first maximal repetition, assuring that the athlete is running at a maximal level before test data collection is initiated, and he is asked to do one repetition maximally after test data collection has stopped. This assures that there will be no drop-out at the beginning and the end of a test sequence, while allowing the athlete the best chance to "get in the groove."

Recovery. Rest periods between test bouts are generally 90 seconds to 3 minutes. These are general guidelines and are used with the understanding that the decision to commence testing is predicated on the individual's cardiovascular response.

NORMATIVE DATA

In extremity isokinetic testing, normative data comparisons invariably consider the uninvolved extremity as the gold standard of an individual's performance. However, in the spine there is no comparable contralateral side. Therefore, for these tests to be useful, normative databases need to be established.[17] Since normative data by its nature needs to be age-, sex-, and activity-specific, criteria for "normal" muscle test results require data from large-scale population-specific samples.[10] In an athletic population, the ideal time to collect normative data is in a preparticipation physical examination.

The preparticipation physical examination is a method of determining an athlete's ability to participate safely in sports.[14] The preseason physicals should be the start of optimizing performance levels. This is done by identifying deviations in muscular strength, flexibility, and balance by testing the area specific to the individual sport.[1] An approach to the preparticipation exam has been described by Kibler et al., including a method of isokinetic testing of upper and lower extremities in a sport-specific approach.[14] Although no mention was made of the use of trunk objective data testing, the approach can be blended with a trunk evaluation approach. An example of how this can be done has been demonstrated by Larry Feeler at Odessa Physical Therapy, Odessa, Texas in preseason screening of a high-school football team. Ten players grouped by position (i.e., defensive back, linemen, etc.) were tested and normative parameters established. Compilation of this data allows not only the individual player to be compared to his previous performance at some point down the line, but also establishes a reference to the parameters that are demonstrated by players excelling in their positions.[11]

In establishing normative data, it is important that the data be adjusted for the effects of gravity and for torque overshoot. Compensating for the effects of gravity is a data-manipulation technique. The individual being tested cannot feel whether the gravity correction is being applied or not. Gravity correction in a flexion/extension test discounts the effects of gravity in the flexion movement and recognizes it as an initial resistance to overcome in the extension movement. This allows more precise data to be calculated and allows ratios such as peak torque and work/repetition to body weight to be used with considerable confidence. Torque "overshoot" is that initial spike that occurs when the dynamometer reacts to the over-speeding lever arm. Although this is found to some extent in all systems, it has been compensated for by the Lido back unit, the system being used at the Texas Back Institute. The additional inertial correction by the Lido system allows for a more accurate evaluation of test results. It has been suggested that this force artifact (torque overshoot) be used as an indicator of the tested individual's willingness to "attack" the movement. This may be true and would have some credibility in the return-to-sport-after-injury determination of willingness to participate rather than in the initial preinjury evaluation or for normative testing. Other factors leading to torque overshoot are (1) a greater trunk mass, (2) a longer lever arm between the center of mass and the axis of rotation, and (3) the mass of the lever arm/carriage itself.

MISCONCEPTIONS ABOUT ISOKINETIC TESTING

Although isokinetics testing, properly used, is a marvelous tool, some aspects of its use have been thought to provide more information than can realistically be expected. For example, it has been suggested that isokinetic testing has the advantage of being able to measure specific muscle output. This is somewhat misleading since no dynamometer has the ability to distinguish between a muscle's torque generation and the contributions of the associated synergists. Parameter values that are generated need to be considered as arising from the total functional unit (i.e., all the components participating in the movement). An example is standing extension testing, which employs not only the back extensor muscles but the pelvic posterior rotators as well. This can be minimized somewhat by firmly stabilizing the pelvis with straps or placing the individual in a seated position, but the effect cannot be eliminated due to the strong forces being developed, the small arcs of motion, and an inability to firmly fix the patient without discomfort.

DATA FROM ISOKINETIC UNITS

Isokinetic units measure torque and the associated range of motion as a function of time. Work can be calculated from the angular movements and the torque values. Power can be derived from the work and time values. These parameters, as well as the associated ratios, form the basis of isokinetic analysis of trunk performance.

Torque. Maximum torque is a measure of the muscular force applied during dynamic conditions. From the standpoint of physics, it is defined as force multiplied by the distance from the axis of rotation to the force application point. Since the large movements of the body and movement around joint centers are essentially rotational, this parameter is the basis for measuring output. Peak torque is a measurement of absolute output at the highest point of force generation during the entire range of motion. This usually takes place at the optimal angle for the biomechanical lever arm. Although it is a single point, it is generally assumed to be representative of the muscle's peak ability to generate force. For comparison purposes based on normative data (unless the individual is being compared against himself), it must be taken in the context of peak torque to body-weight ratio to have any relevance.

Torque exerted during isokinetic movements decreases as velocity increases. This effect has been found in numerous studies of the extremities.[4,19] It has also been documented for the trunk.[9,21] Coyle et al. felt that, since it takes a finite amount of time for the muscle fibers to develop maximum tension, these torque decreases may be indicative of a muscle's inability to develop maximal tension at optimal joint angle.[7] Although these drop-offs are fairly significant in extremity testing, in trunk testing they appear to be much smaller, dropping only 10 to 15% in test speeds ranging from 60 to 150 degrees per second.

Range of Motion. Range of motion in an isokinetic device is the least accurate of all parameters. This is due to the extreme difficulty in maintaining an approximate body axis in line with a precise dynamometer axis. Although it is relatively precise, trunk range of motion from a testing unit should be replaced by a more reliable method of measurement using dual-angle inclinometry[18] or even with a simple goniometer. A dynamic measurement of the range of motion does, however, provide, with some certainty, the range of motion through which the athlete is willing to move at a significant rate of speed. Normative values for range of motion in trunk flexion and extension are approximately 85 to 100 degrees. Beyond this, it becomes somewhat difficult even for athletes to move on any dynamometer with a fixed lever arm due to the inability of the machine to adapt to the changing spinal axis of the athlete.

Time. Time in an isokinetic sense is almost analogous to range of motion. If a device is truly holding an individual isokinetic, the only instances that time can be increased are in the narrow acceleration and deceleration bands at the end of each range of motion and in that finite "turn-around time" when an individual changes from a flexion movement to an extension movement. If the time values are significantly different from what would be anticipated in an isokinetic test, one of the first areas to look at is whether the individual is actually catching the speed of the movement for any significant amount of time. Catching an isokinetic movement will result in the generation of some values, but only in a very narrow portion of the anticipated testing range. It should be noted that isokinetics are designed to prevent an individual from running faster than the preset speed of the movement but not slower.

Ratios. The most commonly used parameters are ratios. The primary comparative ratios are the peak torque to body-weight ratio and the flexion-to-extension ratio.

The peak torque to body-weight ratio is a method of comparing an individual to a representative group. At 60 degrees per second, male body-weight to flexion values in a standing position have been demonstrated to be 94–95%, and extension to body-weight values to be up to 124%. In females, these values are 67–70% in body-weight to flexion values, and 92–95% in body-weight to extension values. Although these values are widely used, caution should be taken in using them in too narrow an application. A wide range of isokinetic peak torque to body-weight ratios may be found in populations.[10] Limited testing of elite athletes indicates that the reported torque to body-weight ratios may be too low for use by some of these groups. For these groups, it was recommended that specific databases be developed.[21] However, testing by Anderson et al. in a comparative study of 57 male elite athletes (soccer players, wrestlers, tennis players, and gymnasts) and 14 elite female gymnasts revealed that although overall mean values for athletes were higher than for normals in pure trunk movements, trunk extension showed no marked differences between male athletes and normals. Note: care must be taken in using data from this study, since the test was done in a side-line, gravity-eliminated position.[2] There are no machines in commercial development that currently use this position.

Another very common parameter that is used is the **flexion-to-extension ratio.** This ratio compares the force generation of flexors to extensors. It is a general rule that in normal individuals extension is stronger than flexion at slow speeds. This is felt to be indicative of the balance in the relationship of the agonist to antagonist complex. If these values are to be used, it is essential that the effects of gravity be accounted for. Beimborn and Morrissey reported that the peak torque extension-to-flexion ratios range between 1.0 and 2.0, with 1.3 being the most commonly cited ratio.[5] The changes in trunk strength that occur during athletic training appear to be similar but opposite to those occurring in patients with back problems. In individuals with back problems, a decrease in extensor strength is the primary disability factor that brings the flexion and extension measures much closer together. In an athletic population (due to increased training), extension strength is very strong, but emphasis on development of anterior trunk musculature again brings the ratio of one to the other much closer.[2] In some studies these extension torques were found to be greater than flexion by values of 1.1 to 1, all the way up to 2.7 to 1.[13,16,21]

Work. Work is defined a force through a range of motion and is truly a quality measure. It has been defined in some references as area under the torque curve.[8] Although this definition serves to give a rough idea of the effect in using work values, the actual calculation of work is based on the torque position overlay curve. This is a torque to position graph that has no time value. However, the concept of work as a volume per repetition does have merit. It accurately conveys that a dip in the torque curve (a concavity, which in itself is never normal) correlates to a decrease in work per repetition. Since work is force through a range of motion, it can truly be used to denote progress, since it takes into account increases not only in force and range of motion, but in the relative ability to generate a higher force through a longer range of motion. Normative values for this complex parameter are difficult to establish and have been developed for groups only on a limited basis. Some studies have shown that the single best indicator for prediction of performance by an individual is work-per-repetition to body-weight ratio.[10]

Endurance. Muscular endurance has been defined as the ability of the contracting muscles to perform repeated contractions against a load.[3] In isokinetics, this is usually determined by having the desired muscle group perform a series of actions against the dynamometer resistance until a predetermined force level decay has been reached. This predetermined level is usually established as 50% of the initial peak torque value. When comparing this to a previously established repetition norm, the method has been shown to be fairly reliable.[6] An alternative method would be to have the individual work over a specific number of repetitions and then compare this to a desired level of work. Although this is an optimal situation, it is somewhat difficult due to the complexities of calculating desired work levels. However, with increased use of isokinetic testing and of back dynamometry in general, the increased use of this method lends itself to a greater and wider ranging application. Initial studies utilizing 50% force-level decay found that many individuals were going as long as 2½ minutes without any significant decrease in endurance. Subsequently, the majority of endurance testing has now been changed to a 25% fatigue index. In the protocols used commonly for isokinetic trunk testing, it has been found that females may have better endurance.[15]

Torque Curves. The use of torque curves in isokinetic testing is promising in the substantiation of diagnostic information.[21] However, there have been no torque curve interpretations that have been shown to reference specific pathologic conditions.[20] Back extension pain with movement cannot be sorted out on any objective data-producing device in a single test. Using different testing positions may somewhat enhance the data, but it is no substitute for a good comprehensive physical examination. It may be that the greatest use of torque curves is to show that there is a drop-off at a particular range of motion. Consistency in the shape and the amount of drop-off would indicate that there is a problem at this particular point in the range of motion and is specific evidence for further investigation.

ISOKINETICS IN REHABILITATION

Isokinetics in rehabilitation offers several advantages. In addition to establishing predictive levels of performance as compared to normative values, it also allows an overall evaluation of treatment progress, efficacy of treatment techniques, and confirmation of suspected weaknesses and imbalances. In a rehabilitation setting, the totally accommodating variable resistance of isokinetics offers optimal dynamic training. Using isokinetics in the treatment of the athlete, one may not have to know specifically what is wrong with the athlete to treat him. An example would be muscle strain versus annular strain in the back. Treatment on an isokinetic device would include: (1) placing the individual in a position of comfort, (2) starting with submaximal exercise, and (3) progressing as tolerated. Concerns of specific weights, adaptation to fatigue, and painful resistance are effectively eliminated. Generally one tries to stay within the guidelines of tissue capacity and tissue integrity; that is, if it is painful, have a good reason before you push through it. In back exercise, a general progression of training from the standpoint of tissue capacity would be isometric repetitions progressing to submaximal short-arc movements, progressing to submaximal full-arc movements, then to maximal short-arc movements, and maximal full-effort. The athlete may then be progressed with eccentric exercise if applicable.

Treatment problems generally can be related into two specific areas: (1) force-related problems, and (2) range of motion-related problems. Force-related problems are signs and symptoms that occur only when increased muscle tension is required; the absence of higher forces allows the individual to move pain-free through a full range of motion. Range of motion-related problems are those that, despite the forces involved, will cause discomfort any time the joint is put in the particular joint angle. Force-related problems are generally treated with submaximal exercise, with progression as tolerated through a full arc, whereas range of motion problems are generally treated by blocking an individual out of that specific range of motion.

Training

Once training through a full arc at maximum effort has been reached, the rationale for specific velocity spectrums comes to the forefront. Velocity spectrums are a procedure of working both slow and fast contractile velocity exercises to help facilitate rehabilitation and conditioning programs based on the specificity of training. This is generally done as demonstrated in Table 1. One

TABLE 1. Data from a Velocity Spectrum

SPEED	60	90	120	150	180		180	150	120	90	60
REPS	10	10	10	10	10		10	10	10	10	10
REST	90 sec	90 sec	90 sec	90 sec	90 sec	3–5 min	90 sec	90 sec	90 sec	90 sec	90 sec

bout constitutes one velocity spectrum. It is theorized that this type of exercise provides the optimal overall environment for stimulation of both fast- and slow-twitch muscles and improves the overall response of the muscle.

RELATIONSHIP OF ISOKINETICS TO FUNCTION

It has been suggested that isokinetic testing is not clinically useful due to the fact that there are no pure isokinetic movements that occur normally. There are no machine-generated tests that can accurately predict function other than by inference. Isokinetics testing is extremely useful in creating an environment in which many parameters are kept constant, with the patient being the variable. This allows an individual to be compared to himself or a representative group that performed the identical test under identical circumstances. The performance in this situation is then used to make generalizations about the tested individual in comparison to the known functional capabilities of the normative group. Ideally, testing should be done in a completely functional manner. However, this is not feasible due to the complexity of motions and the resultant many contributions of motion variables to the end results.

On-axis movements occur when the body movement's axis of rotation is aligned with the dynamometer's axis of rotation. An example of this is shoulder flexion/extension, or trunk flexion/extension. An off-axis movement is one that generally involves a translational force. An example of this is the leg press or functional lifting when the dynamometer does not have a specific axis point from which to measure. Off-axis testing allows a determination of the ability to perform tasks at a specific load but does not allow a determination of where the specific deficit lies. On-axis testing allows the examiner to more clearly identify the area of dysfunction but not to determine the ability of the individual to perform a complex task. Ideally, these two methods should go hand-in-hand in testing determination of function.

RETURN TO SPORT

In knees, the usual range for return-to-sport determinations by isokinetic testing is 80 to 90% of the uninvolved extremity or preinjury state. It is conceivable that a similar finding might be used for the trunk. This could be achieved by dividing the trunk strength of the tested individual by the preinjury values or by the appropriate normative values for the motion tested. The 80 to 90% range is arbitrarily chosen, but with a greater understanding of muscular strength in spinal disorders, isokinetic testing may offer some useful insight on the return to sport determination.[5]

FUTURE PROSPECTS

Isokinetic testing, especially in back dynamometry, is a very young science, but with the advent of active machines the future is very exciting. An active machine is one in which the dynamometer not only has the capacity to receive input (from the patient), but also to generate output (to the patient). This makes it ideal for doing high-level athletic testing, such as the application of eccentrics, which is a predominant trend in the athletic environment. Predictors of athletic performance based on eccentric testing may very well enhance the way we look at parameters in the future. In addition to this, commercial companies are developing equipment that has the means to measure dynamic movements at higher speed ranges and more complex motions than ever before. It may be that some day objective testing of all parameters of an individual will be performed in his own natural environment without any inhibition to his performance. The results generated would truly be indicative of an athlete's ability.

REFERENCES

1. Allman F, McKeag D, Bodner L: Prevention and emergency care of sports injuries. Family Practice Recertification 5:4, 1983.
2. Anderson E, Sward L, Thorstensson: Trunk muscle strength in athletes. Med Sci Sports Exerc 20(6):1988.
3. Baltzopoulos V, Brodie D: Isokinetic dynamometry, applications and limitations. Sports Med 8:101–106, 1989.
4. Barnes W: The relationship of motor unit activation to isokinetic muscular contraction at different contractile velocities. Phys Ther 60:1152–1158, 1980.
5. Beimborn DS, Morrissey MC: A review of the literature related to trunk muscle performance. Spine 13:655–660, 1988.
6. Burdett R, Van Swearingen J: Reliability of isokinetic muscle endurance tests. J Orthop Sports Phys Ther 8:484–488, 1987.
7. Coyle E, Costill D, Lesmes G: Leg extension power and muscle fiber composition. Med Sci Sports Exerc 11:12–15, 1979.
8. Davies G: A Compendium of Isokinetics in Clinical Usage and Rehabilitation Techniques, 2nd ed. S & S Publishers, 1985.
9. Davies G, Gould J: Trunk testing using a prototype Cybex II dynamometer stabilization system. J Orthop Sports Phys Ther 3:164–170, 1982.
10. Delitto A, Crandell CE, Rose SJ: Peak torque-to-body weight ratios in the trunk: A critical analysis. Phys Ther 69:138–143, 1989.
11. Feeler L: Personal communication. Odessa Physical Therapy, 1989.
12. Gracovetsky S, Farfan H: The optimum spine. Spine 11(6):1986.
13. Hasue M, Fujiwara M, Kikuchi S: A new method of quantitative measurement of abdominal and back muscle strength. Spine 2:143–148, 1980.
14. Kibler W, Chandler T, Uhl T, Maddux R: A musculoskeletal approach to the preparticipation physical examination. Am J Sports Med 17:525–531, 1989.
15. Langrana N, Lee C: Isokinetic evaluation of trunk muscles. Spine 91:171–175, 1984.
16. Langrana N, Lee C, Alexander H, Mayott C: Quantitative assessment of back strength using isokinetic testing. Spine 9:287–290, 1984.
17. Mayer T, Smith S, Keeley J, Mooney V: Quantification of lumbar function. Part 2: Sagittal plane trunk strength in chronic low-back pain patients. Spine 10:765–772, 1985.
18. Mayer T, Tencer A, Kristoferson S, Mooney V: Use of noninvasive techniques for quantification of spinal range-of-motion in normal subjects and chronic low-back dysfunction patients. Spine 9:588–595, 1984.
19. Moffroid M, Whipple R, Hofkosh J, et al: A study of isokinetic exercise. Phys Ther 49:735–742, 1969.
20. Rothstein J, Lamb R, Mayhew T: Clinical uses of isokinetic measurements. Phys Ther 67:1840–1844, 1978.
21. Smith S, Mayer T, Gatchel R, Becker T: Quantification of lumbar function. Part 1: Isometric and multispeed isokinetic trunk strength measures in sagittal and axial planes in normal subjects. Spine 10:757–764, 1985.
22. Thistle H, Hislop H, Moffroid M, et al: Isokinetic contraction: A new concept of exercise. Arch Phys Med Rehab 48:279–282, 1967.
23. Thorstensson A, Nilsson J: Trunk muscle strength during constant velocity movements. Scand J Rehab Med 14:61–68, 1982.
24. Walker SM: Delay of twitch relaxation induced by stress and stress relaxation. J Appl Physiol 16:801, 1961.

Chapter 5

THE EFFECT OF NUTRITION ON THE SPINE IN SPORTS

Mary Lynn Mayfield, RN, BSN,
and William J. Stith, PhD

The study of the spine in sports would not be complete without considering the role of nutrition. The focus of sports nutrition is customarily placed on meeting the energy demands involved in sports participation and little attention is given to the spine. The physician treating the spine-injured athlete, however, will need to be cognizant of the athlete's concerns regarding nutrition. Most sports authorities concur that the best nutritional preparation is simply a well-balanced diet. Athletes have the same basic nutritional needs as people who do not exercise. Research indicates that active Americans consume diets that are similar in composition to the diets consumed by their sedentary counterparts. The main difference is that they eat a larger total quantity of food to support the energy demands of training.[38] The four crucial nutritional periods are: (1) nutritional maintenance during training, (2) pre-event nutrition, (3) nutritional support during competition, and (4) post-event nutrition.[27]

NUTRITIONAL MAINTENANCE DURING TRAINING

Nutritional conditioning, as with physical conditioning, is a continuous quest, not something to be practiced a day or two before competition. Optimal training effects cannot be achieved if the athlete does not maintain an adequate nutritional regimen.[27] The athlete's diet should be structured toward his or her individual training requirements for the specific sports endeavor. A basic diet

TABLE 1. Four-Food Group Plan

Food Group	Examples	Main Nutrients	Recommended Serving
1. Milk and milk products*	Milk, cheese, ice cream, sour cream, yogurt	Calcium, protein, riboflavin zinc, vit. B_{12}, thiamine	2
2. Meat and meat alternatives	Meat, fish, poultry, eggs, nuts, legumes	Protein, iron, riboflavin, niacin, vit. B_{12}, thiamine	2
3. Vegetables and fruits	All vegetables and fruits	Vit. A, vit. C, thiamine, iron, riboflavin, folacin, fiber	4
4. Grains, breads, cereals, pasta, and rice	All whole grains, enriched flours, and products	Niacin, iron, thiamine, zinc, fiber	4

* 4 servings for adolescents.

plan that is very simple, yet very effective and a practical approach to sound nutrition, is the Four-Food Group Plan presented in Table 1.[27,38,51]

As long as the recommended number of servings from the variety provided in each group is supplied and cooking and handling are proper, adequate nutrition will be assured. The dietary intake should provide a caloric distribution of approximately 55% from carbohydrates, 30% from fat, and 15% from protein (Table 2).

PROTEIN, CARBOHYDRATES, FATS

Many athletes and coaches believe that a high-protein diet supplies extra energy, enhances physical performance, and increases muscle mass.[25] However, high-protein intakes have never been shown to be uniquely beneficial to athletes.[25,27,65] The RDA for protein intake is 0.8 grams per kilogram (kg) of body weight (BW). Proteins are extremely complex nitrogenous compounds consisting of amino acids. Amino acids supply the materials for repair, growth, and building new tissue. Intakes above requirement are either burned for energy to support activity or converted to fat. Excess protein is wasted protein, since carbohydrates and fats can supply adequate energy.[61] In addition, these processes result in residual nitrogen, which must be discarded through the urine as urea. This requires the loss of water, which can exacerbate the athlete's state of dehydration.[27] As long as the energy intake is sufficient to maintain body weight, the normal dietary intake of protein is adequate.[17] This is particularly true considering that the protein intake of the average American diet exceeds the recommended protein requirement and the average athlete's diet is usually two to three times in excess.[38]

The growing athlete has a greater need for protein relative to body weight than the mature athlete.[8] However, intakes of protein above 15% of total calories

TABLE 2. Dietary Goals for the U.S.

Current Diet	% of Kcal	Recommended Diet	% of Kcal
Fat	42%	Fat	30%
Protein	12%	Protein	12%
Complex CHO	22%	Complex CHO	48%
Sugar	24%	Sugar	10%

cannot be justified on a scientific basis for any athlete.[27] Data suggest that athletes need approximately 1.0 g/protein per kilogram of body weight and may benefit from up to 2.0 grams during periods of prolonged endurance exercise or muscle building.[17,25,27] Endurance exercise results in a protein catabolic state characterized by decreased protein synthesis, increased amino acid oxidation, and increased conversion of amino acids to glucose. Strength exercise or muscle building results in an anabolic state in hypertrophying muscles and the accretion of protein due to increased protein synthesis.[17] The protein requirements for women in hard training may be estimated in a similar fashion to that of men, i.e., 1.0–2.0 grams per kilogram of body weight, but total amounts would be less in relation to their smaller size.[3] The conclusion is that there is little scientific evidence to support the consumption of large protein supplements, and the normal dietary intake of protein is adequate for athletes if the energy intake is sufficient to maintain body weight and to meet the demands of training.[17,25] Furthermore, large intakes of protein or amino acids cause fluid imbalances, calcium loss and liver and kidney hypertrophy, which may put a strain on regulatory mechanisms in these organs.[24]

Fats and carbohydrates are the two major energy sources used during exercise. Either source can be predominant, depending on the duration and intensity of the exercise, the degree of prior physical conditioning, and the composition of the diet in the days prior to the exercise. It is assumed that the average person will use a certain number of kilocalories (Kcal) from protein and then use the remaining Kcal from carbohydrates and fats to meet energy needs.[61]

Work performed under aerobic conditions will favor fat oxidation, whereas work performed under anaerobic conditions will be supported mainly by carbohydrate oxidation. The transition from a carbohydrate to a fat energy source during exercise has been referred to as the "second wind," which seems to result in less laborious work. The second wind probably reflects both elevated levels of free fatty acids and increased muscle blood flow.[1]

A high carbohydrate diet is associated with both a higher initial muscle glycogen concentration and a greater time to exhaustion than a high-fat or mixed diet.[27] Fatigue is highly correlated to glycogen depletion and lactic acid buildup, and the end result is termed "hitting the wall." The higher the level of muscle glycogen when exercise starts, the greater the endurance of the athlete.[27,48,63] Athletes who are in a negative caloric balance compromise their ability to synthesize glycogen. Simple carbohydrates are preferred when insufficient time is available to consume/digest meals containing complex carbohydrates. However, a diet rich in starches will support a greater glycogen repletion than a diet rich in simple sugars.[27] In training prior to competition in specific sports, the carbohydrate intake may be increased above the recommended 50–60% to increase glycogen stores. Specific dietary exercise techniques for glycogen storage will be discussed later. Because of its association to atherosclerotic heart disease, the percentage of fat in the diet should not exceed 30%.

The importance of carbohydrate as the primary fuel source was shown by Connor et al.[9] who, in studying the relatively primitive Tarrahumara Indians of Mexico, found they subsist on a diet that is very high in complex carbohydrates (75% of calories) and low in cholesterol (71 mg/day), fat (12% of calories), and saturated fat (2% of calories). Protein was adequate (13% of calories). These people are noted for their physical endurance. They reportedly run distances of up to 200 miles in competitive soccer-type sports events that last for several days.

There is also a virtual absence of hypertension, obesity, and death from cardiac and circulatory complications.[9,38]

VITAMINS

Vitamins are introduced here and discussed again in the section on "Healing Injuries."

Because of the key role of the B-complex vitamins in energy-yielding reactions during fat and carbohydrate metabolism, it has been speculated that an increase in the intake of these vitamins would enhance energy release and improve physical performance.[38] Numerous studies have been conducted to test this theory by supplementing athletes' diets with thiamine (B_1), riboflavin (B_2), niacin (B_3), pyridoxine (B_6), cyanocobalamin (B_{12}), pantothenic acid, folic acid and biotin. The intent is not to to determine if B-complex vitamins are needed but rather what is the quantity needed for optimum physical performance. The B-complex vitamins are water-soluble and not stored in the body, so a constant supply must be obtained through food or vitamin supplementation. The results of the studies indicate that supplementation with the B-complex vitamins does not generally enhance endurance performance[44] and that an adequate quantity is obtained from a balanced diet.[24,57]

Vitamin C. Vitamin C is necessary for energy metabolism and for tissue repair. Studies of South African mine laborers concluded that a supplement of 100 mg of vitamin C, the amount obtained from two oranges, reduced heat strain from working in the hot, humid mines.[34,55] Also there may be an increased need for vitamin C in athletes as a result of repeated trauma, particularly for endurance runners with heavy training schedules who have an almost continual burden of injured muscle fibers.[3] Anecdotes reporting the beneficial effects of vitamin C for increasing work efficiency, tissue repair, and prevention of colds are common. These may be the results of correcting a prior vitamin deficiency, since a deficiency of vitamin C is common in the American diet.[58] While no scientific proof exists, many trainers and endurance athletes feel that supplemental vitamin C greatly reduces the incidence of muscle and tendon injuries.[6] Vitamin C also has a beneficial effect on iron absorption.[42]

Vitamin E. Vitamin E supplements are also taken by athletes. Studies of vitamin E-deficient animals undergoing exercise tests have demonstrated that low vitamin E content in muscle potentiates damage to skeletal muscle. It seems likely that vitamin E is an essential component in the mechanisms of muscle that prevent exercise-induced damage. Vitamin E is thought to exert its major effect in the body by detoxification of lipid-soluble free radicals. The inference is drawn that free radical production may be increased by exercise. However, there is no proof that vitamin E supplementation of animals or humans to normal vitamin E status has a protective effect.[31] Excess ingestion of vitamin E, as with the other fat-soluble vitamins A, D, and K, may cause cumulative toxic effects. Excess fat-soluble vitamins are stored in the body rather than excreted in the urine as with excess water-soluble vitamins.[7,58]

There seems to be no evidence that supplementation with vitamin B-complex, C, or E enhances physical performance, hastens recovery time, or reduces the rate of injury in healthy, well-nourished adults undergoing physical training.[3,19] A beneficial effect from vitamin supplementation means that the subjects were initially vitamin deficient and the supplementation has restored them to normal.[3]

MINERALS

Whereas vitamins activate chemical processes without becoming part of the products of the reactions, minerals tend to become incorporated within the structures and working chemicals of the body. They provide structure in the formation of bones and teeth, help maintain normal heart rhythm and acid-base balance, and serve as important parts of enzymes and hormones that regulate cellular activity.[38]

Sodium, potassium, magnesium, and chloride are all lost in the sweat, and minimal dietary requirements are greater when there is repeated, heavy daily sweating.[3] Electrolytes lost can be replenished by adding a slight amount of salt to the fluid ingested or to the daily food intake. The ingestion of specific electrolyte supplements is therefore not needed.[51] Minerals are known as micronutrients or trace elements because of small dietary needs; therefore, great care must be exerted in advocating mineral supplements.[38]

Magnesium. Increasing numbers of athletes are supplementing their diets with magnesium to improve athletic performance. According to a review by McDonald and Keen,[39] there is the assumption that athletes have a higher than normal requirement for magnesium and that a marginal deficiency can have a direct effect on athletic performance. There appears to be a positive correlation between magnesium levels and VO_2 max. However, there are no data to support a positive effect of magnesium supplementation on exercise in individuals with normal serum magnesium levels.

Zinc. Low serum levels have been found in athletes. This may be a reflection of poor zinc status due to inadequate dietary zinc intake and/or excessive body zinc losses via urine or sweat. Studies have shown that the muscles of animals fed supplemental zinc took longer to fatigue than control animals. However, zinc supplementation to improve muscle strength needs to be approached with caution because of its effect on the absorption of copper, which can cause copper deficiency.

Excessive zinc supplementation (160 mg/day) seems to result in reduction of high-density lipoprotein (HDL), which is thought to be protective against cardiovascular disease.[39] It is suggested that zinc supplements not exceed the RDA of 15 mg/day.[40]

Calcium. One of the nutritional controversies of the 1980s has been the question of calcium. Can calcium prevent and/or treat osteoporosis? What are the long-term effects of amenorrhea in female athletes? How does this affect the occurrence of stress fractures and their healing? There are no data available demonstrating that high calcium intakes prevent osteoporosis or brittle bones. Instead, the evidence seems to indicate that estrogen deficiency is the primary factor in osteoporosis.[25]

Studies have shown that there is a lower vertebral bone mass in active amenorrheic runners than in eumenorrheic controls.[5,18] In each case, secondary amenorrhea clearly followed the onset of endurance training.[18] Intense exercise may reduce the impact of amenorrhea on bone mass; however, amenorrheic runners remain at high risk for exercise related fractures.[37]

Amenorrheic women have been shown to have decreased estrogen levels.[18] Lack of estrogen may increase the daily calcium requirement. The decrease in calcium absorption and increase in calcium requirement in estrogen-deficient women has led Heaney to recommend a daily intake of 1.5 g of elemental calcium to maintain calcium balance in low estrogen states.[26] Although osteoporosis as a disease of Western culture should not be ignored, overtreating with large calcium supplements should be approached cautiously.[25]

Iron. Iron is important in a variety of biological functions. Seventy percent of the body's iron is found in the red cell as hemoglobin. Hemoglobin is responsible for binding oxygen to the red cell and transporting it to tissues, where it is exchanged for carbon dioxide.

Myoglobin, an iron-containing protein within muscles, may act both to bind oxygen in the muscle as well as to facilitate oxygen transport across the cell membrane.[62] Mitochondria within muscle cells contain many iron-containing proteins that function in the citric acid cycle and electron transport system to produce adenosine triphosphate (ATP) for use in muscle contraction.

Iron deficiency has been judged the most common deficiency in America and may occur even more frequently among adolescent female athletes. Their average dietary intake of 10.5 mg/day fails to meet even the recommended daily allowance of 18 mg/day needed to replace the iron loss through menstrual bleeding.[53] Exercise has also been shown to increase iron loss. Nickerson found a 40% incidence of decreased iron stores in high school cross-country runners who did not receive iron during the running season.[42]

Minimal iron deficiency anemia has been shown to result in high blood lactate levels that can potentially affect performance by increasing acidosis.[46] Studies in nonanemic animals that were iron-depleted demonstrated limited aerobic energy metabolism and resulting concentrations of blood lactate following exercise. These concentrations were greater than normal and caused the onset of muscle fatigue.[20] Studies by Davies et al.[15] and McDonald[39] have shown that maximal work performance is limited by the oxygen-carrying capacity of the blood (hemoglobin) and that submaximal endurance performance is a function of tissue iron proteins.

Given the incidence of iron deficiency reported in women in general (35–58%) and female athletes specifically (15–30%), some clinicians recommend that female athletes undergo biochemical evaluation of their iron status before participation in sports.[19,25,54] It has been recommended that exercising women maintain a hemoglobin concentration of at least 14 mg/d and be evaluated with a serum ferritin test to assess iron deficiency.[32] Routine use of iron supplements by all athletes is not warranted.[25,58]

Minerals are discussed again in the section on "Healing Injuries."

PRE-EVENT NUTRITION

Because muscle glycogen is important to athletic performance, many athletes try to maximize muscle glycogen prior to competition using a loading procedure. The procedure is usually initiated 1 week prior to competition. For the first 2–3 days, the athlete consumes a mixed diet predominantly of fat and protein that contains only 100 g of carbohydrates per day. During this same period an exhaustive training program is followed. For the remaining 3–4 days of the week, a high carbohydrate (60–70% carbohydrate, either simple or complex) diet is fed and exercise is drastically reduced. The result is a twofold or greater increase in muscle glycogen storage, which is localized in the exercising muscle.[27]

This supercombination glycogen loading has some major pitfalls. During the low carbohydrate phase of the program, athletes may find training difficult due to glycogen depletion, which leads to fatigue. Further they are often irritable and experience decreased cognitive response. Exhaustive training prior to competition may result in increased risk of injury or premature physiological peaking.[27] A more moderate regimen can be used that omits the high protein and fat dietary period but utilizes the exhaustive work schedule and high carbohydrate dietary regimen. Some super-compensation can also be obtained simply by increasing carbohydrate intake for 3 days before competition. Carbohydrate loading is most effective for long-term events, when the individual exercises at an intensity between 65–85% of VO_2 max for longer than 80 minutes.

Nutrition immediately prior to competition should be high in carbohydrate (60–70% of total calories), low in fat and protein, low in bulk, low in salt, and it should provide adequate fluid. There should be at least a 2-hour interval between meal ingestion and competition. Ingestion of carbohydrate too close to competition may result in increased insulin output, which decreases mobilization of free fatty acids and lowers glucose release from the liver. The net effect could be premature usage of muscle glycogen stores and an early onset of hypoglycemia, leading to decreased athletic performance.[27,63]

NUTRITIONAL SUPPORT DURING COMPETITION

Liquid meals are available that are emptied rapidly from the stomach, are easily digested, and contain balanced nutrients. These may be particularly beneficial for prolonged competitive events during which the athlete has little time for or interest in food.[27,38,50]

Water and carbohydrates are the major nutrients of concern. Dehydration is the enemy of optimal performance and can be life-threatening. Circulatory and thermoregulatory functions are diminished when more than 2–3% of body weight is lost due to exercise-induced sweating.

It has been documented that male athletes lose more than 2 pounds of water per hour during exercise at high temperature. This amounts to a 1.5% loss, which results in an increase in body temperature and pulse rate, a reduced cardiac stroke volume, and early onset of fatigue, which can significantly compromise athletic performance.

Although sweat loss can be substantial, the loss of electrolytes and minerals is generally considered negligible, and in normal athletes with adequate diet and fluid intake, the losses will not affect performance.[3,7,13,51] Large volumes of fluid (up to 600 ml) empty more rapidly from the stomach than small portions. However, athletes find it uncomfortable to exercise on a full stomach that may interfere with movement of the respiratory muscles. Thus it is recommended that the athlete drink 150 ml to 250 ml at 10- to 15-minute intervals.[10,51]

Fluid losses should be replaced by beverages that leave the stomach promptly. Cold water leaves more promptly than water at room temperature. Gastric emptying is influenced by the osmolarity of the beverage, which is determined by the sugar and electrolytic content. If sugar is used in a sweat replacement beverage, it should be in no greater concentration than 2.5%. If fruit juices, soft drinks, or certain commercially available sports drinks are used, they must be diluted 1:4 or 1:5 to reduce osmolarity.[51] The carbohydrate consumed during the event may enable the athlete to exercise for a longer period at his or her maximum VO_2 by having a glycogen-sparring effect.[60]

POST-EVENT NUTRITION

Studies by Hultman and Bergstrom show that the rate of muscle glycogen resynthesis after depletion is dependent on diet.[29] If a carbohydrate-rich diet was given, muscle glycogen was restored to the predepletion level within 24 hours. Both rest and dietary allowances must be provided to permit total glycogen resynthesis.[11,49] Costill et al.[12] proposed that dietary carbohydrate intake for glycogen replacement be 525–648 g (70% of daily energy replacement). Both simple and complex carbohydrates work equally well for the first 24 hours but subsequently complex carbohydrate produces more glycogen.

Ivy et al.[30] found that providing 2 g of carbohydrate per kg of body weight (23% solution) with water immediately after exercise resulted in a threefold increase in the rate of glycogen synthesis above basal during the first 2 hours of recovery. They found that delaying the ingestion of carbohydrate for 2 hours resulted in a 45% slower rate of glycogen synthesis. They recommend that at least 1.5 g of carbohydrate/kg of body weight be consumed after exercise and again 60 minutes later to ensure rapid replacement of muscle glycogen.

Caution should be taken in the chronic ingestion of high-carbohydrate, low-fat diet. Coulston et al.[14] found that a high-carbohydrate diet (60-80% of calories) as compared to a normal carbohydrate diet led to changes in insulin, triglyceride, and HDL-cholesterol that have been associated with an increased incidence of coronary artery disease.

WEIGHT CONTROL

To compete effectively, athletes must attain their appropriate weight, be well nourished, well hydrated, and have a healthy minimum energy reserve as fat.[7] Too much fat is associated with loss of speed and endurance as well as increased risk of injury in some sports.[50] In the case of spinal injury, excess weight adds stress to the spine.

For the athlete, as well as the nonathlete who wishes to change his or her body weight, a well-planned and supervised weight-control program is emphasized. Weight change should be accomplished gradually (±1 to 2 lb/wk) by adjusting the energy balance:energy intake in relation to energy expenditure.[7,24] Diet modifications for either gaining or losing weight should be based on the Four-Food Group Plan to assure intake of all essential nutrients.[7]

The aim of a weight-gaining program should be to increase lean body mass (muscle as opposed to fat). Muscle mass can only be increased by muscle work with an increase in dietary intake, not by any special food, vitamin, drug, or hormone.[7,25] Monitoring weight gains with skinfold measurements will indicate the type of body weight being added.[24] Increased intakes should not exceed normal requirements by more than 1,000 calories per day.[27]

The ideal method of weight loss is decreasing caloric intake while increasing energy expenditure, i.e., reducing caloric intake by 500–1,000 calories/day and simultaneously adding an energy expenditure of 300–500 calories/day.[50] Starvation or extremely low calorie diets are not recommended.[24] Athletes in limited weight sports such as wrestling must be simultaneously well nourished and hydrated while maintaining minimal body weight. A decrease in performance, as reflected by decreases in aerobic power and capacity, speed, coordination, strength, and judgment, can result from using severely restrictive diets. Prolonged fasting or severely restricted calories result in loss of large amounts of water, electrolytes, minerals, glycogen stores, and lean body mass.[24]

Until recently, it was thought that one pound (0.45 kg) of body-weight loss corresponded to the burning of about 3,500 Kcal. Studies now show that during the first several weeks of dietary restriction, weight loss far exceeds the caloric deficit and reflects primarily water loss. This water loss occurs as the body's stores of glycogen are being depleted. Every gram of protein or glycogen has coupled with it approximately 3 to 4 grams of water. When a deficit of protein or glycogen occurs, water loss will follow.[7]

The majority of problems caused by rapid weight changes can be avoided by a supervised training and controlled diet program well in advance of the competitive season.[27,50]

HEALING INJURIES

The best nutritional preparation for peak performance is a well-balanced diet, but this should be coupled with the prevention and treatment of injury. Painful injuries are stressors.[59] Much of the disability imposed by stress is nutritional.[61]

The injured athlete has increased nutritional demands. When tissues are being repaired, more amino acids, carbohydrates, fats, vitamins, minerals, water, and oxygen are needed than during the normal breakdown and buildup of mature tissue. Yet, when the body is stressed, digestion and absorption of nutrients are impaired. If the stress is prolonged, the nutrient stores are also depleted.[21] There are approximately 50 nutritional factors that have to be continuously available to the cell to sustain life. Some of the biologic compounds are synthesized by the cell from simple compounds or nutrients from outside sources.[41] If these are not being supplied by the athlete's diet after injury, then the question arises whether the athlete should take supplements during periods of stress. The answer should probably be yes. The injured athlete, because of inactivity, will need to reduce caloric intake to avoid weight gain. And reduced caloric intake means a reduced supply of nutrients. Taking a balanced vitamin/mineral supplement, not in mega-doses but in amounts comparable to the RDA, may be necessary.[61] The delivery of nutritional substances to tissue in repair depends upon their availability from exogenous and endogenous sources, the diffusion rates across capillaries, and the distance the substances must travel to their points of use.[43] Due to the biochemical and metabolic changes after injury, the requirement for particular nutrient substances, such as proteins, vitamins, and minerals, is increased.[35]

Spinal Injuries. Central to any discussion of reparative responses on the part of spinal tissue is the question of DNA synthesis and cell replication in the formation of epithelial, connective (cartilage, bone), muscle, and nervous tissue.[36] The tissues to be healed involve principally connective tissues, of which collagen is most abundant. In fact, collagen is the most abundant protein in the body, accounting for over 60% of all proteins, and is the major organic component of the structural and support system of the body.[22,36] Bones, discs, ligaments, tendons, and joint cartilage are classified as connective tissues. They provide mechanical support, transmit forces, and maintain the structural integrity of the body.[22] Collagen serves as the matrix on which bone is formed. It is essential to scar formation; following a wound, collagen glues the separated tissue faces together. The material that holds cells together is largely made of collagen; this function is especially important in the walls of arteries and capillaries.[61] Whether a tissue repairs with a scar, as in the skin, or whether it repairs with a tissue resembling the parent tissue (bone, tendon, synovial membrane, etc.), the response is cellular in the sense that either fibroblasts (which produce the scar) or specific cells (osteoblasts, chondrocytes, etc.) must be present at the local site in order to synthesize the components of the repair tissue.[36]

Collagen synthesis depends on a large number of factors, the final common denominator of all of them being circulation—the infusion of the tissue to be healed. Platelets, thrombin, inflammatory cells, amino acids, vitamins, and minerals all reach the tissue via the microcirculation.[47] This can present a problem after spinal injury in healing of the cartilaginous disc material, since the disc only receives nutrition through the movement of fluid in and out of the disc space, which is enhanced by physical activity.[28,56]

There are no studies showing a relationship between diet and healing in spinal injuries. However, there have been countless studies on the role of nutrition in healing and the effect of nutrient deficiencies on the human body. From this research one can make the assumption that perhaps certain nutrients, when supplied in supplemental amounts, may accelerate or at least prevent delays in healing of low back injuries.

In particular, protein deficiency delays wound healing and produces a wound with diminished tensile strength. The presence of all the essential amino acids is necessary for the synthesis of proteins such as collagen, which comprise the majority of the spinal tissues to be healed.[16,64] Specific amino acids identified as having an influence on wound healing include cysteine, a sulphur-containing amino acid that is thought to be an essential component of the intracellular procollagen molecule and may be required for fibroblastic proliferation. After injury, the requirement for nonessential amino acids, such as arginine, may increase, so a dietary supplement must be provided.[33,45] Studies have shown that disuse after injury causes muscles to atrophy, and this is reflected in an increase in urinary nitrogen content. This muscle catabolism causes a protein loss of 8 grams per day.[2] Food has to replace the protein lost after injury and ensure adequate levels of protein for new tissue formation. The quality of protein is important. Animal protein must be included, for example, milk, eggs, meat, or cheese, to ensure a balance of amino acids.[4]

Vitamin A. Vitamin A deficiency has been shown to retard epithelialization, closure of wounds, rate of collagen synthesis, and the cross-linking of newly formed collagen. Another way in which vitamin A may be used in wound healing relates to its suppressive action on certain infections, probably mediated by the influence of the vitamin on the thymus gland. Patients who have had prolonged interference with food intake or gastrointestinal absorption are at risk of developing vitamin A deficiency.[33,35,43,52,64] Vitamin A is also required for bone remodeling. Some of the cells in bone formation are packed with sacs of degradative enzymes that can take apart the structure of bones. With the help of vitamin A, these cells release their enzymes. Vitamin A also helps maintain the nerve cell sheaths.[61] Only animal foods contain vitamin A, such as milk, butter, cheese, liver, and egg yolk. Dark green leafy and yellow vegetables and yellow fruits contain beta-carotene, the precursor of vitamin A.

Vitamin B. B-complex vitamins serve as cofactors or coenzymes (small protein molecules that associate with enzymes to promote their activity in chemical reactions) in a variety of enzyme systems necessary for normal protein, fat, and carbohydrate metabolism. Although the mechanism by which the B-complex vitamins affect wound healing is poorly understood, it appears that serious deficiency of these vitamins would interfere with repair. Deficiencies of pyridoxine, pantothenic acid, and folic acid are believed to have major effects on antibody and white blood cell formation.[33,43,47] Some of the B-complex vitamins known as stress vitamins for their role in healing nerves are thiamine (B_1), niacin

(B_3), pyridoxine (B_6), cyanocobalamin (B_{12}), folic acid, and pantothenic acid.[61] Meat, milk, and whole grain cereal and breads are food sources of B vitamins.

Vitamin C. The best understood of the vitamins is vitamin C (ascorbic acid), a deficiency of which causes scurvy, notable for abnormal wound healing. Vitamin C has an important role in collagen formation. The amino acid used in abundance to make collagen is proline. After proline is added to the chain of amino acids, an enzyme hydroxylates it (adds an OH group to it) making hydroxyproline. Vitamin C is essential for the hydroxylation step to occur. Vitamin C is also an antioxidant (a bodyguard for oxidizable substances). Because of its antioxidant property, it is sometimes added to food to protect important constituents. In the cells and body fluids, it helps protect other molecules, and in the intestines it protects ferrous iron. It also promotes the absorption of iron, important for its role in the production of red blood cells to carry oxygen. Vitamin C is also involved in the metabolism of several amino acids. The adrenal glands contain a high concentration of vitamin C, and during emotional or physical stress they release larger quantities of the vitamin with the hormones epinephrine and norepinephrine. Vitamin C is also needed for the synthesis of thyroxine, which regulates the rate of metabolism.[61] There is no convincing evidence that wound healing is accelerated by administration of vitamin C when tissue levels are normal. However, seriously ill or injured patients may develop ascorbic acid deficiency rapidly, because it is not stored in appreciable amounts. Consequently, large doses of 1 to 2 g of ascorbic acid daily may be administered for the possibility of aiding in healing of wounds.[33,43,47,52,64] Citrus fruits, tomatoes, potatoes, and leafy green or yellow vegetables are the best food sources of vitamin C.

Vitamin D. Vitamin D is required for normal absorption, transport, and metabolism of calcium and phosphorus. It is also important for normal bone growth and healing.[43,47,52,64] Fortified milk is the best food source, and exposure to sunlight brings about the synthesis of vitamin D.

Calcium. There is much information about the critical role of minerals in wound healing. We know that sodium, potassium, calcium, phosphorus, and chloride are essential for a wide variety of tissue functions, including many that are necessary for tissue repair.[33,43] Calcium regulates the transport of ions in and out of cell membranes. It is essential for muscle action and is required in many enzyme systems that are important in collagen remodeling. Vitamin D and calcium work together in the formation of bones. Calcium wastage is uniformly found in inactivity. Both the mineral content and the matrix of bone deteriorates. Bed rest results in a calcium loss of 1.54 g per week. The Sky Lab astronauts lost appreciable amounts of body calcium in space.[2] Milk products are the outstanding source of calcium in the diet, as well as salmon with bones, sardines, and dark-green leafy vegetables.

Magnesium/Manganese/Copper. Magnesium activates a number of enzymes involved in energy-producing cycles as well as protein synthesis. Its presence is required in all stages of healing, particularly collagen formation. Calcium and magnesium also antagonize each other in normal muscle coordination. Calcium acts as a stimulator, whereas magnesium acts as a relaxer. Vegetables, dry beans, and seeds are good sources of magnesium. Manganese and copper are critical cofactors in collagen metabolism. Copper also is a catalyst in the formation of hemoglobin and helps to maintain the sheath around nerve fibers. Connective tissue synthesis would suffer in the presence of deficiencies of any of the minerals.[43,45,47] Seeds, nuts, legumes, and whole grains are good sources of manganese; organ meats, shellfish, whole grains, legumes, and nuts are the best sources of copper.

Iron. Divalent iron is required for effective collagen synthesis. It has been reported many times in the past that severe anemia seems to interfere with wound healing. However, there is debate about whether the interference in wound healing is due to anemia or to the hypovolemia, vasoconstriction, trauma, and elevated blood viscosity that may impair oxygen transport.

Of all the nutrients, the iron allowance is the most difficult to provide in the diet. Men and boys with their caloric requirements can easily meet their iron needs, but women and girls have difficulty. Lean meats, deep-green leafy vegetables, and whole-grain cereals and breads are the best sources of iron.

Zinc. Clinical evidence of impaired healing due to deficiency of the trace elements mentioned above may be lacking. However, there have been many investigations into the role of zinc in wound healing. It is clear that zinc deficiency has adverse effects on the rate of epithelialization, the rate of gain of wound strength, and causes diminution of collagen strength. Zinc is an important cofactor in a variety of enzyme systems responsible for cellular proliferation, such as biosynthesis of RNA, DNA, and collagen. Zinc deficiency may also interfere with wound healing, because it is needed in the metabolism of vitamin A. There is controversy as to whether administering supplemental zinc can accelerate healing to an above-normal rate. As noted earlier, excessive amounts of zinc may displace copper, which is need in covalent cross-linkages in young collagen. Zinc deficiency is rare but may occur in patients who have suffered severe injury, infections, disorders of the digestive tract, or prolonged unsupplemented intravenous hyperalimentation. Oral zinc sulfate corrects zinc deficiency readily.[43,45,47,52,64]

As with many nutrients, the absorption and utilization of zinc are influenced by the composition of the diet as a whole. Excessive intakes of fiber, such as bran, can reduce the absorption of zinc. Meat is a good source of zinc and enhances its absorption and utilization by the body.[4]

CONCLUSION

In the healing process, emphasis should be on preventive measures. Optimal nutrition is gained by the athlete's following a regimen of eating from the Four-Food Group Plan daily. The athlete should adhere to dietary guidelines that provide 45–55% of the calories from carbohydrates, 12–15% from protein, and 30–40% from fat to meet the athlete's needs for training and competition. Sound nutrition will help the athlete to achieve peak performance, protect the spine from injury, and, when injury does occur, facilitate recovery.

Acknowledgment. The authors would like to thank Barbara Picower for reviewing this manuscript and her very helpful suggestions in its preparation.

REFERENCES

1. Askew E: Role of fat metabolism in exercise. Clin Sports Med 3:605–621, 1984.
2. Bortz W: The disuse syndrome. Western J Med 141:691–694, 1984.
3. Brotherhood J: Nutrition and sports performance. Sports Med 1:350–389, 1984.
4. Burchill P: Wound care: Body builders. Community Outlook Aug:19–22, 1986.
5. Cann CE, Martin MC, Genant HK, Jaffe RB: Decreased spinal mineral content in amenorrheic women. JAMA 251(5):626–629, 1984.

6. Cantu R: Exercise Injuries—Prevention and Treatment. Washington, DC, Stone Wall Press, Inc., 1983.
7. Cantu R: The Exercising Adult. New York, Macmillan Publishing Co., 1987.
8. Coleman E: Protein requirements for athletes. Sports Med Digest 9:6–7, 1987.
9. Connor W, Cerqueira M, Connor R, et al: The plasma, lipids, lipoproteins, and diet of the Tarrahumara Indians of Mexico. Am J Clin Nutrition 31:1131–1142, 1978.
10. Costill D: Water and electrolyte requirements during exercise. Clin Sports Med 3:639–647, 1984.
11. Costill DL, Bowers R, Branam G, Sparks K: Muscle glycogen utilization during prolonged exercise on successive days. J Appl Physiol 31(6):834–838, 1971.
12. Costill DL, Sherman WM, Fink WJ, et al: The role of dietary carbohydrates in muscle glycogen resynthesis after strenuous running. Am J Clin Nutrition 34:1831–1836, 1981.
13. Cotter R: Nutrition, fluid balance, and physical performance. In Thomas J (ed): Drugs, Athletes and Physical Performance. New York, Plenum Medical Book Company, 1988, pp 31–40.
14. Coulston AM, Liu GC, Reaven GM: Plasma glucose, insulin, and lipid responses to high-carbohydrate low-fat diets in normal humans. Metabolism 32:52–66, 1983.
15. Davies KJ, Maguire JJ, Dallman PR, et al: Exercise bioenergetics during dietary iron deficiency and repletion. In Saltman & Hegenquer (eds): The Biochemistry and Physiology of Iron. New York, Elsevier, 1982.
16. Dickhaut S, Delee J, Page C: Nutritional status: Importance in predicting wound-healing after amputation. J Bone Joint Surg 66A:71–75, 1984.
17. Dohm L: Protein nutrition for the athlete. Clin Sports Med 3:595–603, 1984.
18. Drinkwater BL, Wilson K, Chesnut CH III, et al: Bone mineral content of amenorrheic and eumenorrheic athletes. N Engl J Med 311(5):277–281, 1984.
19. Elliot D, Goldberg L: Nutrition and exercise. Med Clin North Am 69:71–82, 1985.
20. Finch CA, et al: Lactic acidosis due to iron deficiency. J Clin Invest 58:447–454, 1979.
21. Fox A, Fox B: DLPA. New York, Pocket Books, 1985, pp 40–45.
22. Gamble J: The Musculoskeletal System. New York, Raven Press, 1988, pp 57, 58, 81.
23. Grandjean A: Nutritional concerns for the woman athlete. Clin Sports Med 3:923–938, 1984.
24. Grandjean A: Nutrition for swimmers. Clin Sports Med 5:65–76, 1986.
25. Grandjean A: Sports nutrition. In Mellion M (ed): Sports Injuries and Athletic Problems. Philadelphia, Hanley and Belfus, 1988, pp 23–36.
26. Heaney RP: Nutrition factors and estrogen in age-related bone loss. Clin Invest Med 5:147–155, 1982.
27. Hecker A: Nutritional conditioning for athletic competition. Clin Sports Med 3:567–582, 1984.
28. Holm S, Nachemson A: Variations in the nutrition of the canine intervertebral disc induced by motion. Spine 8:866–874, 1983.
29. Hultman E, Bergstrom J: Muscle glycogen synthesis in relation to diet studied in normal subjects. Acta Med Scand 82:109–117, 1967.
30. Ivy JL, Katz AL, Cutler CL, et al: Muscle glycogen synthesis after exercise: Effect of carbohydrate ingestion. J Appl Physiol 64(4):1480–1485, 1988.
31. Jackson M: Muscle damage during exercise: Possible role of free radicals and protective effect of vitamin E. Proceedings of the Nutrition Society 46:77–80, 1987.
32. Jaffe R: The female athlete. Del Med J 59:583–586, 1987.
33. Keithley J: Wound healing in malnourished patients. Am Op Room News J 35:1094–1099, 1982.
34. Kotze H, Van der Walt W, Rogers C, Strydom N: Effects of plasma ascorbic acid levels on heat acclimatization in man. J Applied Physiol 42:711–716, 1977.
35. Levenson S, Seiffer E: Dysnutrition, wound healing, and resistance to infection. Clin Plastic Surg 4:375–388, 1977.
36. Mankin H: The articular cartilages, cartilage healing, and osteoorthrosis, In Creuss R, Rennie W (eds): Adult Orthopedics. New York, Churchill Livingstone, 1984, pp 163–270.
37. Marcus R, Cann C, Maduig P, et al: Menstral function and bone mass in elite women distance runners. Ann Intern Med 102:158–163, 1985.
38. McArdle W, Katch F, Katch V: Exercise Physiology. Philadelphia, Lea & Febiger, 1986.
39. McDonald R, Keen CL: Iron, zinc and magnesium nutrition and athletic performance. Sports Med 5:171–1844, 1988.
40. National Research Council: Recommended Dietary Allowances, 9th ed. Washington, DC, National Academy of Sciences, 1980.
41. Navia J, Menaker L: Nutritional implications in wound healing. Dental Clin North Am 20:549–567, 1976.
42. Nickerson HJ, Holubets M, Tripp AD, Pierce WE: Decreased iron stores in high school female runners. Am J Dis Child 139:1115–1119, 1985.

43. Pollack S: Wound healing: A review. III. Nutritional factors affecting wound healing. J Dermatol Surg Oncol 5:615–619, 1979.
44. Read M, McGuffin S: The effect of B-complex supplementation on endurance performance. J Sports Med 23:178–183, 1983.
45. Ruberg R: Role of nutrition in wound healing. Surg Clin North Am 64:705–714, 1984.
46. Schoene RB, Escourron P, Robertson HT, et al: Iron repletion decreases maximal exercise lactate concentrations in female athletes with minimal iron deficiency anemia. J Lab Clin Med 102:306–312, 1983.
47. Schrock T, Cerra F, Hawley P, et al: Wounds and wound healing. Dis Colon Rectum 25:1–15, 1982.
48. Sherman WM: Carbohydrate, muscle glycogen, and improved performance. Phys Sportmed 15:157–164, 1987.
49. Sherman WM, Costill DL, Fink WJ, et al: The effect of a 42.2 km footrace and subsequent rest or exercise on muscle glycogen and enzymes. J Appl Physiol 55:1219–1224, 1983.
50. Smith N: Nutrition and the athlete. Orthop Clin North Am 14:387–396, 1983.
51. Smith N: Pediatric Sports Medicine. Chicago, Yearbook Medical Publishers, 1989.
52. Smith R: Recovery and tissue repair. Br Med Bull 41:295–301, 1985.
53. Squire DL: Female athletes. Pediatrics Rev 9:183–190, 1987.
54. Steinbaugh M: Nutritional needs of female athletes. Clin Sports Med 3:649–669, 1984.
55. Strydom N, Kotze A, Van der Welt W, Rogers C: Effect of ascorbic acid on rate of heat acclimatization. J Appl Physiol 41:202–205, 1976.
56. Urban J, Holm S, Maroudas A, Nachemson A: Nutrition of the intervertebral disc. Clin Orthop 170:296–302, 1982.
57. Vitale J: Nutrition in sports medicine. Orthop Clin North Am 15:158–168, 1985.
58. Vitousek S: Is more better? Nutrition Today. Nov/Dec:10–17, 1979.
59. Weiss M, Troxel R: Psychology of the injured athlete. Athletic Training. Summer:104–154, 1986.
60. Wheeler KB: Sports nutrition for the primary care physician: The importance of carbohydrate. Phys Sportsmed 17:106–117, 1989.
61. Whitney E, Hamilton E: Understanding Nutrition. St. Paul, MN, West Publishing, 1987.
62. Whittenberg BA, Whittenberg JB, Caldwell P: Role of myoglobin in the oxygen supply to red skeletal muscle. JBOL Chem 250:9038–9043, 1975.
63. Williams C: Nutritional aspects of exercise induced fatigue. Proc Nutrition Soc 44:245–256, 1985.
64. Williams C: Wound Healing: A Nutritional Perspective. London, Bailliere Tindall Nursing, 1986, pp 249–251.
65. Williams M: Nutritional Aspects of Human Physical and Athletic Performance. Springfield, IL, Charles C Thomas, 1976.

Chapter 6

OSTEOPOROSIS AND THE SPINE IN SPORTS: THE BENEFITS OF EXERCISE

Richard Sachson, MD, Stanley Feld, MD,
Steven G. Dorfman, MD, and Stephen L. Aronoff, MD

The sophistication of modern medicine has engendered a longer average lifespan and led to the graying of our population. As some of the life-shortening diseases of the past are being controlled, other less dramatic disorders of the elderly, such as Alzheimer's disease and osteoporosis, are entering the scene as major scourges of the older population. The enormity of the problem of osteoporosis is illustrated by the more than 1.2 million fractures that occur annually in the United States. Forty-five percent of these (approximately 540,000) involve the spine. Twenty-five percent of women greater than 70 years of age and 50% of women greater than 80 years of age have evidence of vertebral fractures.[9] The burden of individual suffering, as well as the financial drain (greater than 7 billion dollars annually in the USA), mandate a greater expenditure of resources than is currently allocated toward finding an effective therapy. Our armamentarium at present is ill-equipped to deal with the problem. Available therapy, such as estrogens in menopausal women, appears to allay progression of the disease but does not effectively reverse the loss of bone that has already occurred.

Peak bone density is reached in the third decade of life, with a subsequent inexorable decline of varying rate leading to an almost 50% loss of trabecular bone of the spine over a woman's lifetime.[34] There is ample evidence that the rate of bone turnover becomes negligible in the elderly population.[33] Thus, treatments that decrease the rate of bone breakdown in the elderly but do not increase peak bone density and strength will be of little avail to the elderly. The existing evidence supports early preventive intervention as the major direction of therapy until better means of restoring lost bone are available. We will address the role of exercise as a preventive measure as well as a possible means of restoring lost bone in the elderly. Since peak bone mass is 30% higher in males than females, and 10% higher in blacks than whites, it is no surprise that osteoporosis is predominantly a disease of white females.[10] Most of the available exercise data deal with the effects of exercise in white women.

RISK FACTORS FOR OSTEOPOROSIS

Identification of people at higher risk for osteoporosis would be of value if an effective prophylactic exercise regimen were to be appropriately targeted. A number of risk factors are associated with the development of osteoporosis, some of which are modifiable (Table 1). The high-risk profile that emerges is that of a small-framed, fair-skinned white female with a strong family history of osteoporosis. Substantially increasing the risk of fracture in this prototypical female is an early menopause, either surgical, natural, or exercise-induced.[18]

IMMOBILIZATION AND BONE

The loss of bone mass with increasing age has been shown in some studies to correlate with a parallel loss of muscle mass. At autopsy the ash weight of the third lumbar vertebra has been found to be related to the weight of the left psoas muscle.[12] Sinaki has shown a significant positive correlation between lumbar bone mineral density measured by dual photon absorptiometry and back extensor strength in a cross-sectional study of 68 postmenopausal Caucasian women.[38]

The inevitable loss of bone seen with immobilization is felt to be due either to the absence of tension applied by muscle to bone or the absence or decrease of gravitational pull, based on Wolff's Law. In 1892, Wolff postulated that when a bone is bent under a mechanical load, it modifies its structure by bony apposition in the concavity and resorption in the convexity.[46] Thus, the bone elements increase or decrease their mass to reflect the amount of functional forces exerted upon them.

In 1949, Whedon demonstrated a 51% decrease in the negative calcium balance seen in three immobilized volunteers when they were transferred from a fixed to an oscillating bed.[43] The relative effect of weight-bearing versus muscle tension was demonstrated in an interesting study in which the urinary calcium

TABLE 1. Risk Factors for Osteoporosis

Modifiable	Not Modifiable
Estrogen deficiency of any cause	Female
Inadequate nutrition	Family history of osteoporosis
Excessive consumption of alcohol, caffeine, or nicotine	Northern European ancestry
Glucocorticoid therapy	Fair skin, small stature
Excessive thyroid hormone therapy	
Sedentary lifestyle	

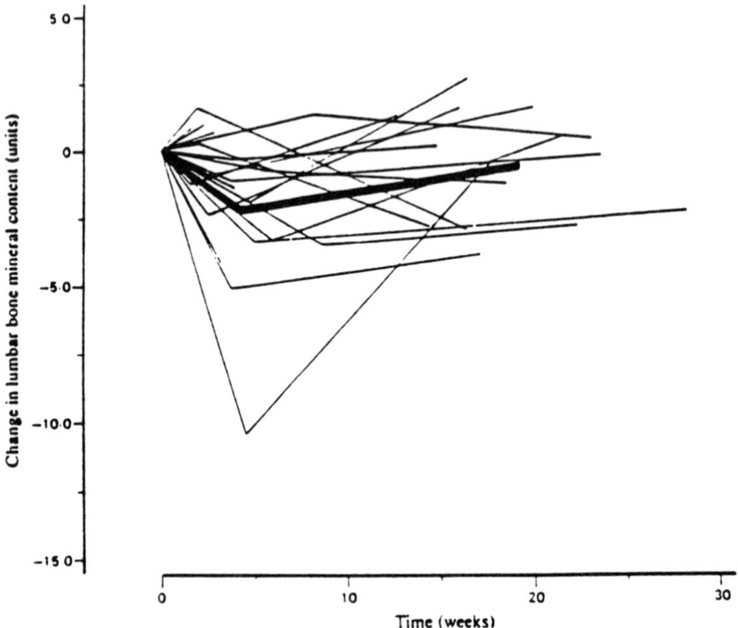

FIGURE 1. Densitometry studies performed on admission after bedrest and after reambulation. A bold line connects mean values. From Krolner B, Toft B: Vertebral bone loss: An unheeded side effect of therapeutic bed rest. Clin Sci 64:537–540, 1983, with permission.

excretion of immobilized subjects was measured after supine exercise on a bicycle ergometer, quiet sitting, or quiet standing.[20] Quiet sitting for 8 hours per day or the use of a bicycle ergometer in the supine position for up to 4 hours per day in five subjects did not produce a change in urinary calcium excretion. However, quiet standing for 3 hours per day produced a significant but slow decline in urinary calcium in four out of five subjects. The conclusion of the authors of this study was that the loss of calcium from bone in immobilized patients was due to the absence of weight-bearing rather than physical inactivity. Krolner followed vertebral bone mineral density by dual photon absorptiometry in 34 otherwise healthy patients (two menopausal) placed at bed rest for the treatment of lumbar disc-induced back pain.[24] Densitometry studies were done on admission, after 27 days at bed rest, and again 15 weeks after reambulation (Fig. 1). There was a mean loss of bone mineral content with bed rest of 0.9% per week. Although there were no control subjects in this study, the generally accepted rate of bone loss in premenopausal adults is approximately 0.3 to 0.9% per year. With reambulation the bone mineral content returned to baseline after approximately 4 months. Bone density studies of 13 adolescent girls immobilized for 3 to 6 weeks for correction of scoliosis revealed a similar rate of vertebral bone loss of 1 to 2% per week. Only four of the subjects regained all lost bone 5 years later.[28]

The weightlessness of space flight has been well demonstrated to produce a loss of bone at a rate similar to bed rest on Earth. This subject has been carefully reviewed by Rambaut in an excellent summary of the calcium and bone

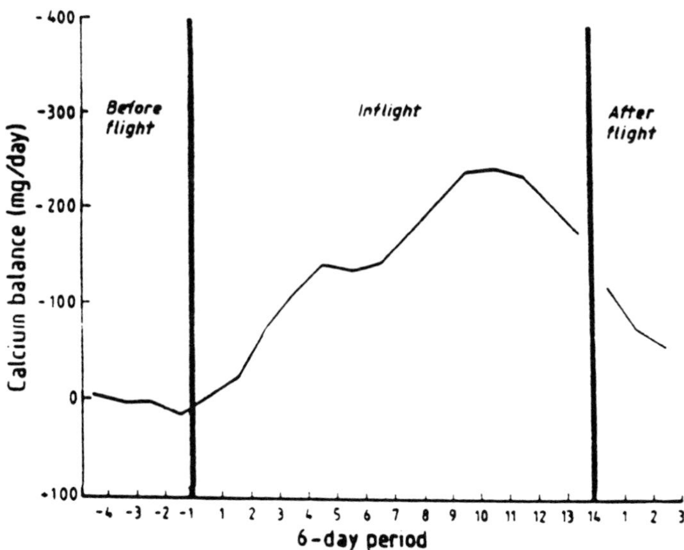

FIGURE 2. Mean calcium balance of all astronauts on Skylab missions. From Rambaut PN, Good A: Skeletal changes during space flight. Lancet ii:1050–1052, 1985, with permission.

metabolic effects of the American and Russian space flight experiences.[32] The best studied U.S. astronauts were the nine who flew the Skylab missions of 28, 59, and 84 days in 1973 and 1974. Urinary calcium losses began to increase as soon as the astronauts became weightless, and mean negative calcium balance progressively increased from 50 mg per day after 1 month to over 200 mg per day at the end of the second month (Fig. 2). The lowest urinary calcium losses were demonstrated in the astronauts on the 84-day flight, presumably because of the greater amount of physical exercise they underwent. The composite data indicates an approximate 25 g calcium loss per astronaut on the 84-day mission. A decrease in bone density of the calcaneus was evident but was not detected in the radius or ulna. Bone density measurements of the calcaneus of the Skylab astronauts remained lower than preflight measurements 5 years after their flights. The loss of bone mineral content of the calcaneus of the Soviet cosmonauts of the Salyut missions was of similar magnitude to the losses in the Skylab astronauts, despite the fact that the Soviets spent more than twice as many days in a state of weightlessness. This decrease in loss of bone is attributable to the 2 to 5 hours of exercise performed daily by the cosmonauts and the presence of restraining elastic straps in their space suits, which placed the astronauts' movements under muscle tension.

Studies in Athletes

The extensive literature on the detrimental effects of immobilization on bone density, as well as the well-documented increases of bone density seen in athletes, strongly suggests that weight-bearing exercise should be beneficial to the strength of the skeleton. Female college varsity athletes who participated in tennis and swimming were studied by single-photon and dual-photon absorptiometry by Jacobson.[21] The radius of the dominant arm of the tennis-playing athletes had a 16% higher bone mineral content than the nondominant arm (the variance in the nonathletic population between dominant and nondominant arms is $\leq$ 3%). The radial bone mineral content in swimmers increased in both arms. The lumbar vertebral density increased in the tennis players but not the swimmers. The authors concluded that the effect of gravitational stress on weight-bearing bones is more apparent in tennis players. Nilson measured distal femoral bone mineral density in 64 athletes, nine world-class, and compared them to those of controls, athletic and nonathletic.[29] The results demonstrated a clear-cut relation between the intensity of training and femoral density, with world-class athletes having greater density than non-world-class athletes, who were followed by nonathletic controls. Nonathletic controls had the lowest femoral bone mineral density, and this did not differ significantly from that of swimmers. The femoral bone mineral density was higher in the leg of preference for the athletes.

Jones measured the cortical thickness of the humerus (with x-ray studies) of 84 professional tennis players, using their nonplaying arm as a control.[22] Every player showed hypertrophy of bone on the playing side, with a 34.9% difference in men and a 28.4% difference in women. Single-photon absorptiometry measurements of the radius of 35 older but still active lifetime tennis players, aged 70 to 84, also revealed a greater mass of the playing arm.[19] The mean bone mineral content for the nonplaying arm was not different from that previously published for the normal male population. The bone mineral content of the playing arms ranged from 4 to 33% (mean: 13%) greater than the nonplaying arm in all but one case—an ambidextrous tennis player. In a later study published in abstract only, Nilson looked at the axial bone mineral content of 24 male weight-lifters and 21 professional ballet dancers.[30] There was a substantial increase in bone mineral content of the radius, tibia, and fibula of both groups, ranging from 19 to 38%, when compared with age-matched controls.

Aloia used the technique of total body neutron activation analysis as well as single-photon absorptiometry of the distal radius to assess total body skeletal mass and bone mineral content of the distal radius, respectively, in 30 male marathon runners.[1] In comparison to 16 sedentary age-matched controls, the marathon runners demonstrated an 11% higher total body calcium, reflecting a significantly greater skeletal mass. However, the bone mineral content of the distal radius of the marathoners, which was 5% greater than that of controls, was not statistically significantly different from the controls. There have been many other cross-sectional studies that demonstrate an increased bone density in athletes.[37] Williams did a short-term longitudinal study of the bone mineral content of the os calcis of a group of 20 male runners at the beginning and end of a 9-month training program for the Honolulu marathon.[45] The age range of the runners was 38 to 68 and that of 10 nonrunner control subjects was 41 to 58. The running group was divided into two subcategories of consistent and inconsistent runners. The consistent runners showed a significant increase of bone mineral content at the end of 9 months, which was not seen in the inconsistent runners and controls. In this study there was a significant relationship between the number of miles run and bone mineral content in the group of consistent runners.

THE EFFECT OF EXERCISE ON BONE IN NONATHLETES

The available data indicate that bed rest or weightlessness leads to a loss of bone that cannot be offset by exercise without weight-bearing. The excessive physical activity of serious athletes can lead to an increase of bone density in the bones that are stressed, but there is no convincing evidence of a systemic effect of exercise on nonstressed bone. Questions remain regarding the beneficial effects of physical training in the young and elderly. Can peak bone mass be increased if exercise begins early enough? Can the rate of the inexorable loss of bone with increasing age be diminished by exercise? Does exercise have lasting effects after it is discontinued or must it be continued forever? Is exercise beneficial to the already-osteoporotic bones of the elderly? The information available at present does not fully answer all of these questions.

A weak correlation between lifetime physical activity assessed by a historical survey and the dimensions of adult bone has recently been demonstrated in a group of 223 postmenopausal women.[23] The bone area, but not density of the radius, measured by CT correlated directly with levels of physical activity from age 22 to 34. The authors state that this is the first study to demonstrate a significant association between historical physical activity and bone area. The results must be viewed with some suspicion, since the historical surveys required recall of levels of activity 35 years in the past. Aloia has assessed physical activity in sedentary premenopausal women by use of a large-scale integrated motion detector worn by each of 24 subjects for 3 days.[2] Bone mass was determined by total body neutron activation analysis, single-photon absorptiometry, and dual-photon absorptiometry to assess total body calcium and the densities of the distal radius and lumbar spine, respectively. A statistically significant correlation was found between levels of exercise, total body calcium, and the bone density of the spine, but not bone density of the radius. Pocock assessed physical activity by means of maximal oxygen uptake determinations in 84 Caucasian women aged 20 to 75 years and correlated this with bone mineral density of the femoral neck, lumbar spine, and the radius.[31] Bone mineral density of the femoral neck and spine but not the radius were correlated with the level of physical fitness in both the pre- and postmenopausal women. As in many other studies, the density of the radius did not correlate well with levels of physical activity. This is probably because the upper limbs are not loaded by the major physical activity of older women—walking. Additionally, the density of the radius reflects predominantly cortical bone, which does not change as rapidly as trabecular bone. Jacobson, in a cross-sectional study, evaluated the effects of athletics in women who exercised at least 1 hour three times per week 8 or more months of the year for a minimum of 3 years.[21] This study did not demonstrate any improvement in lumbar spine bone mineral density in women aged 55 to 75 years, although there was a significant increase in radial bone mineral density. These findings are at variance with almost all other published results. Although none of these studies is a randomized prospective evaluation, they provide a strong indication that antecedent physical activity can produce an increase in bone mass.

Aloia, in another study, demonstrated that aerobic exercise 1 hour daily three times per week in 19 postmenopausal women could prevent the involutional loss of bone mass.[3] Bone mass was measured by nuclear activation analysis and single-photon absorptiometry of the radius in subjects and controls before and after 1 year of exercise. Calcium balance was positive in seven of nine subjects in the exercising group (mean of 42 mg per day) and negative in each of the sedentary controls (mean: 43 mg per day negative). Although the mean bone mineral content of the radius increased in the exercise group and decreased in the controls, this difference was not statistically significant. This lack of effectiveness of exercise on radial bone mineral content was attributed to either the lack of precision of the single-photon absorptiometry in their hands (precision = 3.5%) or the similar findings of many other studies that appendicular bone density may not change in response to aerobic exercises. In another study, 255 menopausal women with an average age of 57 were randomized into a walking (7 miles per week) and control group for a period of 3 years and studied by CT scanning of the radius.[35] There was a comparable loss of bone density of the radius in both groups (–3.74% per year) with no beneficial effect of walking on bone density of the radius. The authors did subdivide the experimental subjects into a group of higher and lower grip strength and showed that there was a very slight increase in radius bone area in those patients with high grip strength who underwent aerobic exercise. The significance of this is unknown. White compared the effects of walking and aerobic dancing for a period of 6 months in 73 recently menopausal females by means of photon absorptiometry of the radius.[44] Patients were randomly assigned to a sedentary control group, to a group that walked 8 miles per week, or to a group performing aerobic dance five times per week. There was a significant decrease in bone mineral content of the control and walking groups (1.6 and 1.7%, respectively). The dancers showed an insignificant 0.8% decrease in bone mineral content. When the groups were further subdivided into those not on estrogen therapy and those who had a greater than 75% exercise compliance, there was no change in the bone mineral content results. The lack of a decrease in radius bone mineral content in the dancing group correlates with the finding that only in this group was there a significant increase in arm strength, implying that dancing does produce loading of the bones in the forearm. Of interest is the observation that exercise produced no change in serum estrogen levels.

The effect of 5 months of dynamic bone-loading exercises on the density of the radius measured by the Compton scattering technique was evaluated in 14 osteoporotic menopausal females by Ayalon.[4] The exercise consisted of 15 to 20 minutes of limb-loading exercise of the distal forearm three times weekly and 40 minutes of warm-up and stretching. In the year preceding the exercise program, both exercise and control groups showed a decline in bone density of 2.0% and 2.8%, respectively. At the end of the exercise period, the control group showed an additional decrease of 1.9% ($P < 0.02$), whereas the exercise group increased by 3.8% ($P < 0.01$).

Chow evaluated changes in bone mass over one year in 58 menopausal volunteers by neutron activation analysis, measuring calcium content in the trunk and upper thighs.[8] Patients were randomized into one of three groups: control, aerobic exercise, and aerobic plus strengthening exercise. Aerobic exercise consisted of stretching warm-ups followed by 30 minutes of aerobic activity such as walking, jogging, or dancing. Strengthening exercises consisted of 10 to 15 minutes of isometric and isotonic contractions of muscle groups of the limbs and trunk using free weights attached to the wrists and ankles. Bone mass diminished in the control group. Both exercise groups showed a significant increase in aerobic capacity and an increase in bone mass that was significantly different from the control group but not from each other. The lack of difference in bone mass between the two exercise groups may be explained by the author's inability to demonstrate any increase in muscle strength in the group that underwent strengthening exercises.

Krolner evaluated a group of 27 women (aged 50 to 73) with previous Colles' fractures using dual-photon absorptiometry of the lumbar spine and distal forearm before and after an 8-month exercise program.[25] Patients were nonrandomly allocated to a control group or a group that did aerobic exercises 1 hour twice weekly. Consistent with many other exercise studies, no significant change in bone mineral density of the radius could be demonstrated. The lumbar bone mineral content in the exercise group increased by an average of 3.5% and in the control group decreased by 2.7%. This was a statistically significant difference.

Smith was able to demonstrate a decreased loss of bone mineral content of the ulna and radius by single-photon absorptiometry in a group of women who underwent both aerobic and upper-body strengthening exercises regularly for 4 years.[40] Sixty-two control subjects (mean age: 50.8) lost bone mineral content of the humerus, radius, and ulna. The 80 exercise subjects (mean age: 50.1) lost significantly less bone mineral content of the radius and ulna bilaterally and the left humerus. Exercise slowed the decline in bone mineral content in both pre- and postmenopausal subjects. An earlier study by the same author is difficult to reconcile with the concept of the need for loading exercises to increase bone mineral content of the radius. Bone mineral content at the distal third of the radius was determined by photon absorptiometry on 29 female nursing home residents aged 69 to 95 (mean age: 82) over a 36-month period.[41] Seventeen patients were used as controls and 12 patients underwent a 30-minute per day, three-day-per-week activity program consisting of unspecified light-to-moderate physical activity. The control patients demonstrated an insignificant 2.5% bone mineral loss, whereas the exercise subjects showed a 4.2% bone mineral increase.

No effect of exercise on lumbar spine bone mineral density could be seen in a study of 17 recently menopausal women (8 exercise, 9 control) who participated in a progressive walking program for 15 to 40 minutes, three times per week, for 1 year.[7] As measured by quantitative CT at baseline, 6 months, and 12 months, there was a 4% loss of bone in the control subjects and a 5.6% loss of bone in the walkers. Although the walkers did work at a target heart rate of 60 to 85% of maximum age-adjusted rate, they demonstrated no change in body fat or postexercise heart rate. It is possible that the amount of exercise done by these subjects was inadequate. This brings up the matter of our total ignorance regarding the specific exercise prescription required to prevent bone loss. Those patients who need the benefits of exercise the most, i.e., those with debilitating osteoporosis, are able to do the least exercise. Just as doses of menopausal estrogen replacement can be too low to be of any effect on bone loss, we need to learn the minimum threshold level of exercise to prescribe to our patients.[16] Sinaki recently evaluated a nonloading exercise program for the axial skeleton.[39] He studied 65 menopausal women randomly allocated to exercise and control groups. None was on estrogen therapy, and patients whose baseline lumbar spine bone mineral density, measured by dual-photon absorptiometry, was below the fifth percentile of the normal range were excluded from the study. The non-weight-bearing exercise consisted of back extension against resistance 5 days per week for 2 years. Despite the fact that back extensor strength increased significantly more in the exercise than the control group, both groups lost lumbar spine density to a similar degree—1.2% per year in the control group and 1.4% per year in the exercise group. The most apparent conclusion of this study is that, as has already been demonstrated in other studies, weight-bearing exercise is necessary to prevent bone loss. It is possible, however, that the exercise used was inadequate because of duration, intensity, or type.

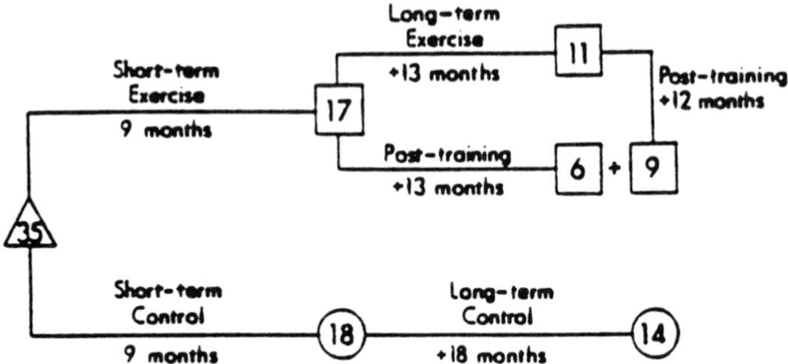

FIGURE 3. Flow chart of the study design. Numbers indicate patients in short-term and long-term exercise groups as well as post-training and control groups. From Dalsky G, Stocke K, Ehsani A, et al: Weight-bearing exercise training and lumbar bone mineral content in postmenopausal women. Ann Intern Med 108:824–828, 1988, with permission.

The most consistent findings of published exercise studies are the apparent increase of the density of trabecular bone of the axial skeleton with aerobic exercise and lack thereof of the predominantly cortical bone of the radius. Dalsky recently demonstrated an increase in spinal bone mineral density with aerobic exercise and also looked at the response to detraining for 1 year after completion of the exercise program.[11] Thirty-five healthy postmenopausal women were nonrandomly allocated to exercise or control groups and followed in a short-term (9-month) and long-term (22-month) protocol, as well as after 13-month post-training-nonexercise period (Fig. 3). Bone mineral content was increased by 5.2% and 6.1% in the short- and long-term exercise group, and decreased by 1.4 and 1.1% in the short- and long-term control groups. Thirteen months after discontinuance of training the final bone mass had fallen to a level 1.1% above the preexercise baseline, indicating no long-term residual effect of exercise.

EXERCISE AND ESTROGEN DEFICIENCY

In the past decade there has been a boom in the interest in aerobics, jogging, and cycling among young men and women. At first glance one should be delighted that all these young women are spending their spare time building up their peak bone mineral content to sustain them through the menopausal years. However, all this exercise is not totally beneficial. In addition to the usual acute and chronic athletic injuries peculiar to each sport, the entity *athletic amenorrhea* has become commonplace among aggressive female athletes. Depending on the intensity of training and the criteria used to define pathologic amenorrhea, the incidence of this entity has been reported to range from 10 to 50%.[18] The menstrual dysfunction is believed to be caused by abnormal hypothalamic function, leading initially to anovulation and subsequently to estrogen deficiency. Whether the hypothalamic dysfunction is related to absolute weight loss, percentage of body fat lost, or some other direct effect of training intensity, such as the release of endorphins in the brain, is unknown. Anorexia nervosa and bulimia are well-accepted causes of amenorrhea, and the incidence of these disorders in young female athletes in the U.S. has been estimated to be as high as 30%.[18] Premature estrogen deficiency (before the age of 40) of many causes, such as surgical castration, prolactinoma, or premature ovarian failure, can cause reduced bone mass.[5,17,36] Thus, young athletic females with amenorrhea and estrogen deficiency present their skeleton with opposing influences. There is ample literature to show that the negative effect of estrogen deficiency on the skeleton is of far greater importance than the positive effects of vigorous exercise and can lead to premature osteopenia and fractures.

Spine bone mass was found to be decreased by 22 to 29% from control values when measured by quantitative CT in a group of women with amenorrhea of various causes.[5] Bone mass of the radius measured by photon absorptiometry was not decreased in the amenorrheic women. Although estradiol levels were decreased in all of the amenorrheic women, the degree of decline in estradiol did not correlate with the degree of decline in bone mineral density. Ten of the 38 women in this study had amenorrhea on the basis of vigorous exercise programs. The exercise did not ameliorate the degree of loss of bone mineral density when compared to other causes of amenorrhea. Drinkwater evaluated bone mineral density at the radius and lumbar spine in 28 female athletes, 14 of whom were amenorrheic and estrogen deficient.[13] Twelve of the 14 amenorrheic women had normal menses prior to initiation of athletic training. The menstruating and nonmenstruating groups did not differ in height, weight, percentage body fat, age at menarche, or length of participation in sports. The only significant differences between the groups were the distance run per week and estrogen levels (41.8 versus 24.9 miles per week, and 38.6 versus 107 picogram/ml in the amenorrheic and menstruating women, respectively). Neither bone mineral content nor bone mineral density of the radius differed between the two groups (Table 2). However, the bone mineral density of the lumbar vertebrae was significantly lower in the amenorrheic, estrogen-deficient athletes (1.12 versus 1.30 g/cm^2). The average lumbar bone mineral density in the amenorrheic athletes, whose mean age was 24.9 years, was equivalent to that of women 51.2 years of age.

To determine whether more intensive exercise training could reverse the negative effects of exercise-induced estrogen deficiency, Marcus evaluated bone mass in a group of amenorrheic elite long-distance runners.[27] Eleven amenorrheic women with a mean age of 20 years and six menstruating women with a mean age of 23.8 years were comparable in all respects other than the age at which intensive athletic training began. The cyclic women began to train intensively 5 years after menarche, whereas amenorrheic women had begun training within 1

TABLE 2. Bone Mineral Content and Density in 14 Amenorrheic and 14 Eumenorrheic Athletes

Site	Amenorrheic	Eumenorrheic	P Value
Radius			
S_1			
Mineral content (g/cm)	0.89 ± 0.03	0.85 ± 0.03	NS
Mineral density (g/cm^2)	0.53 ± 0.02	0.54 ± 0.01	NS
S_2			
Mineral content (g/cm)	0.91 ± 0.02	0.88 ± 0.03	NS
Mineral density (g/cm^2)	0.67 ± 0.02	0.67 ± 0.02	NS
Vertebrae (g/cm^2)	1.12 ± 0.04	1.30 ± 0.03	<0.01

* Plus-minus values are means ± S.E.M. NS denotes not significant. From Drinkwater B, Nilson K, Chestnut C, et al: Bone mineral content of amenorrheic and eumenorrheic athletes. New Engl J Med 311:277–281, 1984, with permission.

year of onset of menses. All of the subjects had completed 10K races within 36 minutes or marathons within 3 hours. Spine density measured by quantitative CT in the amenorrheic women was lower than that in the cyclic women, and lower as well than that in nonathletic age-matched controls (1.51 versus 1.82 versus 1.6 mg/cm^3, respectively). Forearm mineral density was normal in both groups of runners. Spine mineral density was higher in the amenorrheic athletes than among women with secondary amenorrhea of similar duration but who were less active (controls were derived from other studies in the literature[5,13]), leading to the authors' conclusion that extreme weight-bearing exercise partially overcomes the adverse skeletal effects of estrogen deficiency. The loss of bone density does have pathological consequences inasmuch as only one cyclic woman had a single running-related fracture, whereas six amenorrheic women developed fractures. Four of the latter group had several tibial and metatarsal stress fractures.

Ballet dancing is often initiated at a very young age and has been noted to be associated with a high incidence of delayed menarche, secondary amenorrhea, and irregular menstrual periods. The estrogen deficiency in these young women may be caused by their vigorous training schedule, as well as the significant dieting common to ballet dancers. In a survey of 75 professional ballet dancers, the mean age of menarche was delayed by 2 years, and delayed menarche correlated with a 24% prevalence of scoliosis (Fig. 4).[42] The dancers with scoliosis had a greater prevalence of secondary amenorrhea (44 versus 31%), but this association was not statistically significant. The incidence of scoliosis in the families of the dancers with scoliosis was 28% versus an incidence of 4% in the families of the other dancers. Sixty-one percent of the dancers had incurred exercise-related fractures. This did not correlate significantly with delayed menarche. However, the incidence of stress fractures was more than doubled in the groups with secondary amenorrhea. There were no differences between women with and without stress fractures in the number of hours of exercise per week or the ages at which the dancers began their training. An increased incidence of scoliosis has been noted to be associated with delayed puberty and a positive family history.[15,47] Both of these influence most likely played a role in producing the high incidence of scoliosis in this group. Although nutritional deficiency is common among ballet dancers, and the incidence of anorexia nervosa in ballet dancers is reported from 5 to 22%,[42] no biochemical differences related to calcium and vitamin D metabolism could be discerned between those dancers with and without scoliosis.

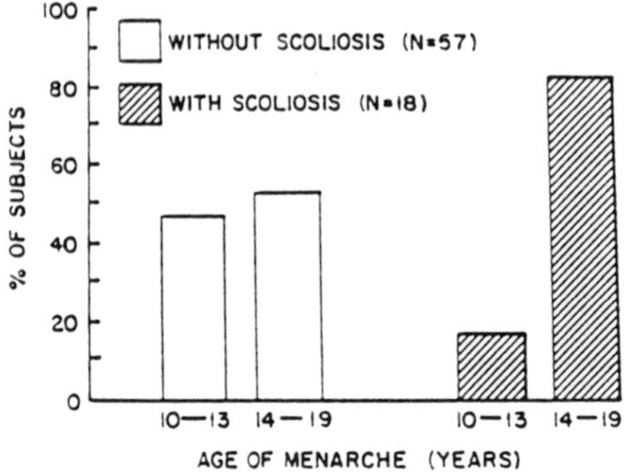

FIGURE 4. Relation between age at menarche and scoliosis. From Warren M, Brooks-Gunn J, Hamilton L, et al: Scoliosis and fractures in young ballet dancers. N Engl J Med 314:1348–1353, 1986, with permission.

Strong circumstantial evidence implicating estrogen deficiency as the causative factor of bone demineralization in athletic amenorrhea is derived from the improvement in bone mineral density seen in athletes who resume menstruation. Drinkwater reevaluated seven of the previously amenorrheic runners she reported in an earlier study[13] when they responded to a follow-up questionnaire indicating they had resumed menses.[14] The formerly amenorrheic runners had cut their mileage by 10% and regained an average of 1.9 kg of body weight. They demonstrated a significant increase in lumbar spine bone mineral density of 0.071 g/cm^2, representing a 6.2% increase in bone mineral density in 14.2 months. During the same period of time, the formerly cyclic runners who remained cyclic maintained a constant bone mineral density, which remained higher than that of the formerly amenorrheic runners (1.369 g/cm^2 versus 1.198 g/cm^2). Two runners who remained amenorrheic showed a further decrease in lumbar bone mineral density (Fig. 5). Further follow-up of the runners who resumed menses will be necessary to ascertain if they are ever able to achieve a completely normal bone mineral density comparable to the continuously cyclic runners. Just as had been demonstrated by Marcus[27] in elite runners, the amenorrheic athletes had a lower bone mineral density (1.198 g/cm^2) than cyclic nonathletes (1.263 g/cm^2), indicating that estrogen deficiency negates the benefit of exercise on bone mineral density. Lindberg was able to demonstrate a similar increase in vertebral bone density in a group of four previously amenorrheic runners who diminished their weekly mileage by 43%, regained 5% of body weight, increased estradiol levels to normal, and resumed menses.[26]

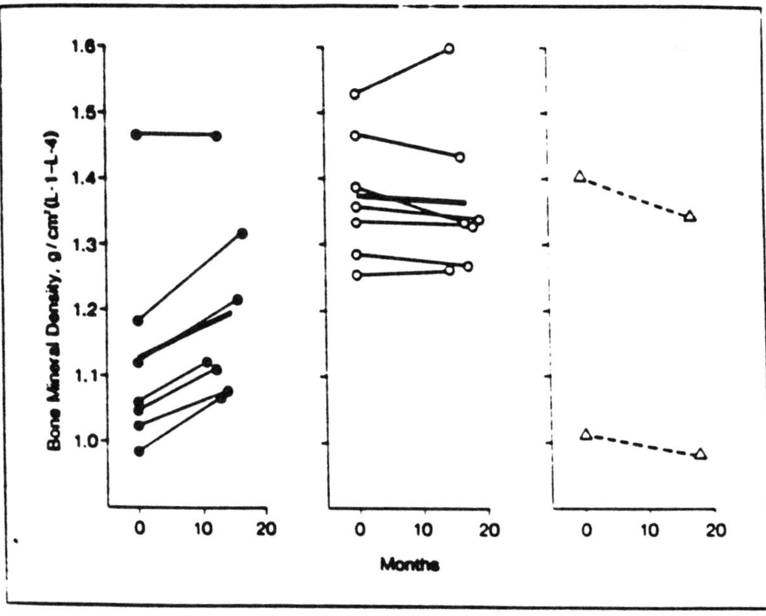

FIGURE 5. Changes in bone mineral density of lumbar spine (L-1 through L-4) with time between test 1 and test 2 for athletes who regained menses (left), athletes who remained cyclic (center), and athletes who remained amenorrheic (right). From Drinkwater B, Nilson K, Ott S, Chestnut III C: Bone mineral density after resumption of menses in amenorrheic athletes. JAMA 256:380–382, 1986, with permission.

It is still unclear if initiation of estrogen replacement therapy in amenorrheic athletes will accomplish the same results as resumption of spontaneous menses, although it seems prudent to do so if the athlete will not cut back on her training schedule enough to resume spontaneous menses. There is also some evidence of a critical window of time for normalization of estrogen levels to have a beneficial effect on bone density. Cann has demonstrated that women with amenorrhea of less than 3 years duration lose bone at a rate of 4.2% per year, but that after 3 years the rate of bone loss diminishes to 0.3% per year.[6] The implications of this study are that if estrogen therapy or resumption of endogenous estradiol production is to have a beneficial effect, it has to happen at the outset of amenorrhea, or the decrease in bone mass may be irreversible. This conclusion is not supported by Drinkwater's findings in previously amenorrheic runners in whom the increase in bone density was not related to the duration of amenorrhea, which ranged from 11 to 84 months.[14]

CONCLUSIONS

It has been clearly established that physical inactivity to the point of immobilization or weightlessness in space can lead to a decrease in bone mineral density. In addition, enhanced physical activity, as seen in athletes, can increase bone density as long as the increased physical activity is not associated with amenorrhea. Bone mineral density begins to decline after the third decade, and the available data indicate that weight-bearing activity can diminish the rate of loss of bone mineral density of the axial skeleton in both pre- and postmenopausal women. The cortical bone of the appendicular skeleton will not respond to exercise unless specific loading of these bones is carried out. The effects of exercise do not appear to be lasting and, based on one study, the mass of bone that is gained with exercise appears to decrease towards that of comparable nonexercising women after discontinuation of exercise programs.[11] Available data indicate that exercise programs can be beneficial even to already osteoporotic bones of the elderly. Young women with exercise-induced amenorrhea must be vigorously encouraged to curtail their exercise programs as soon as possible. If, as is commonly encountered, such women are unwilling to curtail their exercise programs, estrogen replacement therapy needs to be considered. Although there are no available data to indicate that estrogen replacement therapy will prevent loss of bone, the data on endogenous estrogen production in previously amenorrheic athletes and the extrapolation from the data regarding exogenous estrogen replacement therapy in menopausal women lead us to believe that replacement therapy should have beneficial effects in these young, amenorrheic athletes. Most of the available exercise data is derived from cross-sectional, nonrandom, and nonblinded studies. More scientific studies will have to be performed in the future to provide concrete data that will enable us to advise our patients. In addition specific exercise prescriptions will have to be worked out.

REFERENCES

1. Aloia J, Cohn S, Babu T: Skeletal mass and body competition in marathon runners. Metab 27:1793–1796, 1978.
2. Aloia J, Vaswani A, Yeh J, Cohn S: Premenopausal bone mass is related to physical activity. Arch Intern Med 148:121–123, 1988.
3. Aloia J, Cohn S, Ostuni J, et al: Prevention of involutional bone loss by exercise. Ann Intern Med 89:356–358, 1978.

ERGONOMICS

The term *ergonomics* is in common use and refers to a concept of human factors engineering applied to the design of facilities, equipment, tools, and tasks for the purpose of making them compatible with human use. The guiding principle of ergonomics is to potentiate design efficiency while also minimizing adverse consequences to the user. In regard to the lumbar spine, research indicates that if a back support is added to the sitting posture, pressure on the spine can be decreased as much as 35% compared to standing.[8] This is the basic principle behind the use of ergonomic chairs, by which a health-negative situation (sitting) is converted as much as possible, through ergonomics, to a health-neutral situation. This then brings up the interesting question as to whether it might be possible to create a health-positive situation in regard to the low back.

EUGONOMICS

Welcome to the concept of "eugonomics." This term was coined by the author as a means of defining the next logical advance beyond ergonomics. The principle of eugonomics is to achieve, through design, systems intended to potentiate structure, function, and longevity of the body rather than those intended to simply reduce the level of insult and injury. By definition, a eugonomic system is intended to result in the purposeful enhancement of anatomic, physiological, biomechanical, perceptual, and/or behavioral characteristics of humans (relative to the norm). Let us therefore look at the lumbar spine from the eugonomic perspective.

Grieco believes that the *key* to healthy disc metabolism is the alternation between loading and unloading.[9] As Nachemson has demonstrated, loading remains when we are supine.[14] Does this mean that a further potential exists to increase nutrition, matrix synthesis, and healing by the moderation or elimination of load through the creation of negative intradiscal pressures? Are we dealing with the lumbar spine equivalent of the aviation sound barrier? There are most certainly new vistas to be explored in this regard. The challenge is to be able to objectively document such influences. As Ghosh recently stated[10]:

> . . . it could be concluded that there are relatively few therapeutic measures currently available which have been satisfactorily shown to modify the constitution of the intervertebral disc.

At the present time the leading candidate with which we may be able to document such changes is MRI, with which determination of and changes in hydrogen ion concentration are now possible. In addition, research is progressing on the determination of diffusional phenomena.

Lumbar traction is a physical modality that has been in use since the beginning of recorded history for the treatment of deformities and painful conditions. Hippocrates (460–357 BC) used traction tables for the treatment of fractures, dislocations, and other spinal conditions. A most complete review of the subject of lumbar traction and its classic uses has been recently published by Goldish and is worthy of review.[11] When viewed comprehensively, it is evident that many forms of traction have either not produced more unloading of the spine than bed rest alone, or have caused spinal distraction to a degree injurious to soft tissues, or have produced other adverse consequences to the user.

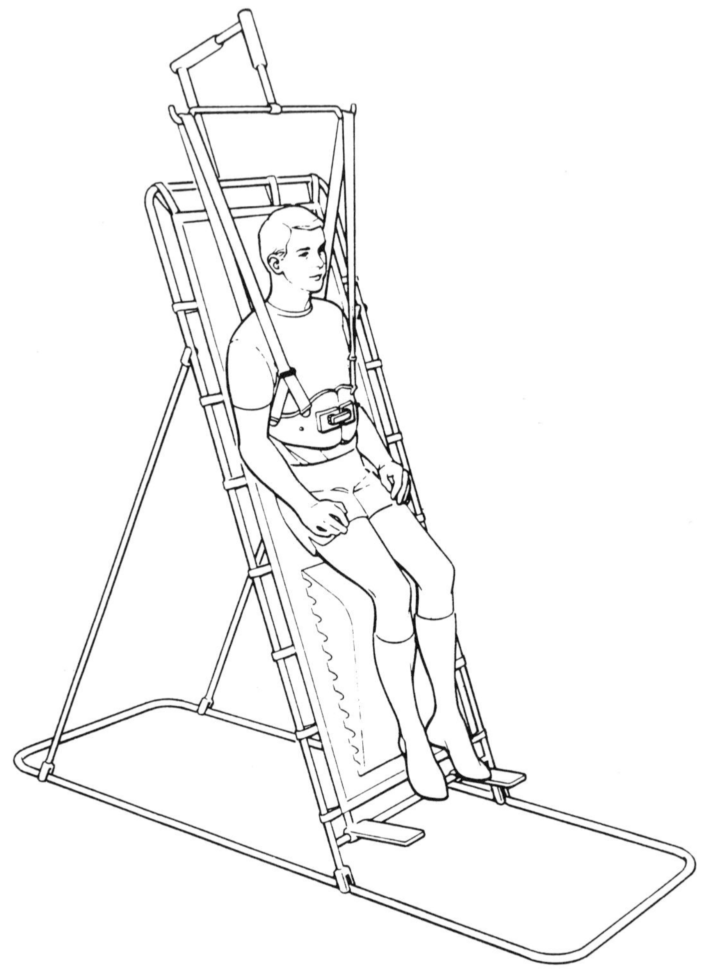

FIGURE 1. The basic equipment for the gravity lumbar reduction program is shown, with the exception of safety straps. The vest supports the rib cage, which serves as the means of supporting body weight. In the Low Back Club at the Institute for Low Back Care, a 5-day outpatient acclimation program, including education and physical therapy evaluation, is offered. Patients with contained disc herniations usually continue traction twice a day for an additional 3 months. Of 163 consecutive patients reviewed, 61% (71) of those not working before the program returned after completion and 100% of those previously working (92) returned immediately.

Lumbar traction is only now being regarded as a direct means of influencing disc physiology and disease. In 1976, the author and his associates at the Sister Kenny Institute in Minneapolis first introduced the gravity lumbar reduction therapy program (GLRTP). This traction system employs 40% of lower body weight as the means of unloading the lumbar spine with the rib cage as the point of fixation (Fig. 1). By not exceeding the normal compliance of muscles or ligaments, GLRTP has attempted to harness more productively

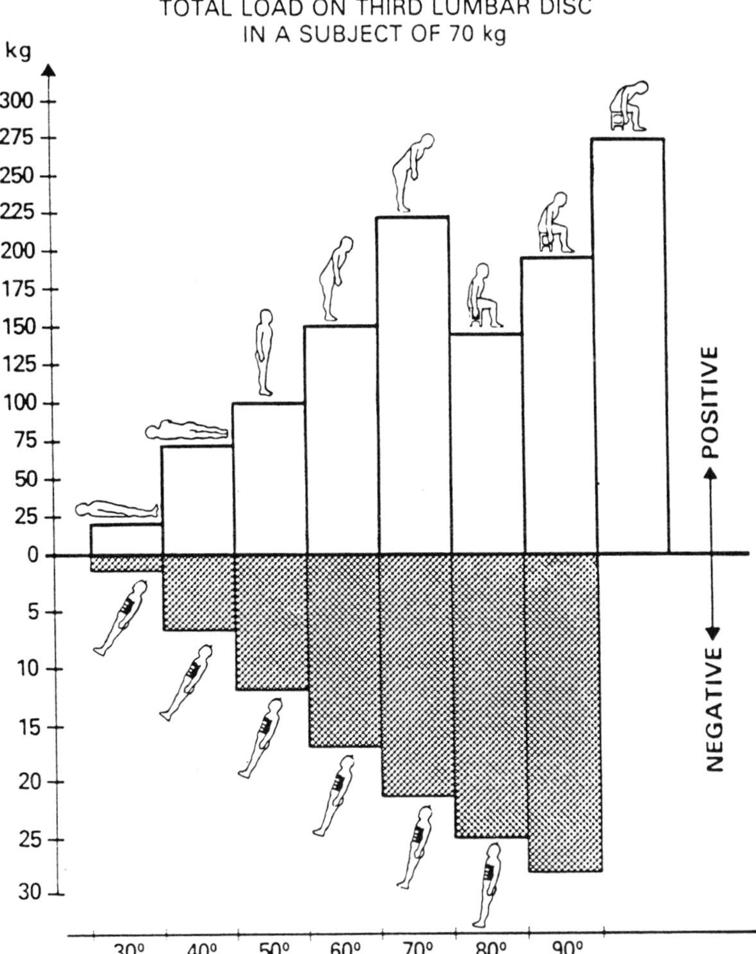

FIGURE 2. This graph includes a redrawing of the figure originally published by Nachemson[14] showing load in kg at the 3rd lumbar level with various body positions. Nachemson's data are based on direct intradiscal pressure recordings in adult volunteers. The gravity traction data are calculated on the basis of Nachemson's work. (Copyright Sister Kenny Institute, Minneapolis, MN. Used with permission.)

gravitational force. Widespread clinical use over a 15-year period has allowed validation of the original expectations, as well as user safety.

During these 15 years, the GLRTP's use has been in therapeutics, usually related to the conservative treatment of acute, contained disc herniations. It is interesting to note that the efficacy in this regard appears to be similar to the nationally reported favorable clinical result rate of 70% for surgical discectomy.[11,12]

Only recently has attention been focused on the GLRTP as a means of influencing acute lumbar musculoligamentous syndromes, as well as nutrition and healing of the disc itself. In Figure 2, a redrawing of Nachemson's lumbar

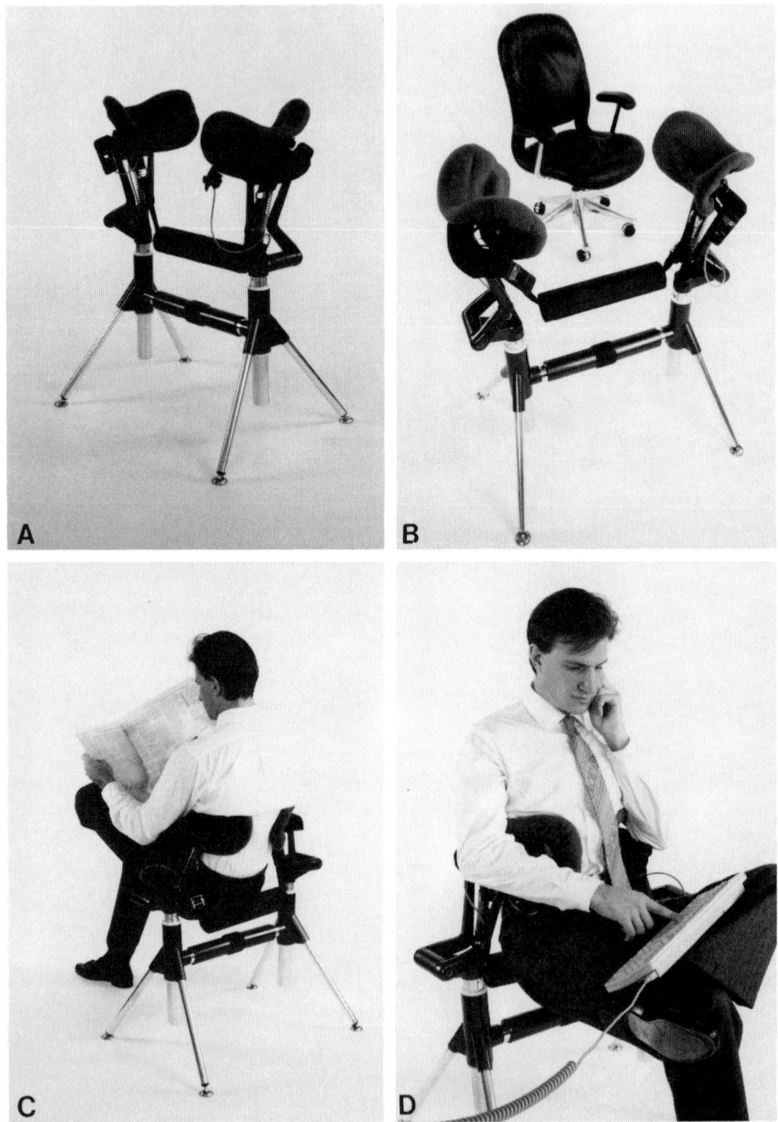

FIGURE 3. In this series of illustrations, the eugonomic seating device is presented (upper left) and then compared with an ergonomic chair (upper right). Front and back views of a subject in the device are illustrated in the lower views. In the examples shown, the roller support has been slipped away from the buttocks to completely unload the back. Loading has been transferred to the rib cage and can be returned to the back (in varying degrees) by engaging the roller component seen behind the buttock. This device is designed to be used in front of a work surface. Preferred use is for 15 minutes three times a day. (SDI Back Chair™, Courtesy of Spinal Designs International, Minneapolis, MN. Copyright 1989. All rights reserved. Patent pending.)

spine-loading data has been presented in order to indicate the calculated negative intradiscal pressures with the GLRTP.[13,14]

Despite the fact that GLRTP is cumbersome, user "unfriendly," and requires time away from work, it has allowed documentation of the successful use of the rib cage as a means of supporting body weight. These appreciations have served to open new vistas of thought regarding the need and the means by which the lumbar spine could be intermittently unloaded and exercised for the expressed purpose of enhancing nutrition, healing, function, and longevity. In order to be able to express this new concept, the term "eugonomic" was coined.

The creation of a low back seating device based on eugonomic principles has been an interdisciplinary and interinstitutional effort. Figure 3 shows such a seating device developed by Spinal Designs International of Minneapolis. Eugonomic philosophy reflects recognition of the modern need to prepare for longer life expectancy and also a higher quality of life. For the athlete, eugonomic low back seating devices represent a means by which unusual occupational stresses may be modified or alleviated using common sense and user-friendly approaches.

SUMMARY

Many athletic endeavors are adversarial to the lumbar spine. It is now appreciated that not all spines are created equal. Those spines that are genetically deficient need to be identified before irreversible injury occurs, and those that are normal require daily enhancement of nutrition and healing so as to avoid what we now understand to be acquired injury due to many factors and influences. The application of eugonomic principles by the athlete provides a means of not only optimizing performance but also achieving potential improvement of later quality of life.

Acknowledgments. The author would like to express his personal appreciation to Gregory Peterson, Elizabeth Hepper, and William Stumpf and his associates for their support and assistance.

REFERENCES

1. Swearingen JJ, Wheelwright DD, et al: An Analysis of Sitting Areas and Pressures of Man (Report No. 62-1). Oklahoma City, U.S. Civil Aero-Medical Research Institute, 1962.
2. Cornell P: The Biomechanics of Sitting, 2nd ed. Grand Rapids, MI, Steelcase Inc., S-065 R289, 1989.
3. Farfan HF, Cossette JW, et al: The effects of torsion in the lumbar intervertebral joints: The role of torsion in the production of disc degeneration. J Bone Joint Surg 52A:568–580, 1970.
4. Kirkaldy-Willis WH: The pathology and pathogenesis of low back pain. In Kirkaldy-Willis WH(ed): Managing Low Back Pain, Vols. I and II. New York, Churchill Livingstone, 1983 and 1988.
5. Urban JPG, Holm S, et al: Diffusion of small solutes into the intervertebral disc. Biorheology 15:203–206, 1978.
6. Holm S, Maroudas A, et al: Nutrition of the intervertebral disc: An in vivo study of solute transport. Clin Orthop Rel Res 178:1977.
7. Heithoff KB: Personal communication.
8. Andersson GBJ, Chaffin DB, et al: Occupational biomechanics of the lumbar spine. In Pope MH, Frymoyer JW, et al (eds): Occupational Low Back Pain. New York, Praeger Scientific, 1984.
9. Grieco A: Sitting posture: An old problem and a new one. Ergonomics 29:345–362, 1986.
10. Ghosh P: Influence of drugs, hormones and other agents on the metabolism of the disc and the sequelae of its degeneration. In The Biology of the Intervertebral Disc, Vol. II. Boca Raton, FL, CRC Press, 1988.

11. Goldish GD: Lumbar traction. In Tollison CD, Kriegel ML (eds): Inter-Disciplinary Rehabilitation of Low Back Pain. Baltimore, Williams & Wilkins, 1989.
12. Burton C: Gravity lumbar reduction. In Kirkaldy-Willis WH (ed): Managing Low Back Pain, Vol. II. New York, Churchill Livingstone, 1988.
13. Burton C, Nida G: The Sister Kenny Institute Gravity Lumbar Reduction Therapy Program. Minneapolis, The Sister Kenny Institute, Publication No. 731, 1982.
14. Nachemson A: The load on lumbar disks in different positions of the body. Clin Orthop 45:107–122, 1966.

Chapter 8

FOOT ORTHOTICS, SPORTS, AND THE SPINE

Bradley T. Britt, MD

In an athlete with back pain, the foot is seldom the primary cause. However, gait and pedal malalignment, which might otherwise be inconsequential, are significant aggravating factors in many instances of back disorders.

The use of pedal modifications to control or modify gait factors affecting the back is effective, noninvasive, and unfortunately often overlooked. Intervention can include devices to modify rotation, pelvic tilt (relative leg length), and impact loading. The biomechanics and specific rationale behind intervention will be discussed in this paper.

GAIT

The normal gait has been well described by many authors. Recapitulation here is meant to emphasize only those elements of gait that affect pelvic tilt and rotation, the factors that most readily play upon the back.

In normal gait, the foot goes through a basic cycle of supination at heel strike, to pronation through midstance, and then back to supination and toe-off. Supination causes the knee to rotate externally and pronation causes internal rotation.

The hemipelvis on the side of the stance-phase leg is essentially fused to the femur by the hip adductors, and therefore the lower limb rotation is to the greatest degree directly translated to the pelvis. The pelvis initially begins internal rotation at heel strike and then progresses through external rotation at toe-off, and just past this into the swing phase.

In supination, the hindfoot is locked and rigid; in pronation, it is soft and flaccid. This locking and unlocking mechanism as the hindfoot cycles through the stance phase is the primary mechanism for the absorption of impact pressures.

ORTHOTICS

The advent of new "sports-specific" shoes has enhanced performance and decreased foot-related injury. Proper running shoes should have good heel-impact protection, rigid heel control (counter), and good flexibility at the site of the natural midfoot break. Court shoes of any variety must have good arch support, good heel (counter) support, and most of all good forefoot fit (for sudden starts and stops). Serious "walkers" should probably be steered toward comfortable running shoes, as much more money is spent on style and less on performance factors in walking shoes.

The shoe must also be capable of accommodating the desired modification, be it depth for inserts or the proper type of sole for external modification. Orthotic management must be initiated slowly and judiciously. A slow break-in period is mandatory, and often multiple adjustments are necessary before the desired effect is obtained.

After careful evaluation of the foot and deciding upon the goal of intervention, a selection of treatment modalities can be made. Many simple padding devices can be stocked and dispensed at the office, but custom orthotic instruction and prescription should only be attempted by one with training in fabrication of these devices.

EVALUATION

Most spine patients have presented with back problems, and the foot portion of the evaluation will be secondary or supplemental. A history and physical examination will already have been done, but the following factors should be considered in terms of the foot and its effect on the presenting back problem.

Specific information to be obtained should include degree of sports participation (mileage, number of tennis sets or golf holes, etc.) and recent changes in the normal pattern. The athlete should be questioned about shoewear (to include recent changes and past history of experiences with good or bad shoes), surfaces (grass, asphalt, clay, hard court, etc.), and recent changes from one to another. Inquiries should be made into foot or leg injuries that might have changed the gait pattern. Finally, one should obtain any history of past use of orthotics or other pedal modifications. Many answers to seemingly complicated questions can be obtained from discussion of changes in an athlete's routine.

Physical examination should begin with a worn pair of shoes, which can provide a good idea of the gait pattern and stresses of the athlete's running or walking motion. Note the heel strike pattern, forefoot wear pattern, and breakdown pattern in the heel counter and arch.

Observation of the patient walking (both in shoes and out of shoes) and running is essential. Pathological factors, such as hamstring or Achilles malfunction, and phasic or positional changes in gait are only observable while the patient is in motion. A gait lab is not always available, but personal observation is.

Have the patient stand facing you and evaluate the status of the pelvis. If it is not level, then use blocks to evaluate the build-up necessary to level the pelvis.

Now lay the patient down and evaluate leg length by measuring from the pelvis to the knee, knee to ankle, and pelvis to ankle. These measurements are certainly less revealing and probably less significant from a functional point of view than information gained from leveling the pelvis on standing.

Now examine the feet in the standing position. Look for symmetry, front and rear, and note the degree and rigidity of arch formation. Observing from the rear, note heel varus and look for Johnson's sign (too many toes), and indications of loss of arch support on the affected side. Ask the patient to stand on tip-toe and again look for heel varus (in the case of pronated feet, the formation of the arch). Sit the patient down and again observe the feet. The presence of an arch whole in tip-toe or in a sitting nonweight-bearing position in a functionally hyperpronated foot is an indication of a supple and functional pes planus. Palpate the foot for rigidity, evaluating for ankle, subtalar, and midfoot motions. Finally note callus formation, which is an excellent indicator of pathological weight-bearing or shoe fit. One must also inquire about the presence of calluses that the patient habitually smooths.

DISORDERS

Leg-length Discrepancy

A large portion of the general population has appreciable leg-length inequality, and most are not symptomatic, even with vigorous athletic pursuits. However, several authors have cited leg-length discrepancy as a possible contributing factor to low back pain, particularly in long-distance runners or those who maintain high weekly mileage. The pelvis is the critical link between the lower extremities and the spine. Therefore, imbalance of the pelvis can affect the vertebral column. Equalizing leg length or leveling the pelvis should be approached with caution, as one can make an asymptomatic situation worse. A good generalization is to correct the calculated deficit 50% initially. Up to about 1/2″ correction may be incorporated in the shoe in the form of a heel pad. Any additional correction should be full-length build-up by either an extra-depth shoe or an orthosis on the outer heel and sole of the shoe. As previously stated, a certain amount of inequality is within physiological limits, so do not be disappointed if a great deal of difference is not appreciated with this treatment.

Rigid Cavus Foot

The main deficit in rigid cavus foot is inability to absorb shock in going through the supination-pronation-supination cycle, with locking and unlocking of the hindfoot. In dealing with this problem, shock absorption and appropriate weight distribution by external means are the goal. A less rigid or flexible full-length orthosis molded to fit the unusual foot shape is appropriate. It can usually be fitted into most good athletic shoes, and some of these devices are reasonably available for stocking the office. In some case a supination or pronation deformity of the forefoot might require medial or lateral wedging, or a "posting," and this should be evaluated at the same time.

Hyperpronated Feet

The main problem with hyperpronation is excessive internal rotation of the lower extremity, with resultant pelvic tilt as well as poor power in toe-off because of the inability to resupinate at that time. A more rigid type of orthosis extending just proximal to the metatarsal heads (3/4 lengths) is most appropriate. A cover can be added for comfort and to regulate shear stresses in the plantar aspect of the foot. With these devices, an extended break-in period and many adjustments are the rule.

Painful Feet

Many feet have a relatively normal configuration, but, owing to various painful situations, gait changes and pain advancing up biomechanical pathways to the spine are possible. Attempts to prevent pain problems are prudent, particularly in athletes participating on a hard court or track. Simply switching to a different shoe with better padding may be all that is necessary. The use of Spinco or other shoe-liners to improve impact-absorption is a very simple and effective means of accomplishing this goal as well. Improving the impact-absorbing properties of athletic shoes may not only decrease foot pain and the development of abnormal gait patterns, but also help decrease the high-impact forces transmitted to the spine in running, when the load generated may be as great as 3 to 4 times the person's body weight.

CONCLUSION

When discussing how to treat runner's knee, Dr. George Sheehan has stated, "You treat the foot." With apologies to Dr. Sheehan, the same thinking should prevail when treating athletes with back pain. Even if not the primary cause of back pain, thorough gait evaluation and, if necessary, recommending shoewear orthotic modification can greatly contribute to the recovery and future well-being of the patient. The selection of shoewear modifications is based largely on experience, and the assistance of a well-established pedorthist can facilitate cost-effective and efficient care of the athlete.

Foot orthotic devices can range from a rigid, custom-molded arch support to in-shoe modification, or indeed the shoe itself can be the orthosis. The best source of information concerning use of and choices in orthotic management are trained and experienced pedorthists, some of whom have developed added expertise in athletic orthotic management. Many top-level athletic shoe companies are quite cooperative and willing to provide information about the specific goals and attributes of their products.

Remember that management in any athletic foot problem begins with the shoe. There is no greater example of the old adage, "You get what you pay for," than with athletic shoes. From golf shoes to running shoes, if they are of poor quality or poorly fitted, then any other intervention attempted is doomed to failure.

REFERENCES

1. Alexander MJL: Biomechanical aspects of lumbar spine injuries in athletes: A review. Canadian J App Sport Sci 10:1–20, 1985.
2. American Academy of Orthopaedic Surgeons: Atlas of Orthotics: Biomechanical Principles and Applications. St. Louis, CV Mosby, 1975.
3. Bordelon RL: Foot first—evolution of man. Foot Ankle 8(3): 1987.
4. Bordelon RL: Surgical and Conservative Foot Care. Thorofare, NJ, Charles B. Slack, 1988.
5. Bordelon RL: Practical guide to foot orthosis. J Musculoskel Med 6(7):71, 1989.
6. D'Ambrosia R, Drez D: Prevention and Treatment of Running Injuries. Thorofare, NH, Charles B. Slack, 1982.

Chapter 9

SPINAL DEFORMITIES AND PARTICIPATION IN SPORTS

Alexis P. Shelokov, MD, and John A. Herring, MD

The 1980s were noted for a renewed interest in sports participation among all segments of the American population. The value of regular exercise has been confirmed by improved cardiac fitness and weight loss, as well as the less tangible benefits of an active lifestyle. Children who develop proficiency in sporting activities also gain a sense of accomplishment and earn the respect of their peers. This is even more important for children with a spine deformity. Limited either by their physiologic condition or the constraints imposed upon them by physicians, these children develop a sense of inferiority or abnormality. Regular exercise and sports participation, within the limits of safety, can help to minimize the "crisis" a child experiences with brace wear or surgery.

The value of exercise as a modality of physical therapy cannot be underestimated. Organized physical therapy is both time-consuming and expensive. Consequently, the actual portion of a day spent doing therapy is necessarily small. Regular exercise and sports participation can be an important addition to regular physical therapy. The child develops and improves muscle tone, increases range of motion of the involved and uninvolved joints, and improves cardiac fitness.

The purpose of this chapter is to help physicians, parents, therapists, and educators reach reasoned decisions to assure safer participation in athletics by children with spine deformity. The chapter is not a cookbook or a simple list that might unnecessarily limit some children while engaging others in an unsafe activity. It is often difficult to determine a safe level of sports participation for an individual, because not enough is known about the biomechanics of many spinal anomalies. The potential risk of injury must be weighed against the physiologic and psychological benefits.

This chapter will discuss some of the common spinal deformities in relation to sports participation. We will begin with scoliosis in some detail and then briefly consider Scheuermann's disease and sway back, as well as certain important aspects of cervical spine disorders in Down's syndrome.

SCOLIOSIS

Scoliosis is one of the most common deformities that brings a child to the physician's office. It is also a diagnosis that causes confusion regarding sports participation. Scoliosis is conveniently divided into cases of either idiopathic or congenital origin. The child with idiopathic scoliosis has a recognizable curve pattern and no neurologic deficit or structural anomaly to explain the curve. The child with congenital scoliosis has a structural vertebral anomaly to account for the alteration in normal growth of the spine.

The initial evaluation of a child with scoliosis requires the search for possible underlying causes. A diagnostic work-up is necessary to exclude tumors, congenital bony anomalies, and neurologic disease, because patients who have structural causes for their scoliosis do require different therapeutic intervention, and their prognosis for sports participation may be different. Bone scan, MRI, and myelography should be used to rule out intradural or extradural masses and tumors of bone origin, such as osteoid osteoma and osteoblastoma, which are known to cause painful scoliosis.

Idiopathic Scoliosis

In general, patients with idiopathic scoliosis and curves of a magnitude less than 20° are managed by regular reassessment. They should be seen every 3 to 4 months for follow-up physical examination and standing radiographs. Bracing is unnecessary unless curve progression is documented. An exercise program is often prescribed to strengthen the paraspinal muscles, stretch contracted ligamentous structures on the concave side of the curve, and increase general flexibility. Bending exercises may be prescribed to dynamically reverse the deformity through active muscle contraction.[14]

Children with scoliosis who have curves of a magnitude greater than 20° when first diagnosed, or those with documented progression of the curvature, usually are started on a bracing and exercise program. Here, however, the benefit of exercise in the long-term management of scoliosis has not been fully established.

Historically, a specific exercise program was initiated for all individuals treated with bracing. Proponents believed that these exercises were responsible, at least in part, for the success of the bracing protocol.[3] Several research studies have failed to substantiate this assertion.[5,18]

While it is therefore unsubstantiated that exercise enhances the curve correction obtained by brace wear, we think that exercise is still important to the bracing program. Bracing can cause generalized deconditioning and a decreased range of motion of the spine by constraining the torso. We feel that it is prudent to promote activity and prevent the disuse atrophy that may result from brace confinement.

Idiopathic scoliosis and brace wear are not, in themselves, a contraindication to a very high level of sports performance, as demonstrated by those individuals in bracing programs who participate in athletic competition at collegiate and national levels. In one study, the brace wear schedule was liberalized to include a 3–4 hour period of aggressive sports participation each day. The clinical outcomes of these patients with regard to curve magnitude at the cessation of treatment were similar to those outcomes in patients treated by more conventional 23-hour-a-day brace-wear programs.[2,11] All forms of exercise and competitive athletics, including contact sports (with the brace removed), are possible for children with conservatively treated idiopathic scoliosis.

One limitation in patients with idiopathic scoliosis was, however, demonstrated by Chong and co-workers, who noted that children with large thoracic curves had a decreased exercise capacity.[6] They found an inverse correlation between the magnitude of the thoracic curve and endurance time for a specific activity. They also showed an inverse relationship between curve magnitude and the maximum aerobic capacity (VO_2 max). Thus, the only true limitation which a child with thoracic scoliosis may experience is that imposed on exercise capacity by chest wall deformity. This re-emphasizes that, although cosmetic considerations are important in scoliosis treatment, one of our primary concerns is the prevention or limitation of chest-wall deformity and the preservation of vital capacity.

Congenital Scoliosis

The determination of activity level for individuals with congenital scoliosis is most difficult. Congenital anomalies cause a decrease in the mechanical strength of the spine and may allow an increased range of motion, both of which can threaten the spinal cord or nerve roots.[14]

The evaluation of a patient with congenital scoliosis must focus on curve magnitude, growth potential, and any abnormal motion of the involved segments. Flexion/extension x-ray studies and tomography can help assess potential instability. When instability is demonstrated, fusion should be undertaken using commonly accepted guidelines for the cervical, thoracic, and lumbar spine. A radiographic survey should also be carried out in patients with congenital scoliosis of the thoracic and lumbar spine, because approximately 25% of these people may have coexisting segmentation defects in the cervical spine.[1] It is also important to remember that congenital scoliosis is only one part of a spectrum of abnormalities that may occur during development. Careful study of the cardiac and renal systems is mandatory.

Restriction of contact sports is appropriate for an individual with a congenital spine abnormality. Even after spine fusion, these patients may engage in strenuous sports, but they should select those activities with a limited potential for collision between participants.

SPORTS PARTICIPATION AFTER SPINAL FUSION

When bracing fails to stabilize a curve and the decision to proceed with spinal fusion has been made, the choices regarding exercise and sports participation become more difficult.

Historically, spinal implants were unable to adequately stabilize the spine in the postsurgical period, and braces or casts were worn until solid fusion was obtained. Athletic participation was limited to ensure solid fusion. With the general availability of more rigid spinal instrumentation, an early return to athletics may be permitted. After discharge from the hospital, patients are now encouraged to perform light exercise until fusion is demonstrated radiographically. Some surgeons allow a return to competitive athletics at 6 months postoperatively, whereas others require waiting 9 or even 12 months.[12] It is known that 6 to 12 months are necessary to obtain solid fusion. This period of time should be used to restore cardiac fitness and to maintain muscle tone. After the demonstration of solid fusion, a return to more normal activities is allowed.

There is considerable disagreement about the level of sports participation for patients following spinal fusion. Many experts are concerned about the possibility of accelerated disc degeneration of unfused segments adjacent to a successful fusion.[11] Patients who have had surgery that included the fourth or fifth lumbar vertebra experience an increased rate of disc degeneration at the lower lumbar levels when compared to individuals with a fusion that ends at the third lumbar vertebra.[7] The importance of this accelerated degeneration is its association with a significant increase in low back pain.[8,9,13,14]

After spinal fusion for congenital scoliosis, a patient should be advised against participating in collision sports. This does not mean, however, that the individual who has undergone fusion cannot maintain an active lifestyle. Swimming, walking, and weight lifting may all be excellent alternatives for these individuals.

What then is an appropriate activity level for a child who has had fusion for scoliosis? The conflicting opinions of the family, the teachers, the patient, and the doctor, as well as potential liability, complicate this issue. In general, patients with thoracic curves and short-segment fusion should be allowed to participate in more vigorous activities than those with longer spine fusions or fusions that extend into the lower lumbar spine. The eventual contribution of fusion to accelerated disc degeneration is not known, but it is presumed that repetitive microtrauma, in addition to the long lever arm created by successful fusion, will accelerate the normal degenerative process. It remains for the well-informed family, the patient, and the physician to decide what risk is acceptable. Even then, the school may be unwilling to allow a child with spinal fusion to engage in contact sports. When considering spine fusion for a child who participates in contact sports, a discussion of these issues prior to surgery with the family and school representative may be reasonable.

SCHEUERMANN'S DISEASE

Scheuermann's disease (or painful juvenile kyphosis) is a disease of unknown etiology that usually affects adolescent males. This condition is not only painful, but may cause progressive thoracic or lumbar kyphosis.

Scheuermann's disease appears as both an idiopathic and acquired traumatic form. The traumatic variant of the disease is associated with a contracted lumbodorsal fascia, which is thought to be a possible precondition. By not allowing adequate flexion of the lumbar spine, the center of rotation of the vertebral body is changed, causing injury to the anterior aspect of the vertebral body and resultant kyphosis. This condition is sometimes responsive to brace treatment—significant correction of kyphosis may be obtained through early Milwaukee bracing if there is growth remaining in the ring apophysis.[16] Bracing can allow reconstitution of the vertebral height and more normal spinal alignment.

At the time of initial diagnosis, and while acutely painful, those individuals with Scheuermann's kyphosis should not be allowed to engage in weight lifting or contact sports. After bracing is instituted, and a specific exercise program to stretch the lumbodorsal fascia has been successful, these patients may return to their previous level of activity but should avoid extreme axial loading activities such as heavy overhead weight lifting. An exacerbation of pain or progression of the kyphosis is an indication to again restrict activity. The management of such a case may require several rounds of activity restriction, specific exercises, and then a judicious increase of activity.

SWAY BACK

Sway back is a lesser known deformity that, unlike scoliosis, occurs among already accomplished young athletes such as gymnasts, figure skaters, and ice hockey players.[11] This condition may be painful. It is associated with tightness of the lumbodorsal fascia and hamstrings. Treatment decisions are based on the physical examination. If the lordosis is noted to be flexible and reversal of the hyperlordotic posture occurs with forward bending, the patient can be managed by an antilordotic exercise program as well as hamstring stretching. However, if the lordosis is fixed, a more aggressive program should be instituted. Fixed lordosis may also require antilordotic bracing. The brace can be worn under clothes and may be used during contact sports if allowed by the regulations of a particular school. Micheli recommends that a prophylactic program of abdominal strengthening and lumbar flattening with emphasis on pelvic tilts be instituted for all children who engage in these potentially high-risk activities.[11]

DOWN'S SYNDROME AND THE SPECIAL OLYMPICS

Individuals in the United States with Down's syndrome have an unusual opportunity to participate in competitive athletics with the Special Olympics. Given the frequency of cervical spine anomalies in Down's syndrome, however, significant concern exists regarding the risks of catastrophic injury due to cervical instability. Semine and co-workers demonstrated a high prevalence of instability and dysplasia of the atlantoaxial junction in patients with Down's syndrome.[15] Eighteen percent of a group of neurologically asymptomatic individuals with Down's syndrome showed some form of cervical anomaly: 12% had abnormal motion between the C1 and C2 vertebrae, whereas the other 6% had an abnormality of the odontoid process, such as hypoplasia, dysplasia, or os odontoidium. The authors point out that any one of these abnormalities has the potential for causing spinal cord injury, and the combination of ligamentous instability and odontoid hypoplasia places the individual with Down's syndrome at an even greater risk for pathologic subluxation. Interestingly, of the ten patients in this study who had an increased atlantodens interval, neurologic deficit was noted in only one individual during the 1-year follow-up.

Burke et al. studied 32 patients with Down's syndrome between 1970 and 1983.[4] They concluded that patients greater than 10 years of age were at significant risk for developing a progressive increase in the atlantodens interval secondary to the intrinsic defect in collagen synthesis peculiar to Down's syndrome. In their study, atlantoaxial instability was defined using the criteria of Martel, who stated that 5 ml is the upper limit of normal in skeletally immature individuals with Down's syndrome.[12] One patient in this study group developed frank atlantoaxial dislocation. There are no other studies that clearly define the risk of neurologic injury in patients with Down's syndrome who have coexistent atlantoaxial instability. Goldberg points out that atlantoaxial instability and odontoid hypoplasia are only one part of the generalized disposition for cervical spine abnormalities in the patients with Down's syndrome.[10] Other important abnormalities in the cervical spine should not be overlooked.

To participate in the Special Olympics, all children must undergo a series of lateral cervical flexion/extension radiographs. If the atlantodens interval is greater than 5 ml in flexion, the patient should not be allowed to participate. Individuals with subluxation of less than 5 ml are allowed to participate in the Special Olympics program, but the neurologic risks are undefined.

The individual with Down's syndrome, once screened for atlantoaxial instability, should be followed on an annual basis. Lateral flexion/extension x-ray studies of the cervical spine and frequent neurologic examination are important because of reported occult development and progression of atlantoaxial subluxation.[4,17]

CONCLUSION

Sports and athletic participation should be an important part of the life of all children with spinal deformity. An active lifestyle can help the child adjust to what is often his or her first encounter with illness. The benefits of an active lifestyle must be carefully weighed against both known and unknown risks for potential neurologic injury. In doing so, the physician can allow patients an important dimension of life that otherwise would be lost.

REFERENCES

1. American Academy of Orthopaedic Surgeons: Orthopedic Knowledge Update. Park Ridge, IL, AAOS.
2. Benson DR, Wolf AW, Shoji H: Can the Milwaukee brace patient participate in competitive athletics? Am J Sports Med 5:7–12, 1977.
3. Blount WP: The Milwaukee Brace. Baltimore, Williams & Wilkins, 1980.
4. Burke SW, French HG, Roberts JM, et al: Chronic atlanto-axial instability in Down syndrome. J Bone Joint Surg 67A:1356–1360, 1985.
5. Carman D, Roach JW, Speck G, et al: Role of exercises in the Milwaukee brace treatment of scoliosis. J Pediatr Orthop 5:65–68, 1985.
6. Chong KC, Letts RM, Cumming GR: Influence of spinal curvature on exercise capacity. J Pediatr Orthop 1:251–254, 1981.
7. Cochran T, Irstam L, Nachemson A: Long-term anatomic and functional changes in patients with adolescent idiopathic scoliosis treated by Harrington rod fusion. Spine 8:576–584, 1983.
8. Edgar MA: Back pain assessment from a long-term follow-up of operated and unoperated patients with adolescent idiopathic scoliosis. Spine 4:519–520, 1979.
9. Ginsburg HH, Goldstein LA, Robinson SC, et al: Back pain in postoperative idiopathic scoliosis: Long-term follow-up study (abstract). Spine 4:518, 1979.
10. Goldberg M: Personal communication. Boston, 1989.
11. Kahanovitz N, Levine DB, Lardone J: The part-time Milwaukee brace treatment of juvenile idiopathic scoliosis. Clin Orthop 167:145–151, 1982.
12. Martel W, Uyham R, Stimson CW: Subluxation of the atlas causion spinal cord compression in a case of Down's syndrome with a "manifestation of an occipital vertebra." Radiology 93:839–840, 1969.
13. Micheli LJ: Spinal deformities and the athlete. In Torg JS, et al: Current Therapy in Sports Medicine. St. Louis, Mosby/BC Decker, 1985, pp 158–164.
14. Micheli LJ, Marotta JJ: Scoliosis and sports. Your Patient & Fitness 2:5–11, 1989.
15. Moskowitz A, Moe JH, Winter RB, Binner H: Long-term follow-up of scoliosis fusion. J Bone Joint Surg 62A:364–376, 1980.
16. Sachs B, Bradford D, Winter R, et al: Scheuermann kyphosis: Follow-up of Milwaukee brace treatment. J Bone Joint Surg 69A:50–57, 1987.
17. Semine AA, Ertel AN, Goldberg MJ, Bull MJ: Cervical-spine instability in children with Down syndrome (trisomy 21). J Bone Joint Surg 60A:649–652, 1978.
18. Slack CM: The spine in sports. Comprehensive Therapy 6:63–74, 1980.

Chapter 10

SPONDYLOLYSIS AND SPONDYLOLISTHESIS IN THE ATHLETE

Jeffrey E. Flemming, MD

Spondylolysis and spondylolisthesis are conditions seen in approximately 5% of the population of the U.S. and are significant causes of back pain in this country.[2,12] It is estimated that 25% of adolescents who present with back pain show radiographic evidence of spondylolysis or spondylolisthesis.[8] In the athlete, this association is even higher. Such sporting activities as diving, gymnastics, wrestling, weight lifting, football, track and field, and athletics in general predispose an individual to spondylolysis.

The defect in the pars interarticularis is felt to be caused by repetitive microtrauma associated with hyperextension of the lumbar spine, ultimately causing a stress or fatigue fracture in the pars.[2,3,10,12]

SPONDYLOLYSIS/SPONDYLOLISTHESIS

The term *spondylolisthesis* was first used by Kilian in 1854 and is derived from the Greek, *spondylo,* meaning vertebrae, and *-olisthesis,* meaning to slide down an incline. The structural defect in the pars interarticularis removes the bony support from the vertebra and allows a forward slippage. With spondylolysis, there is a dissolution of the pars interarticularis, but the vertebra has not slipped forward.

In 1855, Lambl demonstrated anatomically the defect in the pars interarticularis. Later, Naugebauer recognized that the slippage could occur even without a defect in the pars, but simply with elongation of the pars. The etiology of spondylolysis is felt to be due to a stress reaction through the pars interarticularis causing a fatigue fracture that either goes on to a fibrous nonunion or heals in an elongated state. It has been reported that lytic spondylolisthesis occurs only in humans and is not seen in other primates. This is because the lumbar lordosis associated with the standing posture produces the stresses in the pars interarticularis.

The defect has never been shown to be present at birth. The youngest reported case is a 3½-month-old child. Between 5 and 7 years of age, there is a dramatic increase in the incidence of spondylolysis. Frequently this is a "silent" fracture, with the child showing no signs or symptoms. Pain in a child in this age group often indicates an acute stress reaction or fracture. Spondylolisthesis, on the other hand, usually presents at a later date, presumably when the slip has progressed and the soft tissue structures are then being affected by mechanical instability. In the athlete, the lytic defect is associated with repetitive hyperextension maneuvers that occur during the performance of the sport. Unlike the spondylolysis that occurs at an earlier age, those acquired athletically are frequently painful and associated with hyperextension. Some feel the athletically acquired lesion to be a "stable" lesion that will not go on to further slip, despite continued activity.[9] Other authors would dispute this. Commandre found that 3 out of 7 athletes followed until skeletal maturity progressed.[3] Wiltse has found the greatest amount of slippage occurring between the ages of 9 and 14, but seldom after that.[12]

With repetitive hyperextension maneuvers, the vertebral isthmus between the superior and inferior articular processes is subjected to excessive stress. Compressive loads up to 30 kN occur in the hyperextended lumbar spine during weight lifting.[5] This repetitive stress ultimately causes the bone to fail, with development of a fatigue fracture. Lumbar rotation associated with certain sports, such as throwing sports, diving, and wrestling, can cause unilateral spondylolysis to occur (Fig. 1).

There is a definite familial tendency in the development of pars interarticularis defects. The incidence of spondylolysis in the American population is around 5% and is noted to be higher in whites than in blacks, and higher in males than in females. The Eskimo population is noted to have one of the highest incidences of spondylolysis, as high as 50%. This familiality is more commonly noted in spondylolysis that occurs in childhood, as opposed to that acquired athletically. Rossi found that, in the general population, 30% of the cases had a family history of spondylolysis or spondylolisthesis, whereas in the athlete this familiality was much less.[10] Jackson noted in gymnasts a four-fold higher incidence of spondylolysis over the nonathletic population. He felt that, though there is a hereditary factor, the spondylolysis that occurs in athletes is a "different entity."[2]

Rossi noted a definite increase in the rate of spondylolysis/spondylolisthesis in certain types of athletic activities. He found a 63% incidence in divers, which he associated with the hyperextension and twisting maneuvers that occur in performance of this sport. He believed the exaggerated lumbar hyperextension caused by technical mistakes on entry into the water to be the major factor in producing the lytic defect. His study found weight lifting to be associated with a 36% incidence; wrestling, 33%; gymnastics, 32%; and athletics in general with a 22½% incidence (Table 1).[10]

Wiltse has classified spondylolisthesis in five major groups: dysplastic, isthmic, degenerative, post-traumatic, and pathologic. The dysplastic, degenerative, post-traumatic, and pathologic groups are all associated with conditions not

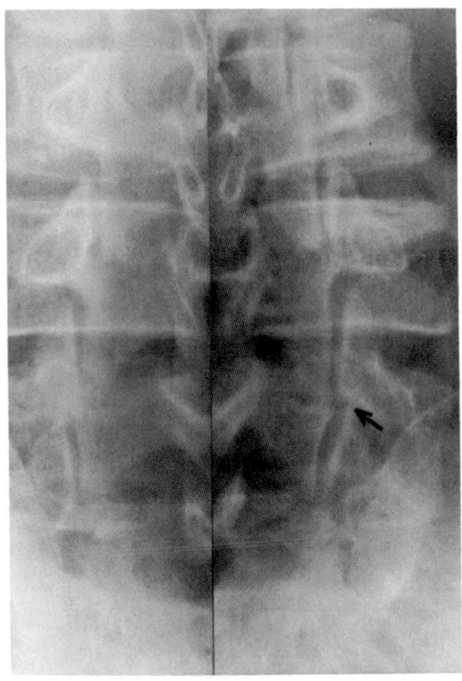

FIGURE 1. X-ray study of a 17-year-old baseball pitcher with lumbar spine pain. Oblique radiographs demonstrate a unilateral lytic defect in the pars interarticularis.

necessarily related to sporting activities. Isthmic spondylolysis is most commonly seen and refers to a defect in the pars interarticularis. Wiltse further subclassified this type into three subtypes: (1) lytic, (2) elongation of the pars, and (3) acute fractures. The lytic defect is felt to be the fatigue or stress fracture through the pars interarticularis that then goes on to a fibrous nonunion, producing the defect we see on oblique radiographs in the so-called "neck of the Scotty dog."

Elongation of the pars is felt to be due to repetitive stress fractures occurring within the pars interarticularis that then go on to heal, but in an elongated position.

Acute fractures of the pars interarticularis can also occur but are very rare and are usually due to severe trauma, often a direct blow to the back with a blunt object, causing acute fracture through the pars and forward-slipping of the vertebral body. The trauma necessary to cause this type of fracture is substantial and more commonly seen in motor vehicle or motorcycle accidents, rather than sporting events.

TABLE 1. Incidence of Spondylolysis in Selected Sports*

Sport	Spondylolysis (%)
Diving	63.3%
Weight lifting	36.2%
Wrestling	33.0%
Gymnastics	32.0%
"Athletics"	22.5%
General Population	5.0%

* From Rossi F: Spondylolysis, spondylolisthesis and sports. J Sports Med Phys Fit 18(4):317–340, 1988.

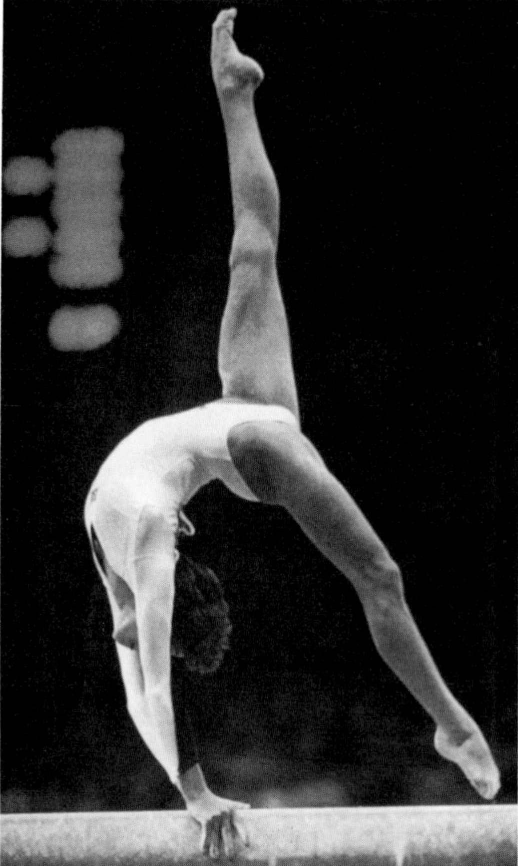

FIGURE 2. Hyperextension of the lumbar spine during athletic training or competition is associated with development of a fatigue fracture through the pars interarticularis.

ATHLETICS AND SPONDYLOLYSIS

As already discussed, the cause of athletically acquired spondylolysis is felt to be secondary to repetitive hyperextension of the lumbar spine that causes microtrauma through the pars and ultimately a fatigue fracture (Fig. 2). The higher incidence in specific sports is felt to be directly related to the type of sporting activity and the maneuvers of the athlete not only in competition but also during the many hours of training that are necessary to obtain success.

Presentation

Athletes will usually note pain with certain maneuvers during their training regimen. These are often associated with the hyperlordotic position. They complain of chronic dull aching in the lumbosacral spine that is exacerbated with hyperextension activities.

On examination, they may demonstrate hamstring tightness and will often have decreased flexibility. Extension of the hip and leg will cause exacerbation of their pain on the side with the defect. Oblique radiographs will frequently show changes in the pars interarticularis, either lytic defects or increased bone density, indicating a stress reaction through the pars. Spina bifida occulta has a 23%

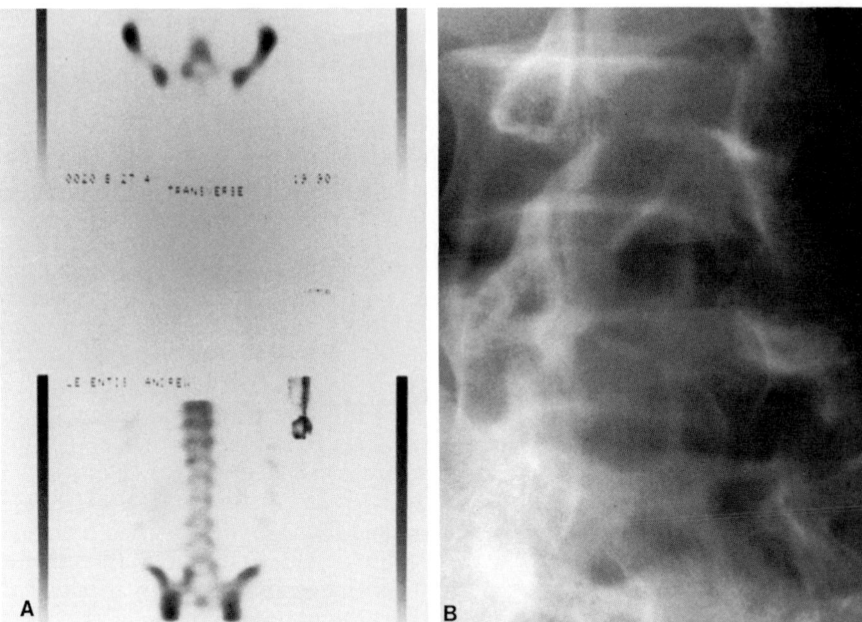

FIGURE 3. *A,* Technetium bone scanning demonstrates increased activity in the pars interarticularis. *B,* Oblique coned-down views are often helpful to localize the area of increased uptake.

association with spondylolysis. In those individuals with normal appearing radiographs, yet with continued lumbar pain, a bone scan is helpful and often diagnostic (Fig. 3).[4] Oblique coned-down views are helpful to adequately visualize the pars interarticularis on the bone scan. The scan will often light up before radiographic evidence is noted. Commandre stated that lumbar pain in the athlete is spondylolysis until proven otherwise.[3] Even a negative radiograph and bone scan do not always rule out the stress reaction, and follow-up studies may be necessary if the patient's pain persists.

Treatment

Various methods of managing athletically acquired spondylolysis have been proposed, from restriction of the athletic activities that cause pain to surgical stabilization. Most patients will respond to conservative management, with restricted activities, bracing, and anti-inflammatory medication.

Micheli treated patients with a zero-degree, lumbar-flexion, polypropylene brace and found that 32% of his patients obtained bony healing of the defect and 88% became symptom-free and were able to resume their sporting activities, even without bony healing.[9] Jackson had several patients in his study that healed despite limited participation in their sport.[7]

Most authors would agree with a regimen of restricted activities, selective bracing, and an exercise program to strengthen the abdominal musculature. Once the athlete becomes asymptomatic, return to athletic competition is permitted. Only in rare instances is surgical stabilization necessary. If surgical treatment is necessary, Bradford has described a technique of wiring the transverse process to the spinous process of the affected level, with bone grafting of the defect.[1] Good results with this technique have been demonstrated, and it is recommended in patients with defects in L1 through L4 who do not respond to adequate conservative management. At the L5 vertebra, fusion of L5 to the sacrum is the procedure of choice for stabilization. In athletes that are skeletally immature, close observation is advised to make sure the spondylolisthesis has not become progressive. If progression is noted, then fusion is often indicated.

If athletes with spondylolisthesis are skeletally immature, and have up to 25% slip (Grade I), they are allowed to participate in sports as long as they remain symptom free. Those with slips of 25% to 50% (Grade II) are allowed to participate in sports that have a low risk for back injury but are discouraged from participation in "stressful" sports. These children must be followed closely for any evidence of progression. Once 50% slippage has occurred, surgical stabilization is recommended. If a child has symptoms that do not respond to 6–12 months of conservative treatment, surgical stabilization may be indicated.[2]

Once the patient is skeletally mature, progression is rare. Spengler studied college football players with known spondylolysis and low back pain versus those without this defect but with low back pain, and found no difference in time loss between the two groups from games or practices.[11] He treated these athletes with heat, rest, anti-inflammatory medication, selective bracing, and an exercise program. Once they demonstrated painless range of motion of the lumbosacral spine, abdominal exercises were stressed and sports were allowed. If pain persists after adequate conservative treatment (6–12 months), then surgical stabilization is an option.

CONCLUSION

Persistent lumbar pain without evidence of nerve root tension in the athlete should raise the possibility of stress fracture in the pars interarticularis. This is further assessed with the history, physical exam, oblique radiographs, and, if necessary, bone scanning to rule out the possibility of a stress reaction or fracture in the pars interarticularis. Many types of athletic endeavors are associated with this problem, specifically those sports that cause repetitive hyperextension of the lumbosacral spine. Torsion associated with hyperextension can predispose the athlete to unilateral spondylolysis.

Treatment is conservative, with restricted activities, rest, anti-inflammatory medication, and selective bracing. Once the athlete becomes asymptomatic and has full range of motion without pain, he or she may once again participate in sporting activities. Surgery is only rarely indicated in the management of these athletic patients. In the skeletally immature athlete, close observation for progression of the spondylolisthesis is advised.

REFERENCES

1. Bradford DS, Iza J: Repair of the defect in spondylolysis or minimal degrees of spondylolisthesis in segmental wire fixation and bone grafting. Spine 7(10):673–679, 1985.
2. Cirillo JV, Jackson DW: Pars interarticularis stress reaction, spondylolysis and spondylolisthesis in gymnasts. Clin Sports Med 4(1):95–110, 1985.
3. Commandre FA, et al: Spondylolysis and spondylolisthesis in young athletes: 28 cases. J Sports Med Phys Fit 28(1):104–107, 1988.
4. Elliott SE, Hutson MA, Wastle ML: Bone scintigraphy in assessment of spondylolysis in patients attending a sports injury clinic. Clin Radiol 39(3):269–272, 1988.

5. Granhed H, Morelli B: Low back pain among retired wrestlers and heavyweight lifters. Am J Sports Med 16(5):530–533, 1988.
6. Joint Committee on Physical Fitness, Recreation, and Sports Medicine: Athletic activities by children with skeletal abnormalities. Pediatrics 51(5):949–951, 1973.
7. Jackson DW, Wiltse LL, Eirincione RJ: Spondylolysis in the female gymnast. Clin Orthop Rel Res 117:68–73, 1976.
8. King HA: Back pain in children. Pediatr Clin North Am 31(5):1083–1095, 1984.
9. Micheli LJ: Back injuries in gymnasts. Clin Sports Med 4(1):85–93, 1985.
10. Rossi F: Spondylolysis, spondylolisthesis and sports. J Sports Med Phys Fit 18(4):317–340, 1988.
11. Semon RL, Spengler D: Significance of lumbar spondylolysis in college football players. Spine 6(2):172–174, 1981.
12. Wiltse LL, Widell EH, Jackson DW: Fatigue fracture: The bone lesion in isthmic spondylolisthesis. J Bone Joint Surg 57:17–22, 1974.

PART II

SPINAL PROBLEMS IN SPECIFIC SPORTS

Chapter 11

BACK PROBLEMS IN THE RUNNER

John J. Regan, MD

The popular idea that exercise is essential to healthy living has given rise to the recent popularity of running. Participation in 10 kilometer, marathon, and triatholon racing has led to increasing numbers of patients calling upon their physicians for advice concerning musculoskeletal problems. For the patient with back problems, physicians have generally discouraged running and promoted swimming and cycling as better forms of exercise. This may not come as welcomed news to the millions who enjoy running as their main form of exercise. The question arises, "Can physicians, from understanding the spinal biomechanics of running and from understanding spinal pathology, make better recommendations to the avid jogger or runner?"

Symptoms related to the spine, restricting running and other strenuous activities, occur most commonly between the ages of 30 and 50. A prospective study of 1,000 consecutive adult runners having disabling musculoskeletal complaints showed only 11 (1.1%) of the complaints were related to the spine.[8] Spinal complaints are infrequent in runners under age 25. The exact incidence of spinal problems in runners is difficult to determine, because most symptoms are of an aching, intermittent nature, and active people often accept their spinal discomfort and never seek formal medical advice. In one study, the incidence of back pain arising in 120 middle-aged adults who participated in a voluntary jogging program was 9%.[3]

BACK MECHANICS AND RUNNING

To explain the patterns of spinal injuries, it is useful to consider the biomechanical aspects of running. Spinal loading occurs in a wide range of sports activities, including running. The insidious onset of back pain may be caused by disc dysfunction.[12] The nucleus of the disc and the epiphyseal plates have no enervation and can be injured without pain. Compressive cyclic loading of the spine occurs as a result of running, which has been described by Slocum and Bowerman as a series of smoothly coordinated jumps.[14] When the compressive load exceeds the interstitial osmotic pressure of the disc tissues, leading to exudation of water through the disc wall,[7] this results in a loss of disc height.

During running, the force generated at the point of heel strike is usually in excess of 2,000 N.[11] This force transmitted to the spine produces significant spinal loading, as demonstrated by the magnitude of intra-abdominal pressure changes with the speed of running.[5] Various factors such as total distance and experience of the runner may influence the intensity of these effects.

Measuring disc height changes during a 6-kilometer run, Neeley found an average loss of 3.2 mm, which increased to 8 mm during a 19-kilometer run. Skill and economy of running motion in experienced runners did not serve to attenuate the spinal loading, as the results were similar between experienced and inexperienced runners. Factors such as selection of appropriate running shoes, the running surface, the distance, and duration of exercise all influenced disc height change, i.e., spinal loading.[13]

Slocum and Bowerman[14] have shown that the position of the pelvis is the key to postural control in running. Therefore, any style of running, such as in a swayback posture, that places the pelvis in an anatomically undersirable position may cause concomitant stresses on the back. Improper running techniques, pelvis asymmetry from scoliosis of leg-length inequality, and increased lumbar lordosis from spondylolisthesis may cause episodes of back pain.

EVALUATION OF THE RUNNER

In the runner, information from the history is of particular clinical benefit in location of pain. Referred pain, particularly radicular pain, often requires more aggressive restriction than localized back complaints. On physical examination, one should note any restriction of range of motion in the spine and lower extremities; reflex, sensory, or motor changes; and signs of nerve root irritation. Leg-length discrepancies become more important in runners. Excessive pronation of one foot may lead to pelvic asymmetry. Length discrepancy in excess of 1 cm should be empirically treated.

Roentgenographic evaluation of the spine is usually of little help. According to Jackson, the incidence of degenerative changes in 71 asymptomatic marathoners was similar to that of the general population.[17] The presence of radiographic changes in the lumbar spine should not preclude the runner from unlimited mileage. Distance runners do not, as a rule, have secondary gains that may interfere with recovery, as is often the case in personal injury or industrial compensation cases. The psychological effects of not being able to run should seldom be inflicted on this patient, as temporary rest and restricted mileage may result in eventual return to unrestricted running.

Flexibility of the Runner

Hyperextension and cyclic loading in the lumbar spine occurs as the hind leg trails in the runner. Unparalleled in any other sport, repetitive hyperextension occurs when the low back moves from the flat-back position with foot strike to an extended lordosis as the trailing leg leaves the ground. Greater extension occurs with faster running.

Although structural changes such as scoliosis, facet tropism, and lumbarization of the vertebral segments usually do not cause back pain in the runner, altered flexibility or degenerative changes in association may result in pain. Asymmetric hamstring tightness may lead to gluteal or thigh pain.

Structural Changes

Spondylolysis, a defect in the pars interarticularis, occurs with an incidence of 5 to 10% in white male runners.[10] Most lumbar pars interarticularis defects develop during childhood and are unrelated to pain in the adult runner. However, localized vertebral instability or slippage (spondylolisthesis) may result in pain.

Runners with pars defects are often unaware of their spondylolisthesis until detected during radiographic examination. Following conservative treatment, most are able to return to running. Painful segmental instability may be aggravated by repetitive extension of the lumbar spine associated with running.

Lumbar Disc Disease

Since the cause of discogenic pain is unknown, most runners receive only symptomatic treatment. Back pain in association with sciatica pain suggests disc herniation. In a series of 1077 consecutive patients with running injuries, only 11 had sciatica.[16] All recovered without surgery and returned to running. Lumbar epidural steroid injection (Depo-Medrol), along with restricted mileage, flexion and extension exercises, and general resumption of running, has been successful in most athletes. In ten runners with acute sciatica from herniated discs, three required laminectomies; two of these resumed running. Overall, eight returned to running and one became a marathon bicyclist. Only one runner was unable to return to sports.[6]

Inflammatory Connective Tissue Disease

For completeness, brief mention should be made of ankylosing spondylitis and Reiter's syndrome. In young runners complaining of persistent sacroiliac pain, a positive bone scan and HLA B27 in association with dramatic response to anti-inflammatory medication should suggest the diagnosis of ankylosing spondylitis. Details of urethritis, conjunctivitis, other joint pain and mucous membrane changes suggest Reiter's syndrome. Treatment of these disorders is better left to the rheumatologist, with resumption of activity depending on the severity of illness and response to treatment.

REHABILITATION

One of the common causes of running injuries is a rapid change in speed, distance, or location. Fixx said that in a given week a runner should not increase his speed or distance by more than 10%.[2]

In treating the herniated lumbar disc, as in less severe ailments of the back, therapists must consider the runner's unwillingness to accept total rest and immobilization. Severe depression may result when the runner is placed at complete bedrest.[4] Controlled rest until the acute symptoms improve gives the runner encouragement for eventual full return to sports participation. Lumbar extension and flexion exercises (McKenzie and Williams) are introduced, supplemented by strengthening and endurance exercises, including aerobic and anaerobic protocols. Hydrotherapy is started early with swimming and light jogging in a pool.

Aspirin and nonsteroidal anti-inflammatory drugs (NSAIDs) are used to relieve acute symptoms. Under this program, narcotics and muscle relaxants are avoided because of their depressing side-effects. As mentioned before, persistent pain after 2 to 3 weeks may indicate the need for an epidural steroid injection, which usually produces rapid relief of pain in the herniated disc syndrome.

One to 2 weeks following subsidence of acute symptoms, nonrunning exercises such as prolonged walking, swimming, and biking may begin. Following this, impact-loading exercises such as indoor running, trampoline, or jumping rope are also permitted, as long as the patient does not land on both feet together. Six weeks into treatment, running on a nonpaved road or indoor track is permitted. A full running program is resumed at 3 months.

SUMMARY

Restrictive lumbar pain syndromes are uncommon in the runner. A temporary period of rest and mileage restriction during symptomatic back pain is the most effective treatment for lumbar spine problems. In the majority, satisfactory resolution and resumption of running occurs. Degenerative changes in the lumbar spine do not preclude one from running per se. However, pain from the repetitive hyperextension demands may preclude some individuals from running. Lumbar disc surgery is rarely performed in the runner, but, when undertaken, it does not necessarily preclude a return to the sport. Selective epidural steroid injection may, in certain instances, hasten recovery and prolong the years of participation in the sport.

Prevention of spinal symptoms in the runner is the goal. Proper stretching before and after running, and avoidance of rapid changes in speed or distance training are important measures. Smith[15] believed that the track athlete runs in a forced extension posture and that the extensor musculature is more developed than the flexor musculature. He felt that it was important for runners to strengthen the abdominal muscles and flatten the lordosis by pelvic tilts, curl-ups, and sit-ups. This concept is also shared by Fairbank, O'Brien, and Davis.[1] Abdominal musculature and hip flexor exercises remain the preferred treatment, although still controversial. Slow progression of training done in a painless fashion remains important if the body is to return to full function.

REFERENCES

1. Fairbank JC, O'Brien DP, Davis PR: Intraabdominal pressure and low back pain. Lancet i:1353, 1979.
2. Fixx J: The Complete Book of Running. New York, Random House, 1977.
3. Glick J, Katch V: Musculoskeletal injuries in jogging. Arch Phys Med Rehabil 51:123–126, 1970.
4. Greist EJ: Antidepressant running. Psychiatr Ann 9:23–30, 1900.
5. Grillner S, Nilsson J. Thorstensson A: Intra-abdominal pressure changes during natural movements in man. Acta Physiol Scand 103:275–283, 1978.
6. Guten G: Herniated lumbar disc associated with running: A review of 10 cases. Am J Sports Med 9:155, 1981.
7. Hersch C: The reaction of intervertebral discs to compressive forces. J Bone Joint Surg 27A:1188–1196, 1955.
8. Jackson DW, Pagliano J: The ultimate study of running injuries. Runners World Nov:42–50, 1980.
9. Jackson DW, Rettig A, Wiltse LL: Epidural cortisone injection in the young athletic adult. Am J Sports Med 8:239, 1980.

10. Jackson DW, Wiltse LL: Sub-roentgenographic stress renetions of the posterior elements in young athletes. Am J Sports Med 9:304, 1981.
11. Lees A, McCullagh PJ: A preliminary investigation into the shock absorbency of running shoes and shoe inserts. J Human Mov Studies 10:95–106, 1984.
12. Nachemson AL: The lumbar spine: An orthopedic challenge. Spine 1:1, 1976.
13. Reilly T, Leatt D, Troup JGD: Spinal loading during circuit weight training and running. Br J Sports Med 20(3):119–124, 1986.
14. Slocum DB, Bowerman W: Biomechanics of running. Clin Orthop 23:39–45, 1962.
15. Smith C: Physical management of muscular low back pain in the athlete. Can Med Assoc J 117:632, 1977.
16. Sutker A, Jackson DW: Low back problems in runners. Chapter 15. In AAOS Symposium on the Foot and Leg in Running Sports. St. Louis, CV Mosby, 1983.
17. Sutker A, Jackson DW: Roentgenographic changes in the lumbar spine in marathon runners (publication pending).

Chapter 12

THE SPINE AND SWIMMING

Stanley V. Paris, PhD, PT

At first thought, one should not suspect that there is enough trauma in swimming to inflict sufficient disability on the spine to interfere with performance and create disabling pain. Swimming does, however, represent hours of training with the spine not only moving into end-range positions but doing so repeatedly. Runners can change style, cyclists can adjust their seating and handle bar position, but swimmers, once their stroke is developed, stay in a consistent pattern of motion over and over again. The spine is, on the one hand, the passive link between the powerhouses of the legs and more especially the arms, but by its contortions it is also the engine that places the limbs in a position to maximally achieve their power. It is the spine that both drives and is driven. Stress fatigue focused in three major areas, i.e., the base of the neck, the low back, and the thoracolumbar junction, is the result. Each of these three areas is known as a transitional zone in the spine, for each represents a juncture between a very mobile section of the spine and one that is less mobile.

Swimming has been considered good therapy for all injured athletes. This assumption must be questioned in view of the specificity of training in sports and the opportunity to further aggravate an injury from an improper pool activity, which is, after all, an alien training environment to most athletes.

THE STRESSES OF SWIMMING

In achieving the preferred reach of the arms or position of the head and trunk, the swimmer thrusts the limbs and spine in and out of a number of end-range positions. The sites of such actions may become the sites of stress and strain that lead from overuse to dysfunction, discomfort, and disabling pain. Examples include forcing the neck backwards for a quick breath, as in breaststroke, or thrusting the low back into hyperlordosis, as in butterfly. It is the repetitive nature of these events—hours a day in training—that takes a toll. By the time symptoms occur in these otherwise fit individuals, the dysfunction/injury is well on the way and immediate attention is required. I term the problems that develop "dysfunctions" rather than injuries, for the term injury implies a single traumatic event, whereas in swimming such is rarely the case. Swimmers suffer from the effects of repetitive motion, i.e., fatigue failure or stress failure of structures placed in repetitive stress.

Stress Dysfunction—Overuse Syndrome

When a metallic structure undergoes repetitive stress, it will fatigue and fracture after so many cycles. Biological tissues are very different. While on the one hand they undergo stress and are prone to fatigue failure, they do have the ability of adapting and of becoming stronger. This property enables muscles, ligaments, and joint capsules to strengthen from moderate and carefully graduated stress. But if training is too hard and too often, especially if suddenly the mileage and/or duration of training is increased, then the risk of overloading the body's ability to adapt to the stress of training rises. Instead of gaining tissue strength, the body fails to recover from the accumulating fatigue, which may then lead to tissue failure. In runners, the stress fracture is a classic example. Swimmers, although not likely to develop stress fractures, do develop stress failure in the joints and ligaments. Swimmers perform toward the end-of-range, whereas runners stay more toward mid-range.

An interesting observation concerning overuse injuries, and even minor strains sustained during an activity, is that they do not hurt at the time. The reason is quite simple to understand: there is just too much else going on. Physical exercise generates a great deal of sensory input to the central nervous system sufficient to block or gate nociception.

AREAS OF OVERUSE STRAIN—THE TRANSITIONAL ZONES

Some of the recommendations that follow, those having to do with suggested stroke and style changes, may not please the swimmer. However the changes need not be permanent, just sufficient to allow adaptation to take place.

Lower Neck (Cervicothoracic Junction)

Perhaps the most vulnerable area of the swimmer's spine is at the junction of the mobile neck with the relatively inflexible thoracic spine.

The breaststroker holding the neck in extension may experience painful cramps. Stretching of the posterior neck muscles (Fig. 1) and strengthening of the anterior neck muscles will give better control over this area (Fig. 2).

The crawl swimmer can usually avoid injury if the neck is kept forward, with the top of the skull to the water rather than the forehead. Keeping the neck forward and rolling with the body as a means of getting air, rather than jerking the head in rotation, inflicts less stress on the neck. Distance swimmers tend to roll the trunk on its long axis, stabilizing with a lateral drift of the contralateral leg, thus controlling neck rotation. Excessive and repeated neck rotation may lead to localized hypermobility and the formation of osteophytes.

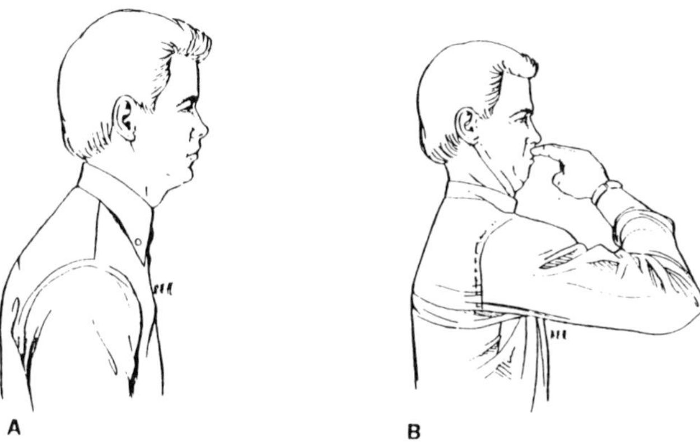

FIGURE 1. **Stretching the posterior neck muscles** is achieved by placing the two middle fingers on the top lip (*B*) and pushing back while keeping the head level. This is also known as axial extension. The movement should be continued until it is felt to take place in the mid-thoracic spine.

In all strokes, the recovery phase places an increased load on the neck. As the arms are thrust forward in breaststroke and thrown overhead in butterfly or in crawl, it is the levators and trapezii pulling down on the neck that initiate the motion. The crawl swimmer can lessen this stress if, just before the hand exits the water for the recovery, it is thrust back and up to create momentum, and then swung in a wider circle during the recovery.

The butterfly swimmer can vary the stress by varying the position of the head during the recovery. The breaststroker is not able to do much to change style, as his or her breathing technique is the most critical. Backstrokers should take additional care to see that the overhead line is in place when training so that they know when to turn and do not have to twist awkwardly to see the end of the pool.

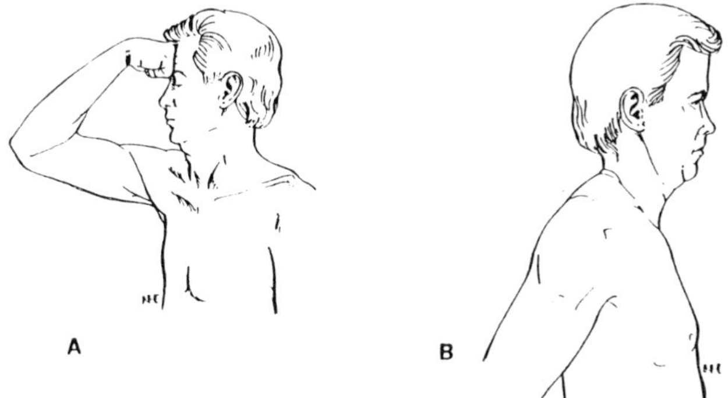

FIGURE 2. **Strengthening the anterior neck muscles:** This is an isometric exercise that is performed with the head in various degrees of rotation in order to bring in all the muscles, both anterior and lateral (*A* and *B*). The resistance is firm and the effort is not to be too forceful. The exercise has the added benefit of inducing reflex relaxation of the posterior neck muscles.

Midback (Thoracolumbar Junction)

Potentially the most painful site, especially in the distance crawl swimmer, is the thoracolumbar spine. This area is at the crossroads of the actions from the arms, which tend to side-bend the upper back, and the restraints of the pelvis, held rather steady by the driving legs. In the butterfly swimmer, the change in the direction of the facets from sagittal in the lumbar to coronal in the thoracic severely limits the ability of the thoracic spine to take the extension movement. It is at this first level of coronal facets that extension stress is most evident. Although pain can be quite acute in this region, signifying a strain, a more insidious onset of instability may give rise to referred pain over the iliac crest and lateral thigh, and thus its origin may go undetected. Clinically, tenderness elicited over the iliac crest, hypersensitivity over the hip, and tenderness with muscle guarding at the thoracolumbar junction suggest this syndrome. Treatment consists of stabilization exercises (Fig. 3). Interestingly, this same syndrome sometimes develops in individuals that have had a one- or two-level spine fusion, who may additionally experience sudden giving-way of the leg.

If the swimmer is a breaststroker, the thoracolumbar junction is more likely to develop a compressive strain of the posterior facets, which commonly leads to muscle guarding (spasm), which again increases the load. Breaststrokers might be better advised to do flexion activities along the lines of the Williams flexion routine (Fig. 4).

Lumbar and Lumbosacral Spine

This area is a common site for back pain in swimmers, owing perhaps to activities outside of swimming. Swimmers develop a great deal of upper body

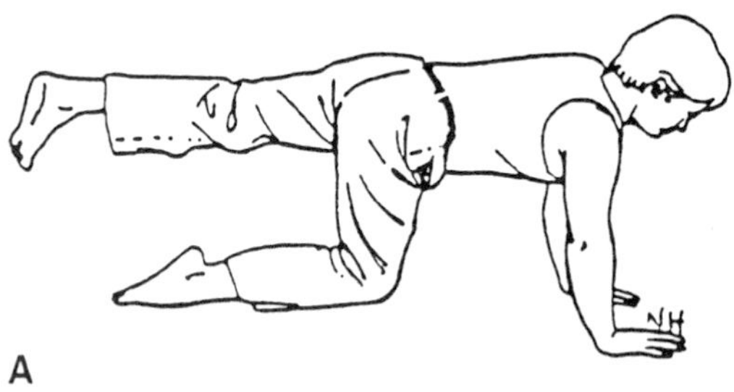

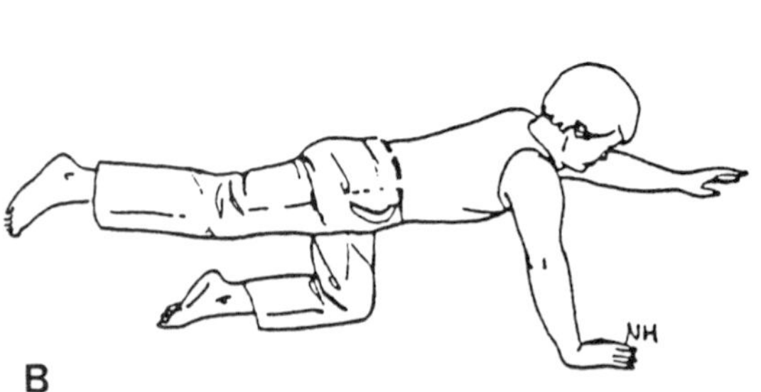

FIGURE 3. **Stabilization for the Lumbar and Thoracic Spines:** In this exercise, first the legs are raised one at a time (*A*), and then together with opposite arms (*B*). It is important not to increase the lumbar lordosis, as such a range of motion appears to bring in the erector spinae and reduce the activity of the more segmentally related, such as the stabilizing multifidus.

FIGURE 4. **Stretching the low back muscles** can be achieved without unduly stressing the lumbar spine by drawing first alternate (*A*) and then both (*B*) knees to the chest. The position should be held for a few seconds to derive maximum benefit.

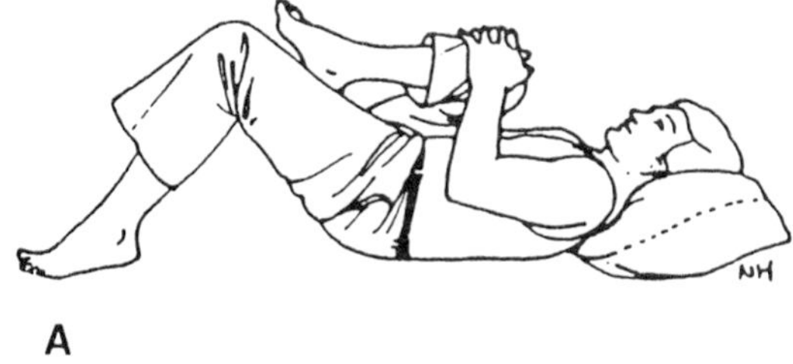

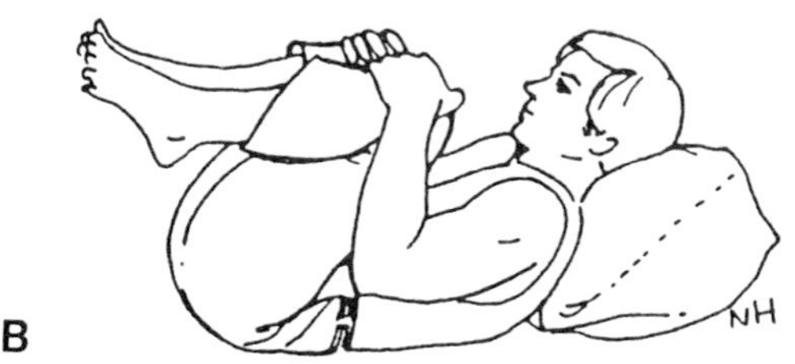

strength, since the principal effort is with the arms. During training the exercise role of the low back is more passive than active. As a result, swimmers, in common with upper-trunk bodybuilders, are able to lift and wrestle with objects that their backs are poorly prepared to handle. The result may be an injury to the low back.

The best treatment is physical therapy, including modalities to help resolve the injury, but in particular exercises to strengthen the lumbar spine.

Thoracic Outlet

The thoracic outlet is in many respects an extension of the spine. The nerves must exit between the scaleni, which attach from the cervical vertebrae to the ribs, and then, in common with the vascular structures, pass over the first rib to go under the subclavius and the pectorals. Aggravation of the neurovascular structures here with or without concomitant cervical dysfunction may make the subject aware of neck and arm pains.

Thoracic outlet syndrome in the case of the swimmer is usually from dynamic factors such as hypertrophy of scaleni and, in particular, the subclavius. But it can also be static, i.e., postural, especially in breaststroke and butterfly swimmers, who tend to develop an imbalance between the anterior chest muscles and the weaker back muscles. The result is a slouch or forward head. This posture, increasing as it does the cervical lordosis, narrows the intervertebral foramen, drops the clavicle with the subclavius muscle towards the first rib, and perhaps allows for adaptive shortening of the pectorals and clavipectoral fascia. In addition, the swimmer tends to have an elevated first rib owing to the unique manner in which he or she breaths—a sudden gasp in using the accessory muscle of respiration.

The swimmer's first experience of thoracic outlet problems may be tingling in the hands early in the season, most notably the little finger. Then, during swimming, the little finger abducts away from the others and seems uncontrollable and weak. If the condition is not attended to at this stage, then semipermanent weakness lasting months may follow. Physical therapy to stretch the muscle and attend to the first rib is called for. If treatment is not available or ineffective, then the swimmer should cut back on training by, say, 50% for 2 weeks. After 2 weeks, the individual should pick up the distance slowly, and most likely the symptoms will not return—presumably because of providing time for the blood vessels to undergo adaptation to the increased loads.

The clinician should examine for the length of all muscles, particularly the scaleni, the pectoralis major and minor, and as best as is possible the subclavius. Tight muscles are best stretched with neuromuscular facilitation techniques. Quick stretches only induce a sharp contraction to protect the muscle spindles, which in turn may further tighten the muscles.

SYMPTOM OF OVERUSE AND BASIC MANAGEMENT

There are three stages of overuse that the responsible athlete should commit to memory. Most serious swimming dysfunctions are preventable provided the swimmer is alert to their early signs and symptoms and takes preventive measures. Prevention here is worth a great deal more than treatment.

Stage One: Minimal Overuse

Symptom: Joint discomfort comes some time *after the activity* and is gone within a few hours.

Management: This is the first warning of matters not being quite right. Give thought to some of the suggestions set out below (see "Avoidance of Overuse Injuries"). Also, have a knowledgeable coach check stroke and style. Perhaps it is time for some subtle changes and improvements that will in turn change the stress to the body.

Physical therapy with heat and/or ice plus massage makes very good sense to rid the area of fatigue and waste products.

Stage Two: Moderate Overuse

Symptom: Discomfort comes on *during the activity* and may last for a full day after the activity.

Management: This might be the stage when the swimmer first seeks medical or physical therapy advise. The problem must be addressed immediately, for if changes are not made, these conditions rapidly progress to disabling pain and altered muscle function. Rest from the activities that stress the area must be undertaken. Pushing on at this stage may cause serious injury. Physical therapy consists of heat and/or ice, massage, and ultrasound to the injured site.

Perhaps if a competitive event is a day or two away, medications, ice, and massage may enable participation without too much additional damage.

Stage Three: Severe Overuse

Symptom: Discomfort and pain are now virtually constant, and although they may change in nature during the activity, they are present practically all of the time. An overuse dysfunction has been changed into a major injury.

Management: A change of attitude is necessary, for the behavior that led to this stage is inexcusable in an intelligent and well-informed individual.

Therapy is made up of rest and modalities, with appropriate retraining by resistive exercises once the subacute stage has been reached. But participation in the activity that caused it should be discontinued for a good 3 to 4 weeks. Try running or cycling to maintain cardiovascular fitness.

Avoidance of Overuse Injuries—Advice to Swimmers

The following is advice that may be given to the swimmer and is written in that style.

The key to avoidance of injuries is to be actively involved in their prevention. Athletes must not think of pain as a reward or warning, rather they should think of pain as saying, "Dummy, you overdid it."

1. **Have a sound stroke,** one that is gentle on the body. Training may involve from 3 to 6 hours a day, and if you attempt the "Channel," you may be there for up to 14 hours. Of course, speed is important in all events, but speed can be achieved without undue stress. Stress your muscles but not your joints.

2. **Don't do anything that hurts.** In the "jock" world of bodybuilding, there has arisen a most unfortunate expression, namely "no pain—no gain." In other words unless the activity hurts, you are not going to benefit. While this may be true in building up muscle bulk to look good or be a power lifter, and it may be part of the hype that goes with football, it is not true in virtually any other sport and most certainly not in the swimmer. It is all right to feel a little fatigued after a swim. It is a good feeling of having worked out. It is healthy for muscles to ache after effort. But let us call that the discomfort or ache of effort and learn how to distinguish that from the pain of over-fatigue or injury.

3. **Resist the temptation to do the occasional sprint when already fatigued.** Trained athletes swim with power and grace. As they fatigue, subtle changes in stroke and motion occur. These changes, caused by fatigue, bring in muscles that are less strong and less trained. The joints are thus not stabilized sufficiently, and joint structures become vulnerable to injury. In racing, sprints are done after a rest. The same should be true when training.

4. **Increase duration and/or mileage gradually.** The body's muscles, joints, and bones take time to train up to full strength and capacity. Use the stimulus of long-distance swimming to help create more muscle bulk and tendon strength and an adequate circulation to the muscle.

5. **Take periods of rest, particularly after increases in distance.** In marathon swimming, one long swim every 2 weeks with the time in between spent getting ready for the next long swim makes the best sense. For most swimmers, training hard every day may not be the wisest method. Two days off once a week or minimal activities on those days is best. Better still is to alternate 3 hard days with 1 easy day in between, and then to rest for 2 days. It is a good approach both mentally and physically, especially for distance swimmers.

6. **Quit when you hit the wall.** In a long day of training, you may run out of muscle energy, which is derived from the glycogens stored in the muscles. Should that happen, then you are not yet ready for sustained training, are not eating right, or are just having a bad day. Back off from becoming fatigued, since it is bad for your stroke and may cause injury.

7. **Do preventive exercises** that help avoid overuse by providing for muscle balance. A physical therapist is well prepared to evaluate muscle function and balance. If he or she also understands swimming, then he or she will be able to assist in preventive routines that help balance out your muscles, loosen tightened structures, and help avoid impingement syndromes, such as swimmer's shoulder.

8. **Remember your old injuries.** By remembering an old injury and especially those activities that either caused or aggravated the injury, it is possible to avoid those actions that caused it.

Proper Warm-up. This should be of a gentle nature, concentrating on shaking and mild stretching of the limbs. A little light jogging on the spot and deep breathing to get the heart and lungs under way is also advisable for the sprinter.

IS SWIMMING GOOD FOR BACK PAIN?

Swimming is all too often recommended as a therapeutic exercise for nonathletes and for athletes. Although swimming is a good form of exercise, it is often a mistake to recommend it as a therapeutic exercise. Most think of swimming as a gentle and peaceful activity, during which the weight of the body is fully supported and cushioned by warm and soft water. In truth the circumstances can be very different and must be carefully matched to the patient.

For the nonathlete, particularly the middle-aged and elderly, the typical community pool is a safety hazard, and the patient should be alerted to its risks, such as children running, slippery surfaces, difficult entrances and exits from the water, and always the possibility of collisions, being jumped on (especially if straying under the diving board), or being nearly drowned if the depth suddenly changes. Then assess the patient's swimming stroke, which may not be smooth and gentle, rather, it may more closely resemble a struggle for survival. So before prescribing swimming, think of environment and the individual's ability. Therapeutic swimming classes would of course be different if conducted by a properly qualified individual. Surf swimming should not be recommended for other than strong and fit swimmers. It is just too easy to be dumped, rolled, twisted, and injured.

For the athlete with back problems, walking in a swimming pool is a sound activity. However, the moment the athlete begins swimming, then many of the concerns expressed in the preceding paragraph may apply. Since swimmers can also have problems in the transitional regions of the spine, any athlete with a problem of a similar nature would gain little if at all from swimming.

Swimming is widely thought of as a good activity to maintain fitness while laying off from another activity due to injury. But this also may not be valid. Fit runners, distance or sprinters, have all experienced the rapid breathlessness that follows even a short unaccustomed swim. The breathing technique and muscles used are so different from those in other sports that one must question the value of swimming to maintain cardiovascular fitness or sports fitness. For the runner, either brisk walking or stationary cycling would appear to be better activities.

Perhaps swimming has been presented too negatively in this section, but then one needs to emphasize the importance of questioning when one should prescribe swimming for spinal problems because of possible negative effects.

CONCLUSION

Swimmers do not experience the impact injuries typical of contact sports. Nor do they tear and rupture muscles as in track and field. Instead they suffer from overuse injuries, most commonly of the spine and shoulders. Since overuse comes on gradually, an awareness of the signs and symptoms can prevent serious disability.

Chapter 13

CONSIDERATIONS IN CYCLING FOR PERSONS WITH LOW BACK PAIN

Chris G. Sheets, BS, and Stephen H. Hochschuler, MD

Cycling is considered to be an effective form of low-impact aerobic activity. In recent years the sport of cycling has become increasingly more popular. In 1980, 27% of the adult population cycled at least once a week.[15] Along with the expanded enthusiasm for cycling has come a preponderance of cycling injuries. These are primarily soft tissue injuries associated with the face, head, wrist, knee, ankle, and foot. However, back injuries are also encountered.[3]

It has been suggested that an adequate level of cardiovascular fitness is associated with a decreased risk and/or extent of back injuries.[4] Since the motion of cycling is low-impact in nature, stationary cycling can be effectively and safely used by many back patients to increase their level of cardiovascular functioning. Even though stationary cycling is generally accepted as a safe activity for back patients, the question remains whether road cycling (recreational and/or competitive) can be safely performed by the patient who has suffered a spine injury. In addition, the problem of back pain and cycling in the uninjured individual needs to be explored and possible solutions postulated.

For these questions to be effectively answered, a number of factors need to be considered. First, an understanding of proper bicycle fit for the cyclist is needed. Second, what, if any, preventive measures can be practiced in order to lessen the risk of injury to the spine while cycling? Finally, what measures can be taken to diminish the amount of stress placed on spinal structures for someone who has already suffered a spinal injury?

PROPER BICYCLE FIT

Many types of bicycles now exist. Some of the most popular types include racing, touring, and all-terrain or mountain bikes. Whatever the type of bicycle, it can be simplified into two general parts, the frame and the components. These two parts are then combined in order to provide proper fit of the rider to the bike. It is imperative for anyone dealing with cycling injuries to have a good understanding of proper bike fit, since many injuries may be directly due to improper fit. For the normal, uninjured cycling participant, a number of standardized guidelines exist that describe the proper set-up of a racing or touring bicycle. There are five basic adjustments that should be considered when fitting a bike to a rider. These include the frame size, seat height, seat position, and handlebar height and reach.[11]

When considering the frame, it is important to realize the differences in the types of material that are used to make the frame. Today's models of bicycles are made from a variety of materials, including chromium-magnesium alloys, aluminum, and carbon fiber compositions. These types of frames are much lighter than those in older generation bikes; they are also stronger and provide better handling. It should also be kept in mind that the different materials used to make the frames are likely to have different shock absorption capabilities, which is an important consideration for people who have suffered a back injury. Whatever type of frame used, the size should be such that there is a 1 to 2 inch clearance between the rider's crotch and the top tube of the bicycle (Fig. 1A).[11]

Seat or saddle height is most commonly defined as the distance from the top of the seat to the center of the axis of the pedal spindle, as measured in a straight line along the seat tube and the crank.[7] As a simple rule of thumb, a seat height that allows slight knee flexion of 10 to 15 degrees with the pedal in the 6 o'clock position is generally recommended (Fig. 1B).[7] To be more specific, physiologic data have been analyzed in two areas. One is the seat height at which the least amount of oxygen will be consumed for a given power output, termed mechanical efficiency. Nordeen-Snyder concluded that the seat height that requires the least amount of oxygen is at a level of 107% of the pubic-symphysis height.[14] However, caution should be used when generalizing this finding, since the subjects were all female and pedaled at a relatively low cadence of 60 rpm. On the other hand, Hamely and Thomas concluded that the saddle height resulting in the greatest short-term power outputs is 109% of the pubic-symphysis height.[10] However, it should be remembered that there is probably no optimal seat height for all riders and probably the best way to maximize performance is to use the above figures as guidelines and then to make small incremental changes in order to find the most comfortable position. It is also important to realize that any adjustment in seat height will change the stress being placed on the lower extremity muscles.[9] EMG studies have been performed to illustrate this point. Increasing the saddle height has been shown to activate the leg muscles sooner and lengthen the time of contraction; however, the magnitude of the forces produced does not change.[5]

Seat position is determined by placing the pedals in the 3 and 9 o'clock positions with the balls of the feet centered on the pedal spindle (Fig. 1C). From this position, a plumb line dropped from the anterior aspect of the patella of the forward knee should intersect the pedal spindle. If it does not, then the seat should be moved either forward or backward until this position is obtained.[11] If

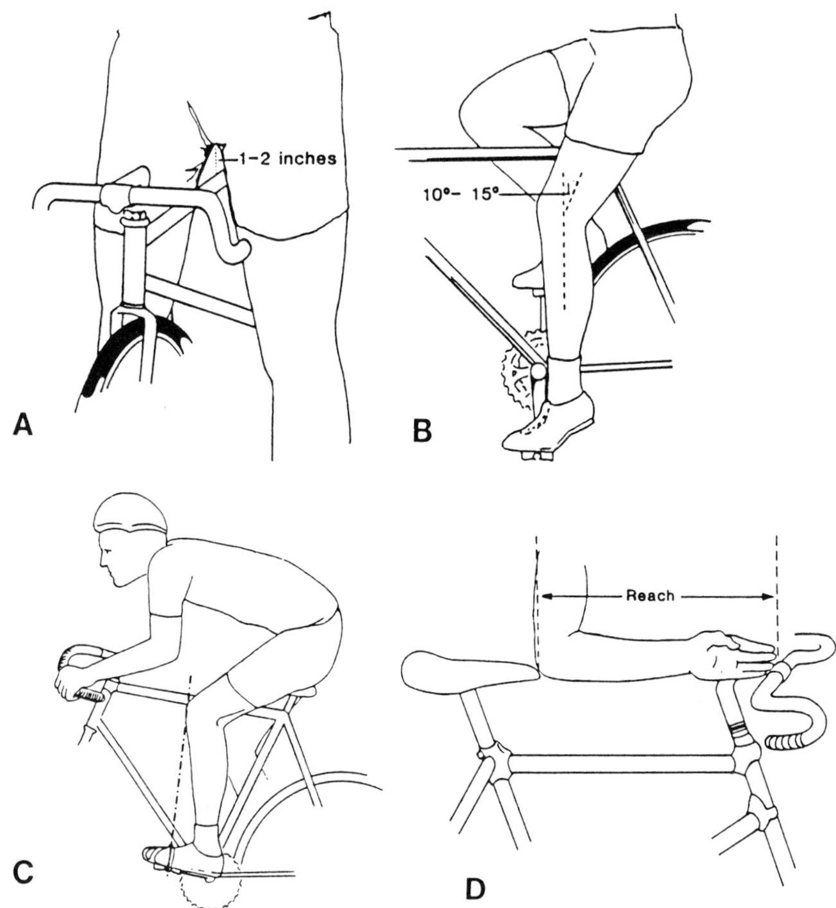

FIGURE 1. *A,* Proper frame size, with 1–2 inches between crotch and top frame tube; *B,* determination of seat height; *C,* seat position relative to the pedals; *D,* determination of proper reach. (From Mellon MB: Office Management of Sports Injuries and Athletic Problems. Philadelphia, Hanley & Belfus, Inc., 1988, with permission.)

the position cannot be obtained in this way, then the crank length may need to be altered. The seat should also be positioned such that it is parallel to the top tube or very slightly angled upward.[11]

The handlebar height should be adjusted so the handlebars are level with or just below the top of the seat. Handlebar reach is the distance from the front tip of the saddle to the horizontal portion of the handlebars. The correct reach can be determined by placing the elbow against the front tip of the seat and extending the arm toward the handlebars (Fig. 1D). Once the forearm is in this position, the extended fingers should just touch the handlebars. If this distance is incorrect, the necessary adjustments may be made by replacing the stem with one that has the proper reach.[11]

PREVENTION OF BACK DISCOMFORT AND PAIN

At this point it should be realized that the proper set-up of the bike is intended to reduce biomechanical stress on the lower body and to maximize performance. For some, these two goals may be realized, but the riders may still experience pain and discomfort of the back. Bohlmann found that out of 20 competitive cyclists, 10% experienced lower back discomfort and pain and another 10% also experienced neck discomfort and pain.[3] In addition, when reviewing 15 cycling accidents, there was one fracture to the coccyx. Therefore, even for these elite cyclists, it can be seen that cycling may affect certain spinal structures. For recreational cyclists these problems may be even more prevalent, since their overall physical condition is doubtless lower. To the knowledge of these authors, no experimental evidence exists that demonstrates any physiologic reasons for increased back pain in direct relation to cycling. However, there are several possible mechanisms for back pain other than direct trauma to this area.

Even if the bike is properly fit using the guidelines outlined above, the positioning of the spine may contribute to increased pain and discomfort of the lumbar region. When a proper riding position is achieved on a racing-style bike, the lumbar region of the spine is in a constant state of flexion. This flexed position is further exaggerated by the use of aero-bars, which enhance the aerodynamics of the rider by enabling the cyclist to assume a tighter tucked position, thus increasing the amount of hip and lumbar flexion. For the spine to be in this position for an extended period of time may cause pain. One source of this pain may be a result of muscular fatigue and/or spasm. However, Houtz and Fischer found that electrical activity of the rectus abdominis and the sacrospinalis muscle was minimal.[12] Desipres also found the electrical activity of the rectus abdominis and the erector spinae to be minimal and variable.[5] On the surface, this would seem to discount lower back pain being due to muscle fatigue, but Houtz and Fischer's subjects were in a fairly upright posture when cycling on a stationary ergometer, and therefore their result would likely be somewhat different if a more traditional racing or touring posture were to be analyzed. In addition, they also stated that when higher workloads were used, the subjects tended to rotate the trunk toward the side of the extremity that was in flexion. Therefore, it is reasonable to assume that increased muscular activity would be necessary for this rotation to occur, which could possibly lead to muscular fatigue at higher workloads. If this is the case, simply using a higher cadence and lower gear ratio may be beneficial. The seat height may also play a role, since a seat that is adjusted too high may cause excessive pelvic rocking, which may lead to increased muscular activity, thus contributing to muscular fatigue.

The cyclist may also experience cervical spine pain. If a normal touring or racing position is maintained, hyperextension of the cervical region is necessary in order for the cyclist to see the road ahead. Cervical hyperextension is further exaggerated if the handlebar drops are used, and even further exaggerated if the new aero-style bars are used. Pain in the cervical region may be due to fatigue of the upper back and neck musculature responsible for cervical extension. In addition, the amount of force the muscles need to exert in this region may be diminished by using a light-weight helmet, thus resulting in less muscular fatigue.

Another possible source of muscular pain in the cervical region may be too much weight being focused on the hands, which then transmit excessive loads to the musculature of the shoulders and upper back. This can occur if the handlebar height in relation to the top of the saddle is too low. The handlebars would simply need to be raised to the proper height to counteract this problem.[11] The cyclist should also concentrate on riding with the elbows slightly flexed, which acts to absorb road shock.

It is important to realize that the types of muscle contractions responsible for holding the cervical and lumbar regions in position are isometric. Isometric contractions restrict blood flow to the area of contraction, thus leading to an ischemic response that may cause muscular spasm and therefore increased pain. In addition, metabolic waste products may also accumulate in the muscles and lead to pain. Periodic dynamic contractions of both the lumbar and cervical musculature when riding should enhance blood flow to these areas, which may result in increased removal of waste products and decreased pain, spasm, and fatigue.

Disc pain may also exist in the uninjured cyclist. Since the adult disc is for the most part avascular, movement of the dynamic segment is relied on to enhance blood supply by diffusion across the endplate. If this movement is not present, the necessary nutrients cannot enter the disc and metabolic wastes cannot leave it. This in itself may cause pain, and again simple movement of the motion segments may remedy the situation.

For the uninjured rider the aforementioned will likely be the extent of the cyclist's complaints. The likelihood of the above problems occurring may be decreased if preventive measures such as stretching, resistive training, and progressive aerobic conditioning are initiated prior to strenuous cycling. Stretching should involve all major muscle groups of the body, but it should concentrate on the lower extremities and trunk muscles. The purpose of the stretching program is to obtain normal range of motion in all joints of the body (see pp. 38–41). Specific to the spine, the muscles and ligaments of the posterior lumbar region must have adequate flexibility to obtain the forward-flexed position used in touring or racing. If flexibility in this region is insufficient, undue stress will be placed on these structures, which can lead to injury and/or increased pain.

Flexibility of the hamstring muscles can also play a role in lumbar posture through the strong ligamentous attachment of the pelvis and sacrum. The same holds true for the hip flexors, which not only affect lumbar posture through the sacroiliac joint but also by direct attachment of the psoas major to the lumbar spine. Since cycling is not a full range of motion activity for these muscle groups, it is very important that they be stretched regularly to inhibit their shortening, which can lead to poor lumbar positioning, thereby placing stress on spinal structures and leading to increased pain.

Resistive training of leg muscles directly involved with cycling is obviously important to maximize performance. However, the postural muscles of the lumbar and cervical region should also be trained for endurance so they will be able to maintain proper trunk position for an extended period of time. This may be best obtained by working at the endurance end of the so-called strength continuum, which would indicate the use of high repetitions and low resistance.[8] It is not within the scope of this paper to outline a weight-training protocol specific to cycling; those interested are referred to Zappe and Bauer.[18]

Progressive aerobic conditioning cannot be stressed enough. If the intensity or duration is increased too quickly, the risk of injury will be greater. The musculoskeletal system needs adequate time for adaptive processes to occur, and if this time is not allowed, injury will more than likely result. For the novice interested in using cycling as a form of exercise, it would be wise to develop an aerobic base with the use of a stationary cycle. This will provide not only cardiovascular conditioning but training of the musculoskeletal system for the movement of cycling. However, the proprioceptive elements necessary for balancing will not be developed. After several months of conditioning on a stationary cycle to establish an appropriate cardiovascular and musculoskeletal base, road cycling can be initiated. Once road cycling is initiated, a low-to-moderate intensity level should be used and duration should be increased progressively to a point that depends on the goals of each individual. Once duration is adequate, intensity should then be progressively increased. Individuals with more competitive ambitions are referred to a chapter by Wells and Pete that outlines a cycling program of a more competitive nature.[16]

CYCLING FOR BACK PATIENTS

Cycling for the apparently healthy is considered to be a fairly safe form of cardiovascular exercise, since it is a low-impact, non-weight-bearing activity. However, for the individual who has had a history of back pain or surgery, a different picture may need to be presented. For those individuals who have suffered from lumbar, cervical, and/or thoracic syndromes, following the above conservative guidelines will prove beneficial. Those individuals who have been diagnosed as having a herniated nucleus pulposus (HNP), spinal canal stenosis, bulging disc, or facet degeneration, or for those individuals who have undergone spinal fusions, special considerations should be addressed.

The patient who has been diagnosed as having an HNP will need to be cautious of riding position. It has been well documented that with flexion in both sitting and standing postures, intradiscal pressure is increased.[2] In addition, one of the most common sites of disc herniation is on the posterior aspect of lumbar discs. Therefore, lumbar flexion as in a traditional touring or racing position may actually be a contraindication in this instance. To avoid this position, it may be necessary to switch to a different style of bike such as a mountain bike. The frame angles and handlebar positioning will allow most individuals to sit in a more upright position, which may relieve disc pressure to some extent. An added benefit of a mountain bike for such individuals may be the dampening of vibration. Vibration, especially in the seated position, has been postulated to worsen disc disruption and therefore may be contraindicated for an individual with HNP.[6] On a road or racing bike, the tires are usually high-pressure tires that do not absorb shock very well. In addition, these cycles are normally designed to handle very responsively, which is beneficial for cornering but also results in a rougher ride. On the other hand, a mountain bike has larger tires that tend to absorb shock better, and the frame design allows for a softer ride. Another possible aid in dampening vibratory effects would be to use a silicone seat cover, which dissipates vibratory stress from the cycle to the cyclist.

The above information, which applies to HNP, also holds true for a disc bulge, since in both instances fissures have somehow developed in annular cartilage, and any position or movement that puts excessive strain on the annulus will probably not be well tolerated in terms of pain. In addition, these situations may also cause further damage to the disc.

Spinal canal stenosis is accepted as a decrease in the ratio between the bony canal and its neural contents.[13] Whatever the cause for the decreased reserve capacity of the spine, it may be beneficial to obtain a flexed position. This type of position tends to open the canal space, thus reducing pressure on the neural contents.[13,17] Therefore, the flexed lumbar position in a racing or touring position may be beneficial, but remember this same position increases the amount of extension in the cervical region and therefore may be contraindicated. If spinal canal stenosis is occurring in the cervical region, it may be of benefit to raise the handlebars to obtain a more upright riding posture or it may be necessary to switch to a mountain-style bike.

For some individuals the degeneration of facet joints may be a source of low back pain. The flexed position of the lumbar region during cycling may actually alleviate pain, since stress on the facet joints is reduced when this position is obtained.[1] On the other hand, if the problem exists in the cervical region, relief may be realized if a more upright riding posture is assumed.

Cycling, due to its relatively non-impact nature, should generally be a safe aerobic activity for the uninjured individual. For those who have had a back injury, simple modifications of the bicycle may be necessary in order to minimize back discomfort. Adequate stretching, muscular strength and endurance, and an established base of cardiovascular endurance are recommended before strenuous road cycling is undertaken. Further research is needed to determine the specific role of the trunk extensors and flexors during cycling. In addition, stresses that are placed on spinal structures such as discs and ligaments during cycling in different positions need to be determined.

REFERENCES

1. Adams MA, Hutton WC: The effect of posture on the role of the apophysial joints in resisting intervertebral compressive forces. J Bone Joint Surg 62B:358–362, 1980.
2. Andersson GB, Ortengren R, Nachemson A: Intradiskal pressure, intra-abdominal pressure and myoelectric back muscle activity related to posture and loading. Clin Orthop 129:156–164, 1977.
3. Bohlmann TJ: Injuries in competitive cycling. Phys Sportsmed 9(5):117–124, 1981.
4. Cady LD, Bischoff DP, O'Connell ER, et al: Strength and fitness and subsequent back injuries in fire fighters. J Occup Med 21:269, 1979.
5. Desipres M: An electromyographic study of competitive road cycling conditions simulated on a treadmill. In Nelson R, Morehouse C (eds): Biomechanics IV. International Series on Biomechanics. Baltimore, University Park Press, 1974, pp 349–355.
6. Dupius H: Biodynamic behavior of the trunk and the abdomen during whole-body vibration. Acta Anaesthesiol Scand 30(suppl 90):34–38, 1989.
7. Ericson M: On the biomechanics of cycling. Scand J Rehab Med Suppl 16, 1986.
8. Fleck SJ, Kraemer WJ: Designing Resistance Training Programs. Champaign, IL, Human Kinetics Publishers, 1987.
9. Gregor RJ, Rugg SG: Effects of saddle height and pedaling cadence on power output and efficiency. In Burke ER (ed): Science and Cycling. Champaign, IL, Human Kinetics Publishers, 1986, pp 69–90.
10. Hamely EJ, Thomas V: Physiologic and postural factors in the calibration of the bicycle ergometer. J Physiol 191:55, 1967.
11. Hill JW, Mellion MB: Bicycle injuries: Prevention, diagnosis, and treatment. In Mellion MB (ed): Sports Injuries and Athletic Problems. Philadelphia, Hanley & Belfus, 1988, pp 257–269.
12. Houtz SJ, Fischer FJ: An analysis of muscle joint excursion during exercise on a stationary bicycle. J Bone Joint Surg 41A:123, 1959.
13. Liyang D, Yinkan X, Wenming Z, Zhihua Z: The effect of flexion-extension motion of the lumbar spine on the capacity of the spinal canal. Spine 14:523–525, 1989.
14. Nordeen-Snyder KS: The effect of bicycle seat height variation upon oxygen consumption and lower limb kinematics. Med Sci Sports 2:113, 1979.
15. Powell B: Correction and prevention of bicycle saddle problems. Phys Sportsmed 10:60–67, 1982.
16. Wells CL, Pate RR: Training for the performance of prolonged exercise. In Lamb R, Murray R (eds): Perspectives in Exercise Science and Sports Medicine, Vol. 1: Prolonged Exercise. Indianapolis, Benchmark Press, 1988, pp 357–408.
17. Weisz GM, Lee PL: Spinal canal stenosis—Concept of spinal reserve capacity: Radiologic measurements and clinical applications. Clin Orthop 179:134–140, 1983.
18. Zappe DH, Bauer T: Cycling: Planning off- and preseason training for road cycling. National Strength and Conditioning Journal 11(2):35–40, 1989.

Chapter 14

WEIGHT LIFTING

Larry C. Feeler, BS, PT

It is hard to imagine that only 50 years ago, weight training was essentially unheard of in this country. Those who participated were considered "muscle bound," implying decreased flexibility and coordination that was hypothesized to decrease athletic performance. Today, weight training is unusual in the fact that it is one of the most frequently utilized cross-training techniques and is associated with virtually all competitive sports activities, industrial and sports medicine rehabilitation programs, and injury prevention programs. Through years of research and development, specific exercise programs have been designed to enhance the performance of competitors in almost every sport—hence, the evolution of superior athletes who are outperforming their predecessors with each passing decade. And the future is even more intriguing. With the advent of technology have come computerized lift-tracking devices and joint-compression indicators, as well as testing and strength programs, all of which can be customized and made sports- and injury-specific. Cahill[4] has revealed that weight programs are safe for adolescents when properly designed and supervised, and programs throughout the world are being developed for "special" youth destined to be the athletes of tomorrow. With diverse input from many different countries, specialties, manufacturers, institutions, research centers, etc., the scope of weight-lifting and strength programs has indeed become complex far beyond the scope of this chapter.

This discussion will address the basic principles and benefits of weight training, the use of abdominal belts, and the proper precautions and warm-up associated with lifting. Furthermore, biomechanical complications, associated injuries, and current treatments as they relate to the spine will be presented, as well as the role of the medical practitioner in the evolution of this wide-ranging activity.

PRECAUTIONS TO WEIGHT LIFTING

As with other forms of exercise, when an individual is just starting a weight-training program, medical clearance is indicated. Katch et al.[27] reveal that most individuals over the age of 35, sedentary individuals, and younger persons prone to risk factors such as obesity, diabetes, cigarette smoking, hypertension, or a family history of coronary heart disease need to see a physician prior to beginning weight lifting. Specifically, straining causes significant increases in blood pressure that could be dangerous, and every precaution should be taken to insure decreased tension and proper breathing techniques. Absolute contraindications include respiratory disease, active infections, fever, cardiovascular disease, anemia, and metabolic or systemic disorders.[46]

PROPER WARM-UP

In order to properly train for any sports activity, it is important to understand the benefits of a proper warm-up. This most often entails 5 minutes of light stretching followed by 5 minutes of active exercises to raise the body temperature at least 2 degrees and produce sweating. This is usually followed by more thorough static stretching and often sports-specific activities such as a light-to-moderate weight for the first set of each exercise. This allows the athlete to get ready both mentally and physiologically for the activity to be undertaken.

Stretching

After the active exercises, thorough stretching of the muscles to be exercised should be performed for 5–10 minutes. Soft tissue stretching involves muscle and connective tissue. When stretching muscle tissue, one must consider the effects of the Golgi tendon reflex, the muscle spindle, and relaxation. Connective tissue is composed of collagen fibers and ground substance that are noncontractile but responsive to sustained stretch. Thus, static stretching of 4–5 repetitions for 30–60 seconds versus bouncing stretches are indicated to avoid reflex muscle contraction and to enhance loosening. It has been shown that ballistic stretching results in almost twice the muscle tension created with static stretching.[49] Since the back is involved in almost all lifting maneuvers, the weight lifter should make a special effort to stretch the low back in flexion (knees to chest), extension (push up with abdomen remaining on floor), and thoracic rotation (sitting with one hand on the small of the back, the other hand on the opposite knee, and pulling the shoulders as close to square with the knees as possible) (Fig. 1).

PRINCIPLES OF WEIGHT TRAINING

Strength. Strength is defined as the "capacity of the muscle to produce the tension necessary for initiating movement, maintaining posture, and controlling movement during conditions of loading on the musculoskeletal system."[43] Strength directly correlates with the cross-sectional size of the muscle,[34,44] even though studies have revealed that it can be improved without hypertrophy of the muscle cell.[7] Strengthening without hypertrophy usually involves high-repetition isotonic[45] and/or isokinetic programs that affect recruitment by firing a greater number of motor units. It should also be noted that the amount of fat cells may influence the speed and degree of the muscle contraction.[16] Other parameters affecting strength are length-tension relations, type and speed of contractions, and of course motivation.

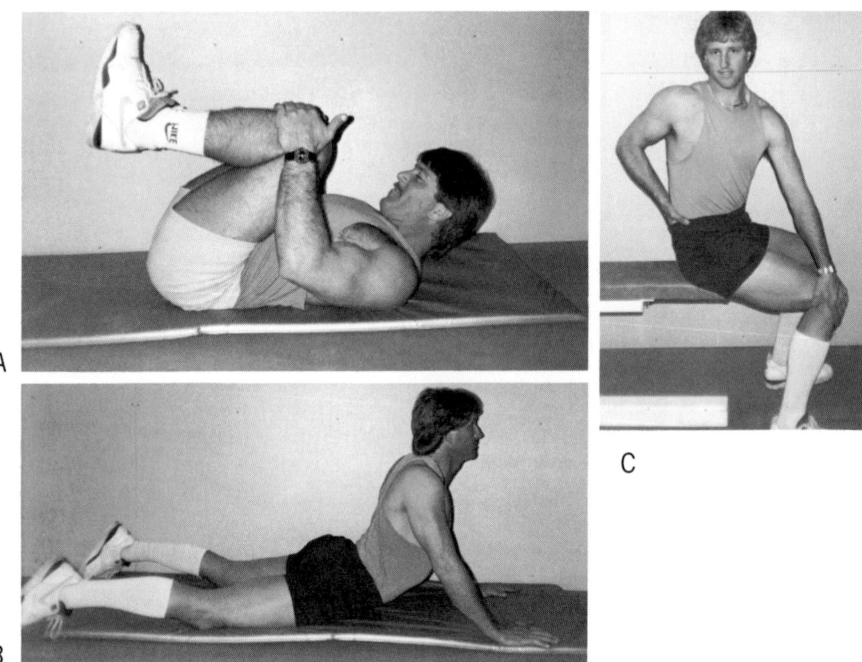

FIGURE 1. Low back stretching exercises for weight lifters: *A,* Knee to chest; *B,* back extension, the most effective exercise to protect the lumbar discs; *C,* back rotation stretch—more complicated and seldom practiced.

Overload Principle. Overload is the development of strength through resistance training that exceeds the metabolic capacity of the muscle, resulting in recruitment or hypertrophy.[23,28] This is most often accomplished with free weights and/or machines used to isolate specific muscle groups to accomplish isotonic concentric (positive) contraction, isotonic eccentric (negative) contraction, and isometric (static) contraction exercises. Isokinetic (same speed, maximum tension) exercises are effective but less readily available, since they consist of computerized training with biofeedback on units that cost an average of $50,000.

Isotonic. DeLorme,[6,7] in the early 1950s, developed the term progressive resisted exercise (PRE) based on the maximum weight that could be lifted or moved 10 times, the 10-repetition maximum (10 RM). The workout includes 10 repetitions at one-half 10 RM, at three-fourths 10 RM, and at a full 10 RM. The weights are increased as the 10 RM weight improves. There have been numerous PRE programs developed since that time with so many variables that their effectiveness has been difficult to assess. However, there are specific parameters that affect the exercise progression and the results with respect to strength gains. These include gradually increasing levels of resistance, working to fatigue, decreasing rest between bouts, and/or increasing the speed or amount of work in a given time. The current trend is to base the percent of maximum overload on a 1-repetition maximum (1 RM). Once the 1 RM is established, 80% of that or above becomes the workout weight, with at least 3 sets of 5 repetitions accomplished before moving up to a heavier weight. This is considered a heavy workout and

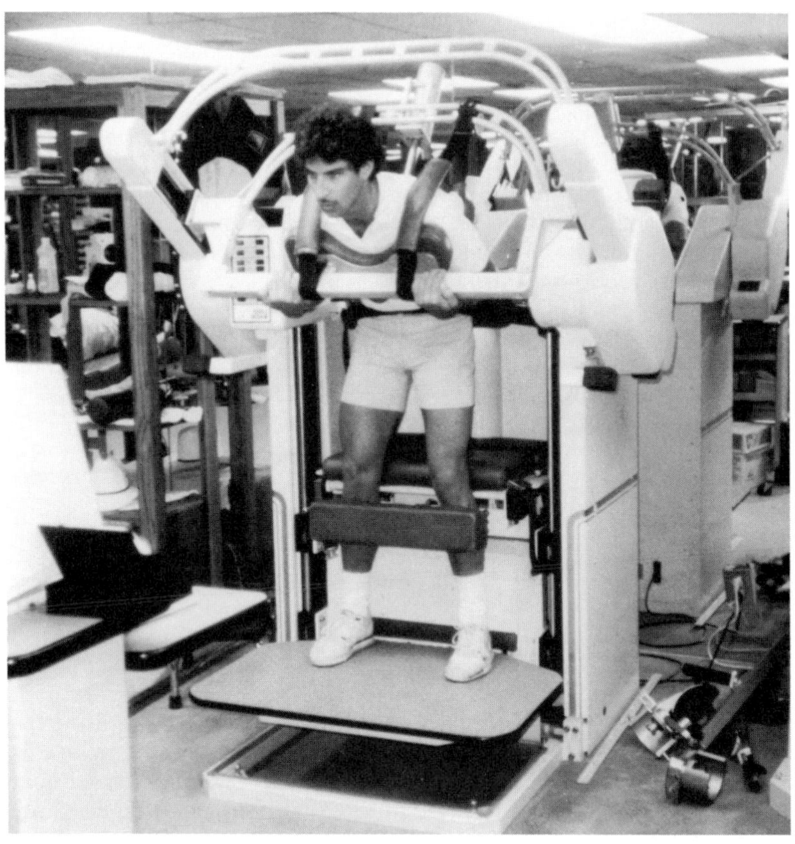

FIGURE 2. Isokinetic trunk flexion/extension on Lido back unit.

is usually alternated with a light (60%) of 1-RM workout every other or every third day. More frequent exercise involves alternating muscle groups to allow for recuperation.

Isometric. In the 1950s, isometric exercises and studies documenting their benefits evolved. Even today, single static contractions held for 6 seconds[26] and multiple brief maximum contractions are recommended to improve strength.[30] Many therapists and trainers have realized the benefits of isometrics performed at 20° increments throughout the active asymptomatic range of motion to improve strength secondary to injury without increasing pain symptoms.

Isokinetic. Isokinetics evolved in 1968 with the advent of computerized testing and strengthening equipment. This type of high-technology exercise equipment (Fig. 2) allows the clinician to set a certain speed and keep all other variables constant to accomplish real-time graphs and computed strength, work, and range-of-motion values. The results are objective and reproducible, with progress reports demonstrating strength, endurance, range of motion, and even in some cases ligament instability of a significant nature. As a result, it is quite simple to do the same number of repetitions and compare the results, e.g., dominant and non-dominant, or injured and uninjured, joints and muscle groups of the trunk and extremities. This tool is expensive but, if available, is the method of choice for clinicians doing research and those needing objective data for possible litigation. Therefore, the medical center setting is the primary location for these units.

Research with computerized isokinetic units has been extensive and reveals significant strength gains, especially in the strongest part of the motion arc at speeds of 30°/second to approximately 100°/second. This is due to increased stimulation caused by maximal tension at each degree of motion being exercised. Higher speed exercises up to 400°/second have been shown to increase total work and power values throughout the range of motion exercised by recruitment and contraction synchrony. Furthermore, multiple-velocity exercise spectrums allow for the alteration of fiber type stimulation.[6,41] One study performed by Frederick Hatfield, Ph.D., a world-champion power lifter, revealed that by gradually increasing the speed of the workout over an 8-week period, dramatic strength gains were accomplished. Hatfield states, "Never have I noticed such marked increases in power through the use of conventional weight training in so short a period of time." He further explains that this method is one of the most important in training for explosive strength in all weight-training athletes and accounts for hundreds of pounds being added to the power lifters' totals.[22]

BIOMECHANICS OF LIFTING

Competitive lifters observed performing maximum squat lifts on videotape have been observed to drop the weight as soon as the force overcomes their ability to maintain the back in lordosis. Numerous authors have supported this lifting posture,[2,5,8,9,17,21,28,50] whereas others advocate lifting with the back in kyphosis.[3,11-15,31,35,37] Those who support the lordotic posture have documented decreased laminar stress,[50] strong back extensors,[1] the ability of contractile tissue to modulate stress, the inability of the posterior ligament complex and bone to modulate stress, the spine buckling without muscular support with loads as low as 2.5 kg,[38] compression force at 53% of the natural stooped lift, ligamentous strain and disc compression at 81% of the kyphotic trunk flexion moment,[21] and uninhibited neurophysiological response to lifting.[28] Supporters of the kyphotic posture have documented a large cross-section of the posterior ligament complex capable of supporting maximal lifts,[10,14,38] the necessity of trunk flexion to place tension on the midline posterior ligaments,[1,11,13] a 25% decrease in compressive stress compared to lordosis,[13] minimized movement at the base of the spine,[31] and better mechanical advantage than muscle with less compressive force.[11]

Obviously there are pros and cons as well as contraindications to both types of lifting. Nachemson[36] has demonstrated decreased posterior disc compression with vertical lifting, whereas the University of Michigan has demonstrated decreased joint compression with forward-bend lifting. Thus, it would seem apparent that patients with adaptive tendencies toward a lordotic posture and with possible degenerative joint changes should lift in a more forward-bent posture to decompress the joints while placing stress on the posterior ligaments. On the other hand, those persons with adaptive tendencies toward kyphosis, those with posterior ligament sprain, or those with disc-compression tendencies should be more efficient in a vertical lifting posture. Regardless, either system should be enhanced by the contraction of the extensor muscles, which will reflexly fire with the head held up in a neutral or extended position. A combination of the two lifts incorporating midline ligamentous support and back extensor muscle contraction, in conjunction with abdominal strength and the effects of intra-abdominal pressure and the thoracolumbar fascia, should contribute to the safety of prolonged repetitive or maximum effort lifting.

DISC DEGENERATION

The disc can be thought of as a sponge squeezing out and soaking up water based on the loads applied to the spine. Through the aging process, this sponge begins to dry out and lose its shape as well as its elasticity, reducing its effectiveness in decreasing stress to and protecting the back. This phenomenon is attributed to the nucleus becoming more fibrotic and to the loss of proteoglycans, which decreases the osmotic properties and the ability of the disc to resist tension.[19]

The degenerative process actually starts in males after the first decade and in females in the second decade.[32] The greatest increase occurs between the ages of 25 and 35 years,[32] when most lifters are constantly increasing the peak of the compressive loads applied to their spines. By age 40, 80% of males and 65% of females demonstrate moderate disc degeneration,[32] and this number seems to be higher in long-term lifters even though weakness is hardly the problem. The most common cause of disc degeneration is thought to be mechanical,[32] with the stress lines actually changing to a biomechanical disadvantage as the disc deteriorates.[24]

Certain risks and genetic[29,48] factors further influence the rate of degeneration. Lifters with early disc degeneration and symptomatic episodes should of course be evaluated for postural predispositions, muscular imbalances, and other biomechanical factors that would affect degenerative changes. Furthermore, back flexibility exercises focusing on extension should be performed routinely three times per day as well as secondary to activities of daily living, such as prolonged sitting, stooping, or bending. Special effort should be made to strengthen the abdominal muscles isometrically or in a short arc "crunch" without contracting the hip flexors. The weight lifter should decrease his training weights to approximately one-third during periods of exacerbation, and then gradually increase based on his symptoms when resting and during periods of inactivity the following day. As discussed previously, a more vertical lifting posture would be indicated. Recurrent episodes with clinical neurological correlation of any significance would contraindicate heavy lifting altogether. Isometrics and extremely light weights with slow, controlled movements could be utilized until the condition stabilizes. Then weight training at no more than 50% of maximum for a higher number of controlled repetitions to fatigue could be accomplished, placing the lifter at low risk of reinjury.

EFFECT OF WEIGHT-LIFTING BELT AND BACK SUPPORTS

There is much controversy as to the benefits of bracing post-injury and the use of a weight-lifting belt to prevent injury. On one extreme, braces are considered to hinder muscle contraction and weaken the supporting structures, whereas the other extreme supports the idea that braces are necessary for all soft tissue and joint-related problems in the acute phase. Some weight lifters feel confident of not injuring their backs while wearing a support, whereas others feel that wearing a support weakens their system, holds the pelvis in a functionally limiting posterior tilt, and does not allow them to feel the weight with the back muscles to insure that they have the strength to control it. Numerous studies have been done to investigate the physiological and biomechanical effects of back supports. With regard to the medical practitioner, Stoddard[47] points out that those who use back supports for all backaches without proper indication and diagnosis are "retrograde and slipshod" in their approach. He reports, to the contrary, that those "that condemn all corsets to the wastepaper basket are also making a mistake." One study revealed no decreased electromyographic or muscle activity to the back extensor muscles, but did show that the abdominal muscle activity was somewhat decreased.[16] Another study suggested that prolonged use could result in atrophy of trunk musculature,[42] while another provided information that wearing a support for up to 5 years did not weaken the trunk musculature.[39] More importantly, several studies have indicated no significant difference with or without lumbar corsets and weight-lifting belts except an elevated intra-abdominal pressure resulting in decreased disc compression.[20,25,40] These findings support the use of a weight-lifting belt as well as the need to strengthen the abdominal muscles to increase intra-abdominal pressure and reduce compression even further. The belt should be worn snugly, especially on heavy workout days, encompassing the lumbosacral junction without significantly restricting pelvis mobility and the ability to feel the weight.

TREATMENT POST-INJURY

The education and treatment of the power lifter or other injured lifter need to be customized to his or her strengths and weaknesses, taking into consideration joint or disc compression based on symptomatology. Muscle flexibility and strength imbalances need to be addressed early, and a progressive exercise program should be customized to meet the needs of the individual. Common problems with chronic injuries include decreased trunk range of motion; decreased hip range of motion; and decreased strength to the abdominals, back extensors, quadriceps, gluteus medius, and quadratus lumborum. These problems should be improved as quickly as possible through static stretching (no less than three times per day) as described above and a progressive strengthening program. This program can be accomplished in three phases: (1) cardiovascular fitness and isometric exercises; (2) progressive resisted isotonic, interval training, slow-speed isokinetic, and functional exercises; and (3) eccentric, high-speed, isokinetic velocity spectrums, isofunctional exercises, and job- or sport-specific exercises. Objective measurements need to be taken, with monthly re-evaluations to assess progress and psychophysical abilities. Upon recovery, the subject, whether injured worker or weight lifter, should be conditioned to hold his or her head up while contracting the extensor muscles of the back, regardless of the degree of trunk flexion, to further develop the protective mechanism involved in lifting.

POWER LIFTING

The sport of power lifting involves extensive training to accomplish three competitive lifts: the bench press, squat, and dead lift (Fig. 3). The total amount of the best weight lifted properly in each position is the lifter's score for his body weight. The current records are phenomenal, with athletes dead lifting, squatting, and occasionally even bench pressing three times their body weight. These lifts must be accomplished by incorporating speed of movement, since without this component Nachemson has documented disc failure at 220 kg and joint destruction between 300 kg and 700 kg.[36] Even so, it is becoming more common to see 1,320 kg bench presses and 2,200 kg squats. Such results have taken their toll, and many lifters' careers are short-term, while significant others have ended with back surgery due to herniations and back instabilities. Nonetheless, to accomplish such feats, the power lifter is an extraordinary individual who focuses

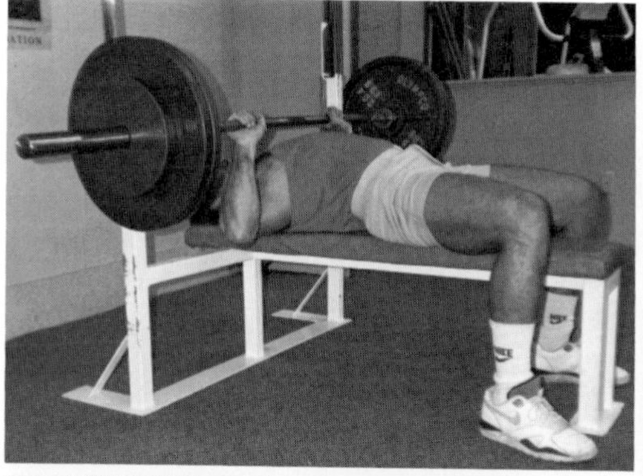
A

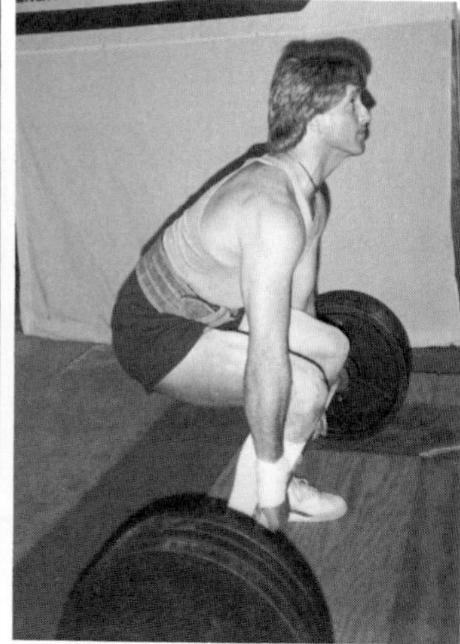
C

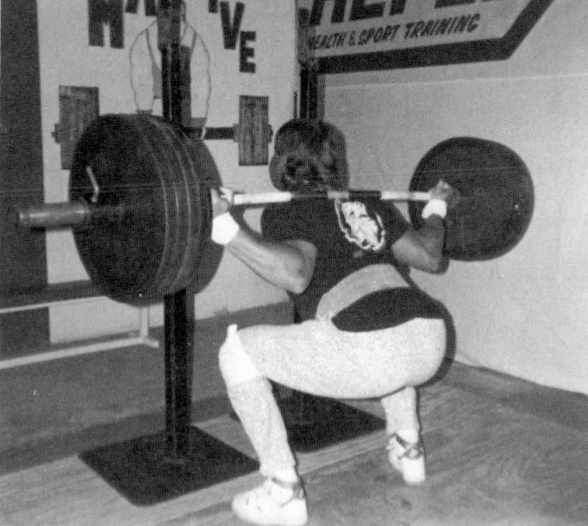
B

FIGURE 3. Three power lifts for competition: *A,* bench press, a very common exercise; *B,* squat—commonly practiced, but not as deeply as is required for competitive lifting; *C,* dead lift—the least practiced exercise for power lifters.

on perfect lifting technique, since the slightest flaw can mean the difference in making or not making that maximum lift. Through continuing education, research, the use of computerized scanning of lifts, specific assistance exercises, and peak strength cycling, the longevity of the sport should continue to improve as well as those phenomenal records.

THE PEAKING CYCLE

This type of training is renowned in the field of weight lifting, especially for power lifters and bodybuilders. The importance of technique to build a strong foundation for lifting is imperative in power lifting, in which athletes are handling weights at plateau levels constantly. In order to avoid injuries, overtraining, and burn-out, the peaking cycle for training has evolved and is the method of choice by most competitors. Briefly described, this method involves studying previous strength gains and using a detailed diary to strategically map out training to accomplish short-, medium-, and long-term goals, all leading up to one main objective—peak strength at the end of the training cycle. The repetitions, percentage of maximum weights, assistance exercises, nutrition, and time of the cycle vary among lifters, but all involve starting at far below maximal lifts, controlling the assistance exercises to avoid overtraining, and gradually increasing the weight while decreasing repetitions to finally surpass one's previous maximum lifts at the end of the cycle. The time frame usually involves an 8–12-week period of training. Then, based on the athlete's mental and injury status, as well as his strength gains, the plan for a new cycle is implemented. One cycle may result in only a 10–15-pound improvement, but a program of 4 cycles a year adds up to an impressive 40–60 pound-per-lift gain.

OVERUSE SYNDROME

Power lifters, bodybuilders, and other serious weight trainers working constantly to increase their strength, power, muscle mass, and definition at plateau levels are most susceptible to overuse syndromes. Many medical practitioners, upon seeing these problems, advocate rest or stopping all activities that aggravate or endanger the condition of the individual. This appears logical but is not realistic. We must realize that these individuals are aggressive and spend most of their waking moments controlling not only their weights but also their lives and those people with whom they are in contact. Most of them are obsessed with their physique and strength, and cannot bear the thought of anything that might weaken what they have worked so hard to achieve. Individuals such as these are willing to train even in life-threatening situations (e.g., steroid abuse) and more than likely will walk out of the physician's office and not return until significant medical intervention is indicated. Therefore, the challenge for the medical practitioner is to become active in understanding these psychophysical behaviors, whether or not the activities are condoned, and to convince the patient that he or she is genuinely concerned and has a plan to return the patient to work and/or sports activities as quickly as possible.

Guidelines for Treating the Overuse Syndrome

Mirkin[33] has documented basic guidelines for the overuse syndrome that are often overlooked by the weight trainer. It is felt that these parameters are relevant for back and extremity pain induced by lifting. The **first stage** involves dull, aching discomfort in the joint or muscle during workouts. Complications can be avoided by reducing the intensity and/or weights to avoid or significantly minimize the discomfort.

The **second stage** involves discomfort that is felt during training and even several hours after training. Complications are imminent unless weight training is avoided for 5–7 days, and then the intensity and weight are slowly reintroduced to maximal levels.

The **third stage** involves discomfort that is felt during and after training as well as persistent pain even when at rest. The athlete obviously should stop training entirely, and if the pain at rest has not dissipated in 2–3 days, should seek medical intervention. While taking a history on the athlete, one can often find that training methods have included increasing the work load too soon, not resting enough between workouts, increasing the intensity of the workout too soon, or even adding new exercises. Problems can be complicated by physical abnormalities, including unequal leg lengths, excessive lordosis or kyphosis of the back, scoliosis, or muscle imbalances. One classic example is the squat lifter who does not have normal hip or ankle flexibility and is required to externally rotate the hips and abduct his legs during this technique. If this same athlete has adductor muscle weakness, he will have extreme difficulty controlling heavy weights without causing undue stress to the back by having to bend forward to accomplish getting his hips down level or below knee height. By working on ankle and hip flexibility as well as adductor muscle strength, the athlete would improve his lifts significantly and more than likely reduce the compressive forces in the back considerably.

The majority of lifters do not have the luxury of someone knowledgeable in the biomechanics of weight training who can customize their imbalances and body composition to their safest and most efficient lift. Most are trained by other lifters who, through trial and error, have learned what seems to work best for them. When the first injury and most subsequent injuries occur, they heal rather quickly. Few practitioners seem concerned with comprehensively assessing, educating, and "training" the athlete to effect structural changes that could deter or alleviate the problem. Through the years, recurrent episodes increase in both intensity and duration, and the lifter, who has by then become less intimidated by pain, does not respond as well to conservative management. It is this degenerative process through which the lifter continues to train that sets him up for surgical intervention owing to significant joint instability and displacement, symptomatic disc herniation, or disc rupture. The role of the medical practitioner is to use the knowledge gained through millions of dollars spent on medical and sports research to provide the weight lifter with a conclusive diagnosis, to discover his or her flexibility and strength imbalances, to teach the most efficient mechanics for the individual's body composition, and most importantly to educate the weight lifter in order to prevent or deter the degenerative process as much as possible, considering the probability that they will continue to train.

REFERENCES

1. Adams MA, Hulton WC: Prolapsed intervertebral disc: A hyperflexion injury. Spine 7:184, 1982.
2. Asmussen E, Poulsen E, Rasmussen B: Quantitative evaluation of the activity of the back muscles in lifting. Comm Dan Assoc Infant Paralysis 21:3–14, 1965.
3. Bartelink DL: The role of abdominal pressure in relieving the pressure on the lumbar intervertebral discs. J Bone Joint Surg 39B:718, 1957.
4. Cahill BA: Personal communication. AOSSM, Orlando, June 1987.
5. Delitto R, Rose SJ, Apts DW: An electromyographic analysis of two techniques for squat lifting. Phys Ther 65:673, 1985.
6. DeLorme TL, Watkins A: Technics of progressive resistance exercise. Arch Phys Med Rehabil 29:263–273, 1948.
7. DeLorme TL, Watson AL: Progressive Resistance Exercise. New York, Appleton-Century, 1951.
8. Eie N: Load capacity of the low back. J Oslo City Hosp 16:75–98, 1966.
9. Eie N, Wehn P: Measurements of the intra-abdominal pressure in relation to weight bearing of the lumbosacral spine. J Oslo City Hosp 12:205, 1962.
10. Farfan H: Muscular mechanism of the lumbar spine and the position of power efficiency. Orthop Clin North Am 6:135–143, 1975.
11. Gracovetsky SA: Letter to the editor. Spine 12:1068–1075, 1987.
12. Gracovetsky S, Farfan H: The mechanism of the lumbar spine. Spine 6:249, 1981.
13. Gracovetsky S, Farfan H: The optimum spine. Spine 11:558, 1986.
14. Gracovetsky S, Farfan H, Lamy C: Mathematical model of the lumbar spine using an optimized system to control muscles and ligaments. Orthop Clin North Am 8:135, 1977.
15. Gracovetsky S, Kary M, Pitcher I, et al: The importance of pelvic tilt in reducing compressive stress in the spine during flexion-extension exercises. Spine 14:452, 1989.
16. Grieve GP: Common Vertebral Joint Problems. New York, Churchill Livingstone, 1988, p 657.
17. Grieve GP: Common Vertebral Joint Problems. New York, Churchill Livingstone, 1988, p 103.
18. Guere DW: Dynamic characteristics of man during crouch and stoop lifting. In Nelson RC, Moorehouse CA (eds): Biomechanics, Vol. IV. Baltimore, University Park Press, 1974, p 19.

19. Guyer RD: Spine: State of the Art Reviews. Philadelphia, Hanley & Belfus, 3(1):15, 1989.
20. Harman EA, Rosenstein RM, Frykman PN, et al: Exercise Physiology Division, US Army Research Institute of Environmental Medicine, Natick. Reported in Med Sci Sports Exerc 21:189–190, 1989.
21. Hart DL, Stobbe TJ, Jaraiedi M: Effect of lumbar posture on lifting. Spine 12:138, 1987.
22. Hatfield F: Activating totally. Powerlifting 11:34, 1989.
23. Hellebrandt RA, Hontz SJ: Mechanisms of muscle training in men: Experimental demonstration of the overload principle. Phys Ther Rev 36:371, 1956.
24. Hedtmann A, Steffen R, Methfessel J, et al: Measurement of human lumbar spine ligaments during loaded and unloaded motion. Spine 14:175–184, 1989.
25. Hemborg B, Moritz U, Holmstom E, Akesson I: Lumbar spinal support and weightlifter's belt: Effect on intra-abdominal and intra-thoracic pressure and trunk muscle activity during lifting. Man Med 1:86, 1985.
26. Hettinger T, Muller EA: Muskelliesturg and muskeltraining. Arbeitsphysiol 15:111, 1953.
27. Katch FI, McArdle WD: Nutrition, Weight, Control, and Exercise. Philadelphia, Lea & Febiger, 1983, pp 190–191.
28. Kugelberg E, Haybarth KE: Spinal mechanism of the abdominal and erector spinae skin reflexes. Brain 81:290, 1958.
29. Lawrence J: Rheumatism in Populations. London, Heinemann, 1977.
30. Liberson WT: Brief isometric exercise. In Basmajan JV (ed): Therapeutic Exercise, 3rd ed. Baltimore, Williams & Wilkins, 1978.
31. Marras WS, King AI, Joynt RL: Measuremens of loads on lumbar spine under isometric and isokinetic conditions. Spine 9:176–187, 1984.
32. Miller JAA, Schmatz BS, Schultz AB: Lumbar disc degeneration: Correlation with age, sex, and spine level in 600 autopsy specimens. Spine 13:178, 1988.
33. Mirkin G, Hoffman M: The Sports Medicine Book. Canada, Little Brown & Co., 1978, p 131.
34. Moritani T, DeVries HK: Neural factors vs. hypertrophy in the time course of muscle strength gain. Am J Phys Med 58:115, 1979.
35. Morris JM, Lucas DB, Breslar B: Role of the trunk in stability of the spine. J Bone Joint Surg 43A:327, 1961.
36. Nachemson A: The influence of spinal movements on the lumbar intradiscal pressure and on the tensile stresses in the annulus fibrosus. Acta Orthop Scand 33, 1963.
37. Nachemson A: The load of lumbar discs in different positions of the body. Clin Orthop 45:107, 1966.
38. Nachemson A, Elfstone G: Intravital dynamic pressure measurements in lumbar disk. Scand J Rehab Med Supplement 1, Stockholm, 1970.
39. Nachemson A, Lindh M: Measurement of abdominal and back muscle strength with and without low back pain. Scand J Rehab Med 1:60, 1969.
40. Nachemson A, Morris JM: In vivo measurements of intradiscal pressure: Discometry, a new method for the determination of pressure on the lower lumbar discs. J Bone Joint Surg 46A:1077–1092, 1964.
41. Osternig L: Isokinetic dynamometry: Implications for muscle testing and rehabilitation. Exerc Sport Sci Rev 14:45–80, 1986.
42. Quintet RJ, Hadler NM: Diagnosis and treatment of backache. Semin Arthritis Rheum 8:126–287, 1979.
43. Smidt GL, Rogers WW: Factors contributing to the regulation and clinical assessment of muscular strength. Phys Ther 62:1283, 1982.
44. Smith MJ: Muscle fiber types: Their relationship to athletic training and rehabilitation. Orthop Clin North Am 14:403, 1983.
45. Smith MJ, Melton P: Isokinetic vs. isotonic variable resistance training. Am J Sports Med 9:275, 1981.
46. Sperryn PN: Sport and Medicine. London, Butterworths, 1983, p 5.
47. Stoddard A: Manual of Osteopathic Practice, 2nd ed. London, Hutchinson, 1983, Appendix 3, p 242.
48. Varlotta GP, Brown MD: Familial predisposition for adolescent disc displacement (abstract). Miami, ISSLS Meeting, 1988, p 4.
49. Walker SM: Delay of twitch relaxation induced by stress and stress relaxation. J Appl Physiol 16:801, 1961.
50. White AA, Panjabi M: Clinical Biomechanics of the Spine. Philadelphia, JB Lippincott, 1978, pp 35–42.

Chapter 15

RACQUET SPORTS

Larry C. Feeler, BS, PT

Racquet sports have grown increasingly popular since the early 1960s, when businessmen became involved in franchising tennis, along with a variety of other sports activities, for profit and social prestige. Tennis has been largely responsible for this growth, but racquetball, handball, squash, and badminton have also made significant gains in participant numbers. According to a National Sporting Goods Association survey, there were over 22 million tennis and racquetball participants in 1987,[1] and estimates exceed 30 million participants for all racquet sports. The U.S. Consumer Products Safety Commission documented 210,000 injuries in racquet sports affecting persons over 14 years of age in 1985. Haas reported that 38% of 148 Men's Professional Tennis Tour players missed at least one tournament because of low back problems.[8] The weekend or recreational athlete in racquet sports is even more susceptible to injury. This pattern, along with the increasing popularity of these sports, has led to a large volume of racquet sports participants with low back problems being attended by medical practitioners. This chapter will review training prior to participation, proper warm-up and stretching, the biomechanical effects of form and body positioning, complications and common injuries associated with spine problems, and treatment of the spine as it relates to racquet sports injuries.

TRAINING PRIOR TO PARTICIPATION IN SPORT

Preparation for competition in racquet sports at all levels has had a significant impact upon the evolution of racquet sports, from games of elegant and graceful form concentrating upon perfect technique to those of overpowering strength, finesse, and stamina, which showcase athletic ability. This change, even amidst surging popularity, has happened during a decline in the number of United States junior tennis players able to perform competitively at international levels.[14] In response, medical and sports research leading to improvements in strength, flexibility, and conditioning programs are precipitating necessary changes to meet the goals of the "new" racquet sports enthusiast. It is becoming more common for the most successful junior tennis players to have trips to sports medicine clinics arranged for them by the United States Tennis Association (USTA), not to work on tennis strokes, but to assess muscle strengths, weaknesses, imbalances, and flexibility limits that affect performance. According to Paul Roetert, coordinator of research for the USTA, "Coaches of the future will be armed with the latest technology in exercise physiology, nutrition, biomechanics, sports medicine, sport psychology, and motor learning. The science of coaching tennis is becoming a reality."[15] In the last 2 years, there have already been more than 20,000 coaches certified in introductory sports science through the American Coaches Effectiveness Program.[15]

Conditioning

Racquet sports usually consist of 200 to 500 anaerobic bursts of exercise with short intermittent rest periods over a 1 to 3 hour time frame, eventually effecting an aerobic response. One study of singles and doubles racquetball players over a 1-hour period showed that both groups met the American College of Sports Medicine criteria for developing aerobic fitness.[19] A study by Kibler et al.[12] of 97 junior tennis players from various countries and training programs over a 2-year period showed 9 significant back injuries (6 male, 3 female), with 6 overload injuries and 3 sprains. A control group of recreational players had an almost identical incidence and type of back injuries. Another study found that 45% of teenagers are estimated to have decreased back flexibility,[11] and it has been documented that the percentage is higher for adults.[18,25] Thus, conditioning for the elite and recreational player is necessary to maintain flexibility, muscle balance, agility, and anaerobic as well as aerobic fitness.

Proper Warm-up

The same principles as those discussed in the previous article on weight lifting apply to racquet sports. Active exercises followed by static stretching and sports-specific exercises such as jogging and light volleying are indicated.

Stretching. Upper extremity and lower extremity stretching exercises,[9,13] as well as proprioceptive neuromuscular facilitation (PNF) techniques,[21,23] are extremely effective for racquet sports players. This discussion is limited to those spine-related exercises that are not so readily available. Special attention should be given to stretching the low back in extension to prepare for serves and overhead volleys. Furthermore, since the coupling motion of trunk flexion and rotation occurs frequently throughout a match, stretching bilateral trunk rotation is imperative. This is easily accomplished by: (1) sitting with one hand on the small of the back and the other on the opposite knee, then pulling the shoulders parallel with the same knee; and (2) the lumbar roll: lying supine with the shoulders kept flat on the floor as the pelvis is stretched in a rotated position (Fig. 1). Another important exercise is the crossed-leg knee to chest (Franquiz stretch, Fig. 2) to stretch the hip extensors and the piriform muscle. When the piriform muscle is tight or in spasm, it may produce pain symptoms with radiculopathy.

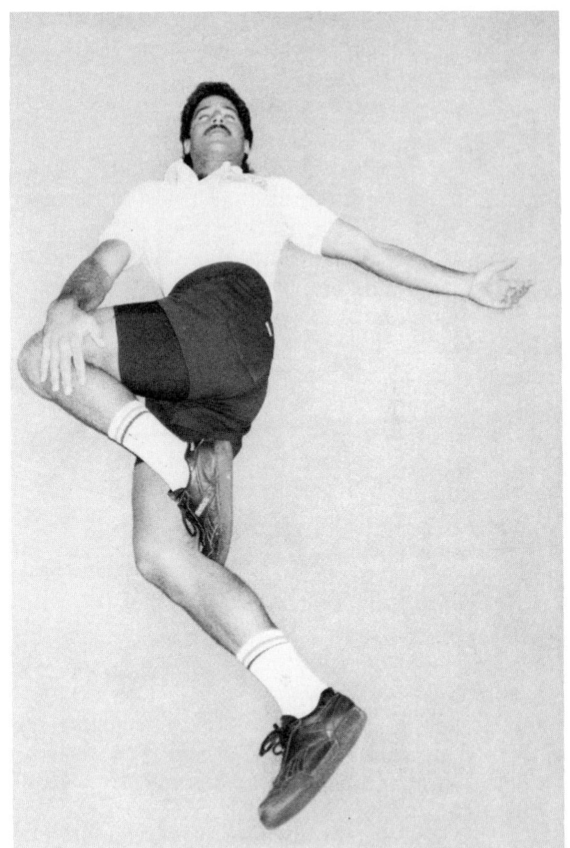

FIGURE 1. The lumbar roll.

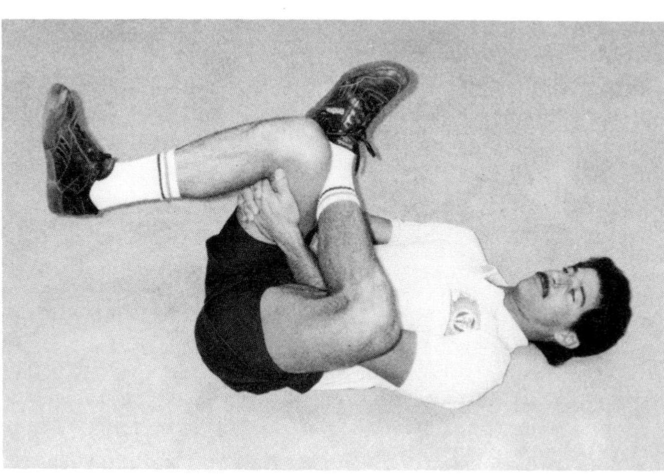

FIGURE 2. Franquiz stretch to stretch hip extensors and the piriform muscle.

RACQUET STROKE MECHANICS AND THEIR EFFECT ON THE SPINE

The basic strokes in all racquet sports consist of the overhead, overhead serve, forehand, and backhand, all of which place certain mechanical stresses on the back that increase the risk of disorders. The dynamic stabilization of the upper body in relation to a constantly changing axis of motion; center of gravity; disposition of trunk, pelvis, and extremities; and the effect of the forces applied to the body by impact from various racquet strokes, places significant demands upon the lumbar region. Even ancillary activities such as repetitious bending to pick up the ball or simply awaiting the next volley poised on the balls of the feet with the trunk flexed to the point that the shoulders are "hanging" over the toes increase the probability of injury.

Overhead. Whether serving or hitting an overhead, the mechanics are the same, with body position and its relation to ball location relaying different stresses to the spine. A ball slightly in front of the body will decrease hyperextension, whereas one behind will increase it. A ball to the side will increase rotation or sidebending in order to make contact. The motion itself involves getting in position perpendicular to the net; rotating away from the net and hyperextending the back completely in preparation for the hit; and finally derotating and following through to approximately 65°–75° of trunk flexion facing the net.

Forehand. The forehand stroke involves standing with the shoulders perpendicular to the net, rotating away from the net to initiate the backswing, and finishing the swing with upper body derotation or uncoiling with follow-through low to high, with very little transition flexion to extension.

Backhand. Backhand stroke mechanics are very similar to the forehand except that the arm holding the racquet crosses the body and increases trunk rotation prior to uncoiling for the hit. A two-handed backhand accentuates this rotation and has been thought to increase the incidence of back trauma.

Variance. It must be noted that the mechanics of the strokes discussed are possible in ideal situations and for persons skilled in their performance. All of the strokes vary in the degree and force of flexion, extension, and rotation of the spine and are dependent upon aerobic and anaerobic fitness. Any variance, whether it be from lack of skill or dictated by circumstances such as an off-balance stroke, if frequent enough, could significantly change the risk of back disorders. Furthermore, the forces generated from the ball to the racquet and from the court to the feet, then to the primary and stabilizing muscle groups, and finally to the spine, all play a part in susceptibility to injury.

SPECIAL BIOMECHANICAL CONSIDERATIONS

Torsion

Since rotation right and left are inherent in every racquet stroke, it is imperative to understand this movement and its effect on back injury. Farfan states that "this motion is probably more dangerous to the disc than any other, except for a combination of axial rotation and lateral bending."[4] During rotation of the back, the ipsilateral erector spinae and the contralateral multifidus and trunk rotators contract. Muscle imbalances, posture, flexibility, and general conditioning all affect the synchrony of controlling this activity at each contributing motion segment. White et al.[28] studied and found 4–12° at each level T2 to T7–8, 6–7° at T8–9, 3–5° at T9–10, 2–3° at T11-to T12–L1, $< 3°$ at L1–2 through L4–5, and < 5° at L5–S1. These findings have been supported by Markholf, who found increasing torsional stiffness from the lower thoracic to the L4 segment and who attributed this phenomenon to the design of the facet joints.[16] Some segments are limited in rotation by ligamentous tension and rib articulation, whereas others, e.g., the T12–L1 motion segment, are limited by orientation of the articulating facets.[27]

Farfan[4] has shown significant joint injury under static loading with as little as 3.5° of axial rotation. He has also shown that the torque strength of the joint is stronger when the rate of axial rotation is increased. This could account for the racquet sports player's ability to withstand joint problems associated with torsion. Even so, this motion increases intradiscal pressure,[24] has been shown to damage the facets, and, if carried beyond the physiologic limits noted, results in circumferential tears in the annulus fibrosus.[3,5] These problems can be made worse through trauma, degeneration, and/or the aging process. Studies have revealed an increase in back flexibility in rotation between the ages of 15–24 followed by a gradual decline in motion to as much as 50% in advancing years.[18,25]

Hysteresis

In relation to racquet sports, one must consider the effects of hysteresis caused by repetitive impacting throughout the match. Repetitive loading and unloading results in gradual deformation of the disc and distortion of its ability to dissipate the energy transmitted to the spine. The lower lumbar discs have a greater loss of energy than those of the thoracic and upper lumbar motion segments, and are therefore less protected and more susceptible to fatigue and concurrent injury.[7,27] This phenomenon has furthermore been shown to vary based on age, the rate of loading, the force of loading, and permanence of deformation due to trauma.[26]

COMMON BACK PROBLEMS

Numerous top athletes attribute their successes to mental and physical preparation on and off the court. Racquet sports, especially performed in an intense manner without proper maintenance and conditioning, will inevitably lead to mechanical back and/or disc symptoms. The symptoms may be predisposed by the same risk factors, e.g., posture, that are discussed in the previous chapter on weight lifting, but the etiology most often includes trauma, mechanical dysfunction, and/or degenerative changes.

The Elite Athlete

In reference to the elite racquet sports athlete, long hours of practice, tournament play, and travel result in microtraumas, fatigue, and resultant decreased strength without ample time for repair, eventually leading to overuse syndromes affecting the spine. Common problems and their causes are as follows:

1. Muscle strain—e.g., rectus abdominis tear due to overexertion on overhead volleys or serves.

2. Ligament sprain—hyperflexion and/or forced torsion resulting in microtrauma to the posterior longitudinal ligament and/or ligamentum flavum.

3. Back extensor and/or abdominal muscle weakness due to microtrauma and nonspecific training.

4. Disc symptoms due to static long-term trunk flexion and repetitive rotation, with an increase in posterior disc pressure.[27] Typical characteristics

include being of tall stature, being moderately deconditioned, having a kyphotic low-back posture, and following through in racquet strokes with the trunk rotated over the pelvis.

5. Disc symptoms due to decreased thoracic rotation and excessive force and number of repetitions in trunk flexion-rotation coupling motions. This problem appears to be magnified when the athlete uses a two-handed backhand volley.

6. Degenerative joints due to repetitive compression and gradual hypertrophic changes affecting the facets. Long-term changes can result in spinal stenosis.

7. Joint irritation due to decreased back extension flexibility amidst repetitive forced hyperextension with overhead volleys and serves.

8. Hyperlordosis due to strong back extensors and weak abdominals, as well as excessive hip flexor strength and tightness. This often predisposes to spondylosis or spondylolisthesis.

The Recreational Athlete

The recreational athlete, especially if only a part-time sportsman, usually suffers generalized deconditioning and poor muscle tone to the muscles that support the spine. The typical injured person is a slightly to moderately obese and deconditioned, yet aggressive, 25–40-year-old who participates in racquet sports on an irregular basis. Our observations of the most common back problems associated with this type of racquet sport enthusiast are as follows:

1. Sprain and strain are due to trauma, poor form, poor tensile strength, decreased flexibility, improper warm-up, improper equipment, muscle imbalances, overexertion, etc.

2. Facet impingement or locking occurs with trunk flexion and slight rotation, causing the facet joints to "shift out of their normal congruous relationship triggering a reflex muscle spasm."[22] This patient presents with the trunk flexed and deviated to one side and with the knees and hips slightly flexed during ambulation. Significant guarding and intense subjective pain are noted, but there are no neurological symptoms.

3. Disc herniation or disruption are due to a straight-legged, bent-back posture, coupled with repetitive forced rotations and predisposed by decreased spine stability and deconditioning. This person usually has a history of recurrent progressive trauma, and in the subacute or chronic stage, presents with a similar posture to the previous example, but has varying yet consistent degrees of neurological involvement based on the severity of the lesion.

PHYSICAL THERAPY AND RACQUET SPORTS

It is somewhat unfortunate that most athletes, whether elite or recreational, seldom have consultations regarding posture, form, etc. until an actual injury occurs. In the acute phase, especially with disc symptoms, bed rest may be indicated, but no longer than 2 days.[2] It has been our own experience that bed rest and extension exercises are more beneficial than bed rest alone. One such experience involves a 31-year-old male hospital administrative assistant whose father was the attending radiologist. This patient was playing racquetball and ruptured a disc, with a CT scan confirming an inferior disc fragment of 1–2 cm at the L5–S1 segment. This patient was in excruciating discomfort for 2 days and wanted to have surgery to stop his left hip and lower extremity pain. He had no change in symptoms until the third day, when he was started on prone lying and gentle back extension exercises 5 minutes every half hour. After only 4–5 hours, the patient's radicular pain began to subside slightly. Continuing this course, he was able to make transitional movements and begin ambulation the following day. Even though he was improving, the patient was encouraged to have surgery, as in his father's experience this was definitely a surgical lesion due to the large extrusion noted. His CT scan and a report of his clinical presentation from the physical therapist were forwarded to a spine specialist (the editor of this book), who agreed that conservative measures should continue as long as the patient was improving. The patient progressed at a dramatic pace with conservative modalities, intermittent pelvic traction, body mechanics instruction, and progressive exercises, including the McKenzie[17] protocol, flexibility exercises, stabilization exercises, and strengthening exercises. The patient went back to work 2 hours on the 15th day post-injury, progressing to 8-hour work days by 3 weeks. The patient was completely asymptomatic by 4 weeks and was dismissed from supervised medical care in 5 weeks. This patient's recovery was remarkable, and 2 years later the patient has had no further problems except his retirement from racquetball.

This patient's anatomical structures were capable of accommodating the disc extrusion without complication once the initial physiological response to trauma dissipated. This patient and others like him are fortunate enough to have large enough disc spaces and nerve root foramen to accommodate even a ruptured disc. On the other hand, it is possible for other individuals to have very small disc and nerve root spaces that are easily compromised with a slight herniation, resulting in significant discomfort. Such information compounds the need to correlate diagnostic studies and clinical symptoms, as well as short-term progress to differentiate a true surgical lesion.

Mechanical and disc problems may be helped by a variety of physical modalities and customized exercise programs. Low back schools and other education programs have been shown to help with the understanding of back anatomy and body mechanics to prevent recurrent problems.[10,20] In the subacute stage, active trunk movements, back and pelvic flexibility limits, aerobic fitness level, postural deficits, and muscle imbalances can be assessed with a plan implemented to address problem areas. In the chronic or symptom-free stage of recovery, the racquet sport participant must continue to address dysfunction from the subacute stage, but special emphasis should be placed upon increasing flexibility in trunk rotation, to hamstring and multifidus length, as well as in strengthening the abdominals, quadratus lumborum, and gluteus medius muscles.

Prior to participation, our clinic utilizes back stabilization exercises performing multifidus strengthening (opposite arm and leg raise with weights) on all fours, moving in diagonal patterns (Fig. 3). The multifidus muscle is the "major negative sagittal rotator of the spine"[6] and must be strong to counter the forces of decelerating trunk rotation. Isokinetic exercises are also incorporated to stabilize the trunk over the pelvis. These exercises isolate the back extensors and are performed in a progressive sequence, starting in a sitting posture working on straight plane trunk rotation (Fig. 4) and sidebending, progressing to standing diagonal patterns. Isofunctional exercises include resistance with rubber tubing in diagonal patterns of trunk movement, as well as static body positioning with resistance applied to the racquet in a variety of pre- and post-ball impact postures for the different strokes. Return to sport is gradual, with asymptomatic match play in practice important before actual competition.

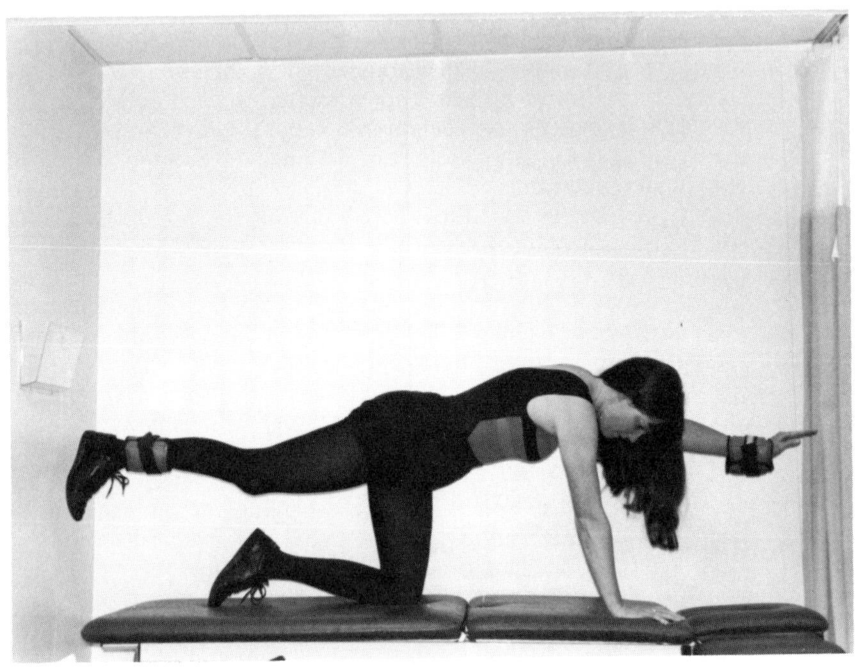

FIGURE 3. Multifidus strengthening exercises with weights

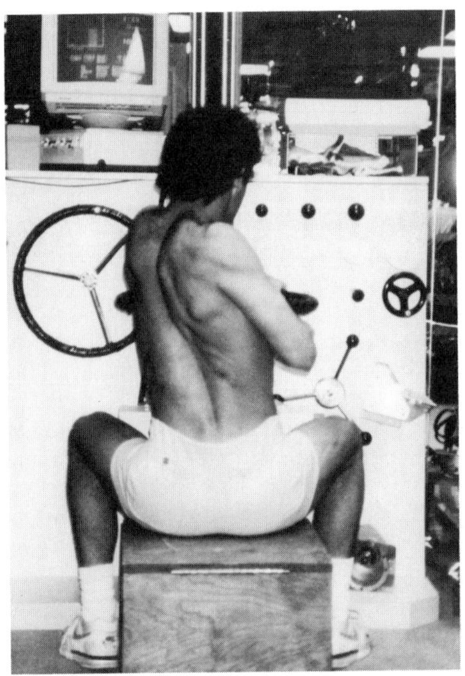

FIGURE 4. Back stabilization: trunk rotation, lumbar spine held neutral, on the Lido Workset isokinetic unit.

CONTRAINDICATIONS TO RETURN TO RACQUET SPORTS ACTIVITIES

Ideally the medical practitioner's goal is for all elite and recreational athletes to return to racquet sports participation. Those participants who should avoid the complications associated with racquet sports and repetitive twisting secondary to injury are patients with significant degenerative joint and disc disease, ruptured discs, herniated discs with symptomology, chronic pain that disturbs sleep, surgical intervention, gross ligament instability, progressive spondylolisthesis, and stenosis.

REFERENCES

1. Bureau of the Census: National Sporting Goods Association sports participation survey in 1987. National Data Book and Guide to Sources Statistical Abstract of the United States. US Dept of Commerce, 1989, pp 227–228.
2. Deyo AL, Diehl AK, Rosenthal M: How many days of bedrest for acute low back pain? A randomized clinical trial. N Engl J Med 315:1064–1070, 1986.
3. Eie N: Load capacity of the low back. J Oslo City Hosp 16:73–98, 1966.
4. Farfan HF: Mechanical Disorder of the Low Back. Philadelphia, Lea & Febiger, 1973.
5. Farfan HF, Cossette JW, Robertson GH, et al: The effects of torsion on the lumbar intervertebral joints: The role of torsion in the production of disc degeneration. J Bone Joint Surg 52A:468–497, 1970.
6. Grieve GP: Common Vertebral Joint Problems. New York, Churchill Livingstone, 1988, p 102.
7. Grieve GP: Common Vertebral Joint Problems. New York, Churchill Livingstone, 1988, p 106.
8. Haas SS, MacCartee CC, Wells JR: Medical Aspects of the Men's Professional Tennis Tour (in preparation).
9. Hageman CE, Lehman RC: Stretching, strengthening and conditioning for the competitive tennis player. Sports Med 7:211–216, 1988.
10. Hall H, Iceton JA: Back school: An overview with specific reference to the Canadian Back Education Units. Clin Orthop 179:10, 1983.
11. Johnson TR: Children Are Different. Columbus, OH, Ross Laboratories, 1978.
12. Kibler WB, McQueen C, Uhl T: Fitness evaluations and fitness findings in competitive junior tennis players. Sports Med 7:403–416, 1988.
13. Kisner C, Colby LA: Therapeutic Exercise Foundations and Techniques. Philadelphia, FA Davis, pp 261–267.
14. Lehman RC: Sports Medicine: Racquet Sports. Philadelphia, WB Saunders, 1988, xi.
15. Loehr J: Test of a champion. World Tennis pp 30–32. Sept 1989.
16. Markolf KL: Deformation of the thoracolumbar intervertebral joint in response to external load. J Bone Joint Surg 54A:511–533, 1972.
17. McKenzie IA: The Lumbar Spine, Mechanical Diagnosis and Therapy. Waikanae, New Zealand, Spinal Publications, 1981.
18. Moll JMH, Wright V: Normal range of spinal mobility. Ann Rheum Dis 30:381, 1971.
19. Morgans LF, Scovil JA, Bass KM: Heart rate responses during singles and doubles competition in racquetball. Phys Sports Med 12:64–72, 1984.
20. Nachemson A: Work for all: For those with low back pain as well. Clin Orthop 179:77–85, 1983.
21. Prentice WE: Comparison of static stretching and PNF stretching for improved hip joint flexibility. Athletic Training 18:56–59, 1983.
22. Seimon LP: Low Back Pain: Clinical Diagnosis and Management. New York, Appleton-Century-Crofts, 1983.
23. Surberg PR: Flexibility exercise re-examined. Athletic Training 18:37–40, 1983.
24. Troup JDG: Biomechanics of the vertebral column. Physiology 65:238, 1979.
25. Twomey LT, Taylor JR: Factors influencing ranges of movement in the lumbar spine. In Grieve GP (ed): Modern Manual Therapy of the Vertebral Column. Edinburgh, Churchill Livingstone, 1986, p 112.
26. Twomey LT, Taylor JR: Flexion creep deformation and hysteresis in the lumbar vertebral column. Spine 7:116, 1982.
27. White AA, Panjabi MM: Clinical Biomechanics of the Spine. Philadelphia, JB Lippincott, 1978, pp 35–42.
28. White AA, Panjabi MM: The basic kinematics of the human spine. Spine 3:12, 1978.

Chapter 16

THE LUMBAR SPINE IN FOOTBALL

F. Alan Barber, MD, FACS

The lumbar spine is the part of the spine most susceptible to injury.[1] Due to the collision nature of the game of American football, the player can expect to sustain impacts and stresses from a variety of directions. The type of lumbar spine injury is consequently dependent upon the variations in magnitude, direction, and point of impact. Wooden reports 6% of high school players sustain lower back injuries.[23] Twenty-seven percent of 506 consecutive college players developed lower back problems during their careers.[19] The incidence of spondylolisthesis in professional interior linemen is reported to be one in three,[5] which is not surprising since half of college interior linemen have back pain.[7]

Most acute back injuries are the result of the hyperextension commonly seen as the lineman drives forward pushing against his opponent. The extension of the lumbar spine transmits this force and applies a shear stress that can lead to a pars interarticularis injury.[3]

Compression in line with the axis of the spine (usually produced by the normal body's weight while standing) is greatly increased by head-on impacts normally occurring during blocking or tackling. These forces are often in combination with torsional loads from twisting and spinning of the players' bodies as they try to redirect the opposing players' movement or down the ball carrier.

Tension forces resulting from distraction of various elements of the lumbar spine can occur by themselves, as when the player is stopped by tackling the legs while the upper body continues its forward motion, or in combination with compressive forces, as with bending. Forward flexion on the trunk, for example, places compressive forces on the anterior vertebral body and tension on the posterior elements.

A third force to be considered is a shear force applied parallel to the horizontal plane of the spine. This force is increased by the tilt of the lumbosacral angle. As the tilt increases, so does the shear force. Rotational stresses, as might be applied by a tackler trying to bring down a ball carrier, are limited by the lumbar facets. Forces that exceed the lumbar facet joints' ability to withstand the stress result in fractures in this area.

PRESEASON SCREENING

In order to forestall many of the more obvious potential problems that may occur in a football season, a thorough preseason screening examination should be made of each participant. In the absence of any complaints or history of injury, this may be rather brief. However, should the player indicate a history of back injury, the athlete should be questioned as to whether the injury required treatment, how long he was unable to play, and if recovery was full. An examination should look for excessive lumbar lordosis and scoliosis. While evaluating the athlete for scoliosis, palpation of the iliac crests from the back will help identify potential pelvic obliquity and leg length discrepancy. At this point palpation of the lumbar spine can be done to look for a "step off" that may suggest spondylolisthesis.[23]

General flexibility tests should include both forward bending, the patient attempting to touch fingertips to the floor with the knees extended, and side bending to both sides. If forward flexibility is reduced, a sitting straight-leg-raising test will better assess hamstring tightness that might suggest spondylolisthesis. Pressing on both anterior superior iliac spines in the supine athlete will distract and quickly assess the sacroiliac joints. Abdominal muscle strength should be sufficient to perform a bent-knee sit-up that holds the chest about 6 inches off the mat at least 10 seconds. For this test, the arms should be crossed on the chest.[23]

STRAINS AND SPRAINS

Lower back injuries are common in football and usually are due to a contusion from the bruising effects of a direct blow, a strain from tearing or stretching of the muscles or tendons, or a sprain from injury to the ligamentous structures. These are commonly due to blows to the back, lifting, or twisting. In the adolescent, a predisposing factor to ligmentous and musculotendinous injury is the growth spurt.[16] During this phase, if the paraspinous tissues do not grow at the same rate as bone, the resultant tight lumbodorsal fascia and hamstrings combine with weak abdominal muscles to place the athlete at greater risk for back pain. Emphasis on maintaining flexibility as well as judicious strength training will mitigate this situation.

Regardless of the cause, tight hamstrings, weak abdominal muscles, and hip flexion contractures increase lumbar lordosis. If there is coexisting degenerative disc disease and facet joint disease, the increased lordotic position creates a relative spinal stenosis or foraminal encroachment that can produce symptoms.[20]

FRACTURES

Fractures in the lumbar spine can be divided into those that affect the vertebral body and those that affect the posterior elements. The most common type of vertebral body fracture is the compression type. This occurs primarily at the anterior vertebral body, which is the weakest site in the lumbar vertebra due to the lack of horizontal trabeculations.[11] Rapid flexion, especially associated with vertebral compression, can cause these injuries.

Young athletes with open growth plates can develop fractures of the vertebral endplate in which the nucleus pulposis herniates into the vertebral body. The compressive strength of the nucleus pulposis is greater than that of the cartilaginous endplate and consequently, with excessive compressive forces, the endplate is more likely to fracture. This may occur by a gradual weakening of the endplate, and as the endplate becomes worn and fractured, the disc may dehydrate at an accelerated rate.[14] Under vertical compression the vertebral endplate bulges in toward the vertebral body and decreases the blood in the cancellous bone.[6] The normal disc is stronger than bone, and the normal nucleus pulposis is noncompressible and tends to maintain its shape whereas the vertebral endplate will fail at loads greater than 2300 N.[6]

Some athletic injuries result in a horizontal fracture of the vertebral body when there is rapid and forceful rotation of the trunk beyond the normal range of rotation.[6] This injury is often associated with tearing of the supporting lumbar spine ligaments, including both the anterior and posterior ligamentous support. A forceful flexion or flexion rotation injury, such as occurs when the feet are fixed with cleated shoes to the ground, can result in this fracture.

Other common fractures of the lumbar spine include fractures of the transverse processes or the spinous processes. These may result from a direct blow.[18] A sudden strong contraction by the psoas and quadratus lumborum can also cause this type of injury. These fractures can also be the result of forceful movements of the trunk avulsing the attachments of the muscles. In one study, four of six lumbar fractures involved the transverse processes. All of these were found in either offensive halfbacks or offensive ends. The other two fractures were vertebral body compression fractures in defensive linemen.[2]

DISC HERNIATIONS

Many different types of forces can cause injury to the lumbar disc, but are most probably aggravated by anterior shear forces during conditioning by weight lifting. The lumbosacral angle is increased by forward flexion, consequently increasing the shear component of the compressive forces. It has been hypothesized that disc injury is initiated by such a shearing force, which separates the cartilaginous endplate from the adjacent vertebral bodies, and with further fissuring and weakness of the annulus, nucleus pulposis protrudes through the annulus afterward.

In one study of 12 college players treated for clinical symptoms and signs of herniated disc disease, 6 failed conservative care and underwent surgery. Clinically, the symptoms were confined to one extremity, with radiculopathy confined to the thigh. Surgically, 2 of the 6 were found to have a fracture of the superior facet of L5 that was compressing the L5 root. Also, only 2 of the 6 who underwent surgery ever returned to play football.[4]

Herniated discs can cause back pain in adolescents as well. This group may be more difficult to diagnose, with the presenting signs confined to hamstring and lumbodorsal fascia tightness. Whether the symptoms are obscure or have a typical sciatic pain distribution, initial treatment should be rest and analgesics.[20] Epidural cortisone has been reported to be useful in chronic cases.[10]

NEURAL ARCH DEFECTS

Neural arch defects have been variously reported as existing in 5% to 20% of athletes. Hoshini reported a 20% incidence of spondylolysis in the lumbar spine of 677 Japanese high school and university athletes.[8] Spondylosis can occur in as many as 50% of interior linemen.[7]

It has been suggested that this defect in the pars interarticularis results from repeated trauma, and fatigue fractures occur due to repeated stress.[22] The athlete often complains of low back pain with spasm and hamstring tightness. Some authors believe that these stress fractures occur more commonly in athletic activities that place heavy loads on the spine while in hyperlordosis.[17] Such activities would include weight lifting and other training techniques associated with football and wrestling.[13] It has also been suggested that a relationship exists between spondylolysis and heavier athletes and those with stronger back musculature.[8] However, in a group of college football players followed for all 4 years of college play, only 2.4% developed spondylolysis while in college.[13] Another study found that a player with low back pain and spondylolysis had no significant increase in time lost from practices and games when compared to a player with low back pain but no spondylolysis.[19]

Spondylolysis occurs most frequently at L5. The pars interarticularis is the weakest part of the neural arch. However, a defect at this site is unlikely to curtail a football career.[13] Repeated stresses in hyperflexion and hyperextension, as well as doing rapid rotational movement, are thought to be the cause of fatigue fracture in the pars interarticularis.[21] Although spondylolysis is asymptomatic in many individuals after an injury, the fibrous tissue present in the defect may be uncomfortable from stretching. This discomfort can persist for weeks to months. If treatment such as rest, medication, and physical therapy does not clear the problem, and radiographs are normal, a bone scan may be positive for a fatigue fracture in the acute stage.[13] McCarroll recommends bracing to allow the fracture to heal in this situation.

SPONDYLOLISTHESIS

Bilateral defects in the pars interarticularis can lead to slippage of one vertebral body in relation to the vertebral segment immediately below it. This is spondylolisthesis. Spondylolisthesis has been reported to occur in approximately 2% of adults.[15] This is usually at L5–S1. Various classifications exist to grade the degree of a slippage, but it is most commonly agreed that first-degree spondylolisthesis results when a superior vertebra exhibits a forward slip of not more than 30% of the diameter of the inferior vertebra. A second-degree slip is one in which the vertebra slips forward 30% to 50% of the diameter of the inferior vertebra. A third-degree slip is between 50% and 75%, and a fourth-degree slip of the vertebra slips completely over the vertebra below.

Jackson et al. feel that the major cause of pars defects in athletes is repeated trauma to the lumbar spine.[10] There is a greater incidence of these defects in contact sports such as football and the martial arts. Interior linemen who repeatedly hyperextend the spine in a 3-point stance place additional stress on this area. Wiltse et al. suggested that spondylolysis is a fatigue fracture primarily caused by repeated trauma and stress, rather than an isolated single traumatic event.[22] These authors also suggest that pars interarticularis defects differ from other fatigue fractures because they develop at an earlier age, have a hereditary predisposition expressed because of minor trauma, and do not seem to heal in contrast to other fatigue fractures in other sites that almost always heal.

A typical history of a young athlete with spondylolisthesis starts with low back pain at age 15 or 16. The pain will radiate into both thighs and is worse during activity and decreased by rest.[12] The forces that act to displace one vertebra into spondylolisthesis include the effect of gravity above the level of the slip, the activity of spinal muscles, and movement.[21]

CONCLUSION

Although these are the most common causes of lumbar spine problems, other conditions such as neoplasms and infection must be considered when the athlete with persistent low back pain does not respond to conservative care and modifications in activity. Pain into the leg can be the result of vascular claudication and should be considered if the symptoms resolve rapidly with rest. Urologic and gastrointestinal conditions can also present as low back pain and should be part of the differential diagnosis.

REFERENCES

1. Alexander MJL: Biomechanical aspects of lumbar spine injuries in athletes: A review. Can J Appl Sport Sci 10:1–20, 1985.
2. Bowerman JW, McDonnell EJ: Radiology of athletic injuries—football. Radiology 117:33–36, 1975.
3. Cantu RC: Lumbar spine injuries. In Cantu RC (ed): The Exercising Adult. Lexington, MA, Collamore Press, 1980.
4. Day AL, Friedman WA, Indelicato PA: Observations on the treatment of lumbar disk disease in college football players. Am J Sports Med 15:72–75, 1987.
5. Dominquez RH: The Complete Book of Sports Medicine. New York, Charles Scribner, 1979.
6. Evans DC: Biomechanics of spinal injury. In Gonza ER, Harrington IJ (eds): Biomechanics of Musculo-skeletal Injury. Baltimore, Williams and Wilkins, 1982.
7. Ferguson RJ, McMaster JH, Staniski CL: Low back pain in college football linemen. J Sports Med 2:63–69, 1974.
8. Hoshina H: Spondylolysis in athletes. Physician Sportsmed 8(9):75–79, 1980.
9. Jackson DW, Wiltse L, Cirincione R: Spondylolysis in the female gymnast. Clin Orthop Rel Res 117:68–73, 1976.
10. Jackson DW: Low back pain in young athletes: Evaluation of stress reaction and discogenic problems. Am J Sports Med 7:364–366, 1979.
11. Kapandji IA: The Physiology of the Joints. Vol 3, The Trunk and Vertebral Column. New York, Churchill Livingstone, 1974.
12. Leach RE: Disc disease, spondylolysis and spondylolisthesis. Athletic Training 12(1):13–17, 1977.
13. McCarroll JR, Miller JM, Ritter MA: Lumbar spondylolysis and spondylolisthesis in college football players. A prospective study. Am J Sports Med 14:404–406, 1986.
14. McIntosh A: Lower back problems—the engineer's viewpoint. Future Health 5(2):4–5 Summer, 1983.
15. Magora A: Conservative treatment in spondylolisthesis. Clin Orthop Rel Res 117:74–79, 1976.
16. Micheli LJ: Low back pain in the adolescent: Differential diagnosis. Am J Sports Med 7:362–364, 1979.
17. Monticelli G, Ascani B: Spondylolysis and spondylolisthesis. Acta Orthop Scand 46:498–506, 1975.
18. Roy S, Irvin R: Sports Medicine—Prevention, Evaluation, Management and Rehabilitation. Englewood Cliffs, NJ, Prentice Hall, 1983.
19. Semon RL, Spengler D: Significance of lumbar spondylolysis in college football players. Spine 6:172–174, 1981.
20. Slack CM: The spine in sports. Compr Ther 6(9):68–74, 1980.
21. Troup JDG: Mechanical factors in spondylolisthesis and spondylolysis. Clin Orthop Rel Res 117:59–67, 1976.
22. Wiltse LL, Widell EH Jr, Jackson DW: Fatigue fracture: The basic lesion in isthmic spondylolisthesis. J Bone Joint Surg 57A:17–22, 1975.
23. Wooden MJ: Preseason screening of the lumbar spine. J Orthop Sport Phys Ther 3:6–10, 1981.

Chapter 17

CERVICAL SPINE INJURIES IN FOOTBALL PLAYERS

Robert G. Watkins, MD, William H. Dillin, MD, and James Maxwell, MD

There is probably no more difficult a decision for the football team physician or the practitioner treating an amateur or professional football player in the office than the decision regarding the player's return to play following a neck injury. Football is a unique sport, involving (1) high-velocity collisions, sometimes between players of various sizes, skill, and preparation; (2) use of the helmet and head for spearing, face tackling, and blocking; and (3) unexpected deforming loads on the head/shoulder alignment.

Over the past several decades, neck injuries in football have been on the rise, but more information has become available due to the increasing awareness and attention of team physicians. Albright,[3] for example, found a neck injury incidence causing 4% *lost* time, nearly one-half of the cases with neurologic involvement. He also found that 50% of high school football players had had significant neck pain preceding any documented neck injury. It has been our experience that the majority of football players at all levels have had neck pain to some degree, though there is probably no predilection in the offensive or defensive player. Serious neck injuries are uncommon, but once injuries occur, recurrences are common.

It is incumbent upon the physician who undertakes care of cervical spine injuries to understand the syndromes; the gravity and breadth of the problems; and their prevention, treatment, and care. He should be well-versed in their immediate care, be familiar with the transport of the injured player, and be able to adequately work up the case so that an intelligent assessment of future risk can be made. Recommendations for the adolescent player and the professional may differ, but every effort must be undertaken to make decisions based on the medical facts of the case. Contract provisions, disability contracts, the player's desire to play, the desires of others (coaches, team owner, wife, girlfriend, mother, father) are factors to be avoided in the decision making. Everyone, regardless of what is said, is looking to the doctor for *medical* advice only. Trying to do someone a "favor" can be disastrous. There is an old orthopedic surgical admonition to "stay close to the bone." Stay as close to the medical facts as possible in cervical spine injuries.

THE BURNER SYNDROME

The **burner** or **stinger** is the prototypical neck injury sustained in this setting and is seen a number of times by most team physicians. Typically, the player will complain of transient loss of function accompanied by searing, lancinating pain down an arm. There is temporary paralysis, but symptoms usually last only up to 10 to 15 minutes. Trace neurologic deficit may persist for months. The mechanism for injury may either be a distraction-type stretch injury, with the head having been knocked to the opposite side of the painful arm and the ipsilateral shoulder knocked down, or cervical spine extension-compression and rotation toward the arm with the burner. The latter mechanism is essentially the Spurling maneuver, in which the head is extended and rotated toward the involved arm, and compression is applied to the forehead.

The upper trunk of the brachial plexus is taut when the head is flexed away from the depressed shoulder, thus easily explaining one of the known mechanisms but not the one seen clinically. Beginning inside the canal, cervical nerves are supported by the dentate ligaments. They are relatively free from attachment in the medial foramina but are attached by fibrous tissue to the vertebral artery and at the distal intervertebral foramina. The narrowing of the foramina with extension, compression, and ipsilateral rotation must affect nerve roots at the intervertebral foramen, accounting for the second mechanism of injury. A positive Spurling maneuver produces radiating pain down the ipsilateral arm in cervical radiculopathy, owing to foraminal stenosis or a herniated cervical disc.

Initially, the player complains of total arm weakness and burning. As the symptoms resolve, a C6 distribution numbness (thumb, index finger) persists, and motor deficit may be found in shoulder abduction and wrist and finger extension, strength then returning from proximal to distal. The player cranes his neck forward and resists extension and rotation. Head compression maneuver or the Spurling maneuver at this point would produce the symptoms.

PREVENTION OF BURNERS

The primary preventive rule for burners is wearing properly fitted shoulder pads. Shoulder pads should accomplish four basic functions: (1) absorb the shock; (2) protect the shoulders; (3) fit the chest; and (4) fix the midcervical spine to the trunk. The typical shoulder pad (Fig. 1) is a soft-arc, very thin-padded material that has questionable shock-absorbing properties and fits the chest in a semi-arc-type of configuration. The fixation to the chest is less than ideal and allows sliding of the shoulder pads on the shoulder during contact. In order to fit the chest properly, the pad should be a more of an A-frame with very rigid and

FIGURE 1. Typical shoulder pad of a professional defensive end.

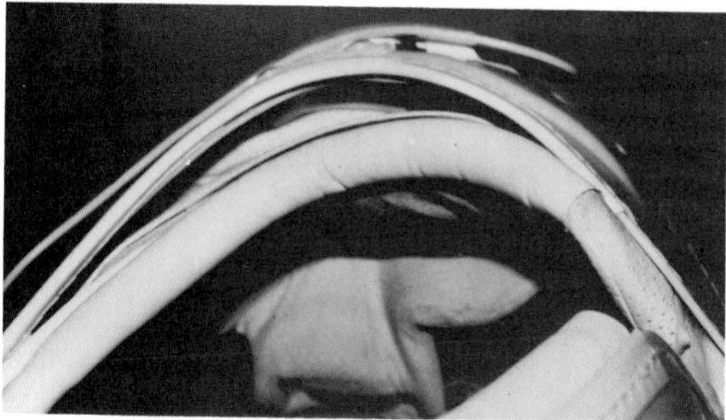

long anterior and posterior panels. The shoulder pads should contour well to the subxiphoid portion of the chest and fit snugly around the chest. A proper shoulder pad should incorporate many of the characteristics of a proper cervicothoracic orthosis. Because fixing the head to the chest is impossible in a football player, modification to the ideal must be made.

Immobilization of the cervical spine in any type of cervical brace requires rigid fixation to the chest. All studies evaluating fixation methods that include only the neck, such as a hard or soft cervical collar, demonstrate poor fixation and limitation of cervical spine motion. It is only when the base is extended and firmly fixed to the chest, as in a proper cervicothoracic orthosis, that restriction of cervical spine motion occurs. Some support, however, can be provided between chest and base of neck by the use of properly fitting neck pads, which effectively elevate the shoulder pad at the base of the neck, thereby "supporting" the lower cervical segments.

The majority of neck rolls are inadequate in that they are attached at the top of the shoulder pads and rotate away from the neck approximately 6 inches at the moment of contact. This rolling back of the shoulder pads further decreases protection for the cervical spine, especially in resisting compression. This mechanism is commonly seen in serious neck injuries and plays a major role in the burner syndrome. As the shoulder pad rolls back, the head coils into the hole in the shoulder pad. There is no protection against head compression in the extension, compression, and rotation mechanism of a burner. It is very difficult to place a collar roll on the back of the shoulder pads that can block extension during contact. One professional veteran used a stiff cervical collar that was tied tightly around his neck posteriorly and attached to shoulder pads by strings to the laces on the front of the pads. This was an attempt to prevent the extension seen with collar rolls.

Thick, comfortable, stiff pads at the base of the neck are the key. It is this support laterally at the base of the neck that offers fixation to the cervical spine. Some posterior support could be helpful but is very difficult to obtain. Higher, thicker, lateral pads that are tighter at the base of the neck can improve fixation of the cervical spine (Fig. 2), especially when the pad fits the chest and shoulders well.

A common method of adapting pads is to add lifters (Fig. 3). The lifters provide a pad at the base of the neck that supplements the typical shoulder pad. Often, the combination of lifters, the pre-existing pads, and the neck roll will all add to the improved fit of the pad laterally at the base of the neck (Fig. 4). Because most of the rotation of the cervical spine occurs at C1–2, it is believed

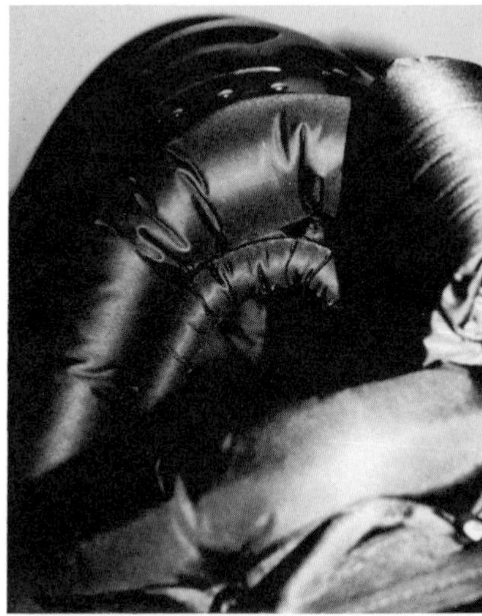

FIGURE 2. Well-constructed shoulder pad.

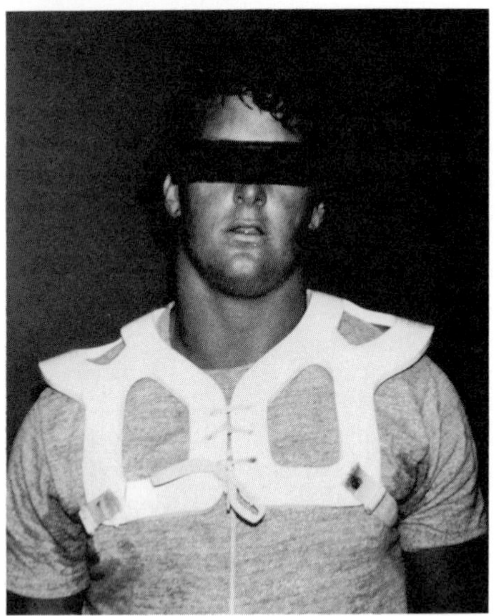

FIGURE 3. Lifters to provide additional neck support.

that this support should not limit the player's visibility and should provide some added support in the mid- and lower portion of the cervical spine. Figure 2 shows a shoulder pad that provides good padding for the base of the neck. Also, the tighter fit to the chest can be seen in the shape of the shoulder portion of this pad.

Regarding the shock-absorbing capability of the shoulder pad, proper fit to the chest is important in distributing the shock to the shoulders evenly over the pads and into the thorax. Better resistive padding and better plastics in the outer shoulder pads will absorb shock and allow the use of the shoulder in proper blocking and tackling techniques. Better shoulder protection should allow one to deemphasize the use of the head as a blocking and tackling instrument.

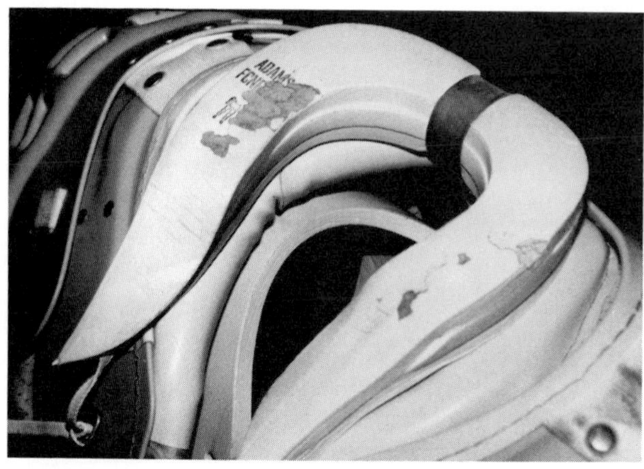

FIGURE 4. Modified shoulder pads.

TREATMENT OF BURNERS

When a player has a burner complaint during play, the physician needs to be aware of on-the-field care, proper transport of the player, initial history-taking and physical examination, radiographic techniques, and the need for additional tests. All of this must occur before short- and long-term recommendations can be made.

Initial Care

The decision-making process begins the moment the player injuries his neck. If the patient is conscious and up and running toward the bench, take him to the bench, sit him down on the bench, question him, and complete the evaluation on the bench. This is certainly the most common way in which people are evaluated for neck and arm pain during the game. If the player is lying down on the field, it is standard practice for the trainer to reach the player, start the evaluation, and call for the doctor.

The chief diagnostic obligation of a clinician involved in situations of this type is to diagnose a potentially unstable cervical spine that could lead to a major neurologic deficit after an initial injury. This diagnosis begins with the player down on the field. The doctor determines if there is a potential for an unstable spine and assesses the patient's condition. This leads to a therapeutic plan, beginning with assurances of vital function and protective transportation.

The player down on the field with neck and arm pain should be examined closely to determine first whether there is cervical spine injury. An unconscious player is treated as having an unstable cervical spine injury until proven otherwise. If his symptoms totally resolve, the player is usually walked to the sidelines and then reexamined on the bench or removed to the locker room for an x-ray study at that time. If he is not *totally* asymptomatic, it is important to insure a proper airway. This can usually be done regardless of position without moving the player inappropriately. If the airway is a problem—if there is choking, or evidence of swallowed tongue, or if the mouth is not clear—then clear the player's mouth and turn him onto his back as one does for an unstable spinal cord injury.

Start the diagnostic evaluation by determining whether the patient has or just had motor-sensory loss. Does he have spinal pain? Was he unconscious? Is there neck or arm pain? Is there spine and leg pain?

The initial history and physical are critically important. Many times continue-to-play decisions made months later depend on the facts obtained in this crucial initial period. The patient must be carefully questioned as to what sensations he felt; whether he had or has weakness, numbness, tingling, inability to move his legs, move his toes, squeeze his hands, or move his arms. The length of time of involvement of the symptoms must be carefully documented. Stiffness can be a sign of an occult fracture.

Transportation

Cervical pain, cervical tenderness, and neurologic symptoms in the extremities are all criteria for spinal cord injury transport. **When in doubt, do it.** If the technique is a standard, well-practiced one, it should take only a few minutes. Then, re-evaluate on the sidelines.

The turning technique involves first having five or six people to move the patient. Trying to move the patient with three is inappropriate. The most frequent error in transport is not having enough people available who know how to transport a player with a potentially unstable cervical spine injury. The most important key to the technique is to have one person controlling the head and shoulders, who is not responsible for any weight of the transfer (Fig. 5). Therefore, there are at least four people, one on each side of the shoulders and one on each side of the waist, possibly a fifth one at the feet, who are handling the weight of the transfer, and one key person responsible for the head and neck, fixing the head to the shoulders during the transfer (Fig. 6).

The person on the head and neck is the chief and calls the moves. Having the chief person holding *only* the head is very dangerous. Holding only the head and trying to keep it aligned with the body is very difficult to do. Try it on an awake subject. Have someone hold his head only and let the subject tell you how much he felt his neck move during that period of time. The best way is for the chief person to clasp the trapezius, clavicle, and scapula if possible. Grabbing the inside of the shoulder pads and the trapezius is second best. The chief should cradle the forearms along the side of the head and neck, holding the head

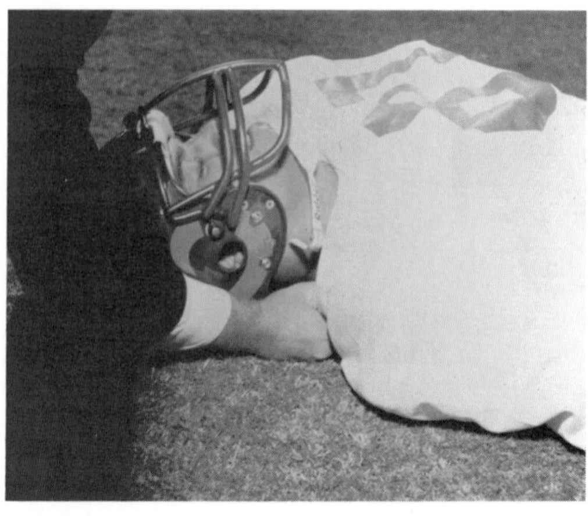

FIGURE 5. The method of immobilizing the head to the trunk. The person in charge holds the trapezius-clavicle-scapula area with his hands and holds the head between his forearms.

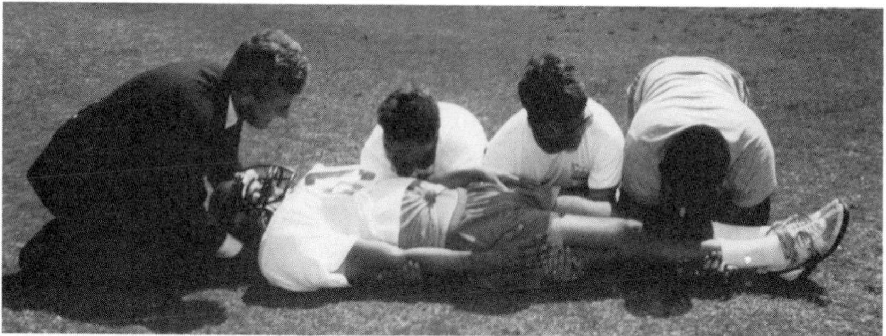

FIGURE 6. Multiman carry. The chief immobilizes the head and neck and calls the signals. Three men on each side of the body (the three on the near side are not pictured) join hands and lift. The spine board is introduced underneath.

between the forearms. Simultaneously, an additional person in the transport team can hold the head to the forearms of the chief. With the head held between the chief's forearms and fixed to the shoulders and pads, the other members position themselves on each side of the player, reach underneath, clasp hands, and lift. A back board can then be placed under the player. The chief calls every move and controls the head and shoulders. The patient can be moved very safely with this method.

If the player is face down, the chief rotates his arms and takes a similar hold. The additional man to hold the head to the chief's forearms is imperative in this circumstance. As the others turn the patient over, the chief's arms will rotate into the standard position.

Do not remove the helmet on the field. There should be equipment available for removal of the face mask on an emergency basis as quickly as possible. By cutting away the face mask quickly, the airway can be cleared and there should be no reason for removing the helmet. Removing the helmet is very difficult to do without producing neck flexion. Move the patient onto the stretcher and have the chief maintain control of the head and neck during transport off the field to the locker room. Remember, the shoulders are very large and bulky and the head has a tendency to hyperextend; therefore, the head should be supported.

Secondary Evaluation

At the bench or in the locker room, decisions must be made and are dependent upon an adequate history (discussed above) and the key physical findings. For example, players are not returned to play with any symptoms or motor weakness in the arms. Physical examination should consist of a complete neurologic examination, head compression test, Spurling's and Adson's maneuvers, resistive head pressure, and cervical range of motion. If there is any doubt, it is far safer to leave the helmet in place, pending satisfactory lateral radiograph. If suspicion of serious cervical spine injury remains, take the helmet off in the hospital, with definitive treatment modalities available. If it is safe to remove the helmet locally, then remove it just as you would with an unstable spine. If not already done, cut the face mask off. The chief reaches inside the helmet-shoulder interval from the anterior and holds the occiput to the trapezius with his hands.

Two assistants pull out the sides of the helmet and remove it in a cephalad direction as the chief's hands are moved into the standard position.

Stadium x-ray facilities available to professional teams allow detailed radiographic evaluation. Without these facilities, and when there are indications for an emergency x-ray exam, such as significant neurologic deficit and severe neck tenderness, then transport as one does for a spinal cord injury.

When is it prudent to remove a player from the game? The decision hinges upon two key criteria. The first criterion is radiating arm pain and loss of function, such as paresthesias and weakness. Radiating arm pain and neurologic deficit can be indicators of a more serious problem, such as spinal instability, that can lead to a permanent neurologic deficit, either cord or radicular in nature. For this reason alone, until complete diagnostic evaluation is carried out, the player should not play.

Loss of cervical range of motion is the second key finding that should disallow return to play. This finding could be the only residual sign of the unstable cervical spine lesion. Pain perception may be altered by the emotion of the game, but experienced sideline clinicians will restrict the player from playing if he has a stiff neck or a stiff painful neck. This may indicate an occult fracture. Other signs of fracture can be neck pain with head compression and pain when resisting hand pressure to the head. Any lower extremity involvement at the time of head or neck injury can be difficult to interpret.

"Numb all over" may be loss of consciousness, a transitory quadriplegia, or nothing. Usually, if it lasts 1 to 5 seconds and there are no residual symptoms, the player walks off the field. Any lingering symptoms or persistent lower extremity weakness or numbness should be examined closely and the patient transported as one does for a spine injury. Lower extremity numbness and tingling or abnormal gait should eliminate the player from competition until diagnostic evaluation can be obtained. If there is lower extremity involvement (even transitory) that can definitely be identified as characteristic of myelopathy, the player should not be allowed to return to the game that day. If there is transitory neurapraxia in the arm, the player can return. Loss of cervical range of motion and/or neurologic deficit are the chief criteria for removing a player from the game; no return should be permitted as long as these symptoms persist.

X-ray Evaluation

When locker room x-ray studies are available, this evaluation should consist of anteroposterior, lateral, two oblique (when possible), and flexion-extension films. In a patient with residual stiffness in his neck, the flexion-extension films may be worthless. They could fail to disclose a subtle ligamentous instability and/or partial subluxation owing to a facet fracture. The flexion-extension x-ray study should be considered valid only if full range of flexion-extension motion is seen on the film (Case I). It is important to see the entire cervical spine, including C7. This can be difficult in football players. Boger straps are passive stretch straps that have few equals in terms of their ability to demonstrate a full x-ray view of the cervical spine in patients with shoulder pads and large shoulders. We have not found a circumstance in which the Boger straps did not show C7 under these emergency conditions (Fig. 7).

If Boger straps are not available, an assistant standing at the foot of the x-ray table can place the patient's feet onto his chest and grasp the patient's hands. By pulling distally on the hands against the resistive force of his own chest to the

CASE I. A, B, Flexion-extension films of a 17-year-old high school football player; flexion films show the V-shaped displacement of the ring of C-1 on the odontoid. A 5-mm displacement at the top of the ring and a 2-mm displacement at the base of the ring should be treated as a partial transverse ligament tear.

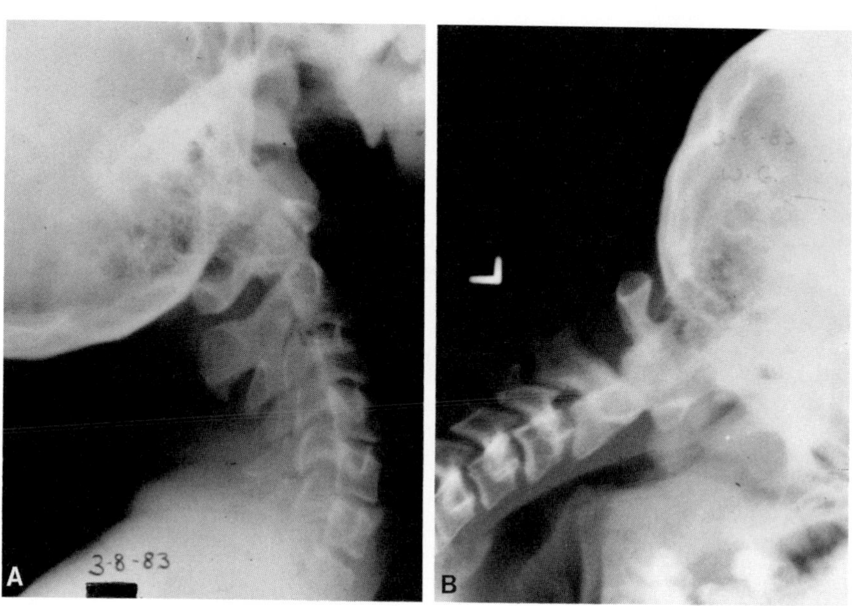

patient's lower extremities, the assistant can be effective in uncovering the C7 segment otherwise hidden from radiographic view. With adequate results from flexion-extension films and plain x-rays, and normal cervical range of motion and some mild residual neck pain, the patient can return to the game. Players are not sent back into the game with residual numbness, tingling, dysesthesias, weakness, or pain radiating into the arm.

Measure for ligamentous instability on the flexion-extension lateral films by drawing lines parallel to the inferior endplates of each vertebral body. The angle between any two adjacent lines should not be 11 degrees greater than the angle measured between the pair above *or* below. Horizontal translation greater than 3.5 mm may be another indication of ligamentous instability. Dynamic instability may also be noted in that only the flexion films show translation. This may be due to facet fracture, pillar fracture, or major ligamentous injury.

One difficult aspect of the radiographic evaluation is to determine whether the problem is an acute injury, an old injury, or an asymptomatic finding. One complicating factor is the presence of a hypermobile segment over stiff, arthritic segments. Many athletes who do neck strengthening exercises on a regular, consistent basis, especially starting at a young age, have relative osteoarthritic changes at certain lower cervical levels. The stiffness of these levels produces a relative increase in mobility at levels just above these stiffened segments (Fig. 8).

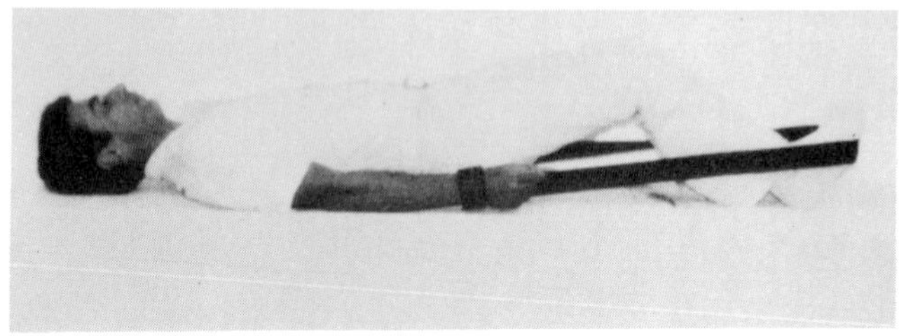

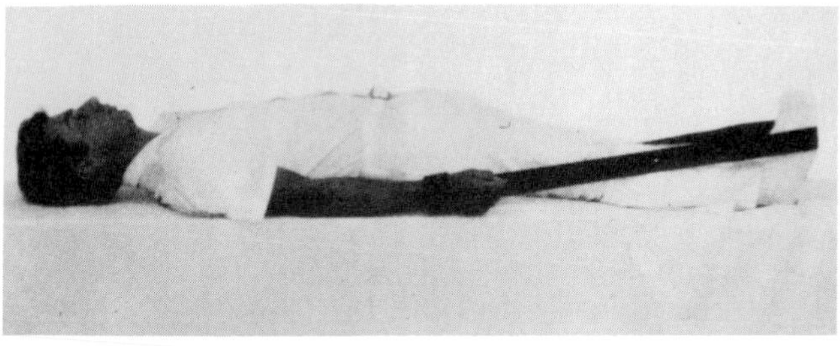

FIGURE 7. Boger straps. The Velcro adjustments make the length adjustable. The straps can be used in an unconscious patient by pushing down on the knees and holding them down with a sandbag.

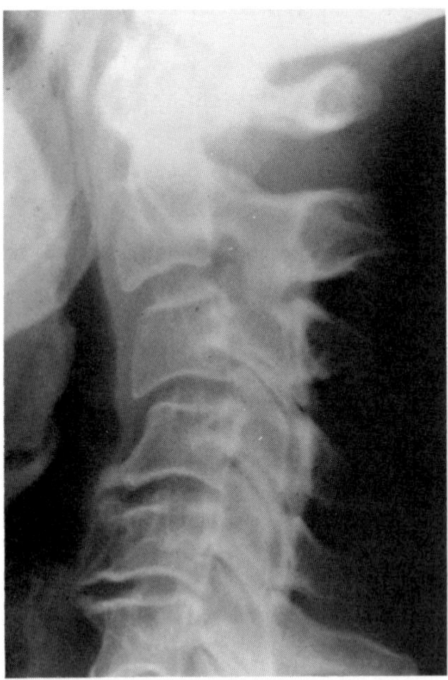

FIGURE 8. Flexion-extension films often indicate only which segment has the most motion and do not indicate an acute ligamentous injury. This x-ray study from a 52-year-old ex-wrestler and football player demonstrates a hypermobile segment above the level of an osteoarthritic stiff segment. Pain from a neck of this type may very well be at the hypermobile segment or the stiff osteoarthritic segment. If he was involved in a traumatic episode, it would be very difficult to distinguish this from an acute ligamentous injury. Currently, active professional football players will have more subtle amounts of arthritis and stiffness in certain spinal segments. There will often be hypermobile and stiff segments that must be evaluated for acute injuries.

Of course, the ideal x-ray study would help identify an area of ligamentous instability owing to a recent injury. Because this is seldom possible, it must be determined whether the hypermobile segment is the result of a recent injury. An excellent way of determining this is using the averaging technique for the amount of kyphotic displacement; that is, if there is no motion in the lower segments, it should be even harder to produce a dynamic instability measuring greater than 11 degrees differences on film. A fixed deformity rarely meets criteria for instability.

Additional Tests

Order a CT scan if temporary quadriplegia persists beyond the briefest sensation of "the quadriburner." Order a CT scan if radicular dysfunction persists beyond 7 to 10 days. Of course, myelopathy should be worked up by a spinal consultant as soon as possible.

If you order the study, be prepared to deal with the consequences. The key to the importance of certain findings, such as CT changes, requires relating the studies as specifically as possible to the patient's clinical findings. Remember that in the general population at least 30% of CT scans will have abnormalities, and cervical CT scans in football players inevitably show abnormalities.

Ordering diagnostic tests for football players is similar to ordering diagnostic tests for anyone else. If there is reason for concern about danger to the patient, order the tests every time. When in doubt, order them. There is no reason for x-ray studies if the results will not change the diagnosis, the treatment, or the prognosis. An x-ray finding that does not affect the treatment plan is seldom a medical necessity. Any diagnostic study may reveal totally asymptomatic lesions that have nothing to do with the current problem but necessitate in themselves serious decision making concerning their implications to the patient. The clinician should be prepared to treat lesions found on diagnostic studies and to make recommendations about potentially symptomatic lesions that do not match the clinical syndrome. Changes found on x-ray studies can affect the future of a football player. Professional football players hurt during play are employees injured at work, and recommendations about future disability and compensation must be made about every anatomic lesion and symptom present. Often, the prognosis is extremely important in athletes. Teams need to know as precisely as possible how long the patient will be disabled in order to make appropriate roster adjustments. The player, agent, and team often need to know what can be expected for the future, that is, what level of play can be possible or expected based on a certain injury. The safest way to order diagnostic studies is as described initially; order according to the best medical diagnostic and treatment plan for the patient involved.

The diagnosis upon which the treatment is based is very important. A common problem involves referring to a symptom complex as a strain, such as cervical or lumbar strain, and subsequently having a diagnostic study such as a CT scan read out as a disc herniation. This can be a difficult situation for the clinician and the patient. In order to prevent this sequence of events, it is necessary either to report an open, flexible clinical diagnosis or to pinpoint the exact anatomic problem prior to giving any diagnosis.

A direct chain of communication is important to avoid diagnostic and treatment conflicts. Just as the spinal consultant reports to the orthopedic surgeon or the medical director, he or she has a primary obligation to the player as a patient. Again, open, frank discussion with the player about diagnosis, prognosis, treatment, risks, and future problems is of maximum importance. The proper way to do it is always to tell the player and the team the same thing.

CERVICAL STENOSIS IN FOOTBALL PLAYERS

At times, the diagnostic workup will demonstrate stenosis of the cervical canal, previously asymptomatic.

Congenital stenosis is typified by short pedicles in a funnel-shaped canal.

Developmental stenosis is not uncommon in strength-sport players. The cervical bony anatomy thickens in response to stress just as do the ligaments, capsular structures, and muscles, thereby causing spinal canal narrowing.

Acquired stenosis can be due to cervical spondylosis, bone spurs, disc bulges, bulges of the ligamentum flavum occurring with disc-space narrowing, and osteophytes on the facet joints, all contributing to the cervical stenosis.

Measurement of Cervical Stenosis

There are different techniques for measuring the size of the spinal canal in order to assess the presence and degree of cervical stenosis. Pavlov and Torg[10] described a ratio of the central canal sagittal diameter to the vertebral body sagittal diameter measured on a lateral x-ray film in order to correct for x-ray magnification. Torg[10–14] determined that a ratio of 0.8 or less is indicative of cervical stenosis, but the determination was based on symptoms of transient cord neuropraxia in people with 0.8 or less and a lack of symptoms in people with ratios higher than that. In a group of myelopathic and radiculopathic non-football patients, Odor et al.[8] compared the ratio to CT scan central canal diameters and found the 0.8 ratio to be extremely sensitive but not as specific a measurement. Every patient who had a 0.8 ratio or less had 10 mm or less of central canal diameter, but there were patients with 10 mm or less who had a higher than a 0.8 ratio. With 17 ± 5 mm considered by most to be the normal sagittal diameter, 10 mm is considered to be abnormally small.

The contrast CT scan used in this study is the definitive technique for measuring central canal diameter and allows one to measure not only the central canal diameter but also a functional central canal diameter. The functional central canal diameter in the sagittal plane can be defined as the amount of canal available for the dural sac and spinal cord. The trefoil-shaped canal and the canal with a small, peaked, empty space, exactly in the midline, are canal shapes that do not allow full expansion of the dural sac and cord throughout its central diameter. Including a small, peaked area of space of possibly 2 mm when measuring the central canal diameter, when it will not accommodate the dural sac, is an incremental measurement of little consequence to cord function. This is certainly true in the lumbar spine, where lateral recess stenosis very commonly produces a major compression on the entire sac, leaving an empty dorsal portion of the spinal canal.

Matsuura et al.,[7] at Rancho Los Amigos Hospital, found strong correlation between the shape of the spinal canal and the predisposition to spinal cord injury from trauma. They used the ratio of sagittal to transverse diameter and found a strong positive correlation between this ratio and spinal cord injury when compared to controls. While the transverse diameter was inversely proportional and the sagittal diameter was directly proportional to the spinal cord injury, the area of the spinal canal was not. The exact mean ratio varied at different levels but was best correlated at the three most important levels, C4, C5, and C6. The control mean was approximately 0.6 and the spinal cord injury mean was 0.5. In this paper, the Torg ratio was stated to be not as powerful a discriminator as the sagittal diameter. Ogino et al.[9] used the sagittal to transverse "compression" ratio as an indicator of cord damage in myelopathy patients. This study, done on cadaveric specimens, shows a relationship between compression ratio and the degree of cord damage in people with cervical stenosis and myelopathy.

Although it may not be as "powerful an indicator" of risk of cord injury, the 0.8 Torg ratio may be more useful as a predictor of who will have recurrent episodes of transient neuropraxia. Also, the Torg ratio is measured on plain x-rays, whereas a CT scan must be used for the compression ratio. An entire team can be screened with one lateral x-ray per player using the Torg ratio.

The area of the canal as related to the area of the body has been found to be important in radiculopathy and myelopathy. Measuring surface area of the dural sac vs. the canal determines the surface area of canal available for the sac. The lateral portions of the canal and the area of the nerve root sleeves that will not accommodate much dural expansion should not be included in the area available for dural expansion.

There are individuals with a larger spinal cord or a smaller cord/sac ratio. Measuring exact cord shapes is dependent upon exacting radiological techniques. The presence of a large volume of dye circumferentially around the cord is a helpful sign, and the obliteration of dye ventrally can be an important sign of ventral compression.

Dynamic MRI has been used to demonstrate the narrowing of the cervical canal that occurs with extension. It is well known that the cervical spinal canal can narrow up to 2 mm in full extension as compared to neutral or flexion. Neurological tissue in the spine becomes slack and loose in extension and taut in flexion, and the spinal canal narrows in extension and opens in flexion. Numerous clinical syndromes are defined based upon how these dynamic factors affect spinal cord and nerve root function, in addition to exact central canal measurements and ratios. The biomechanics of the spinal column and neurological tissue motion must be considered in continue-to-play decisions when cervical stenosis is present.

Several facts are known about cervical stenosis in non-football players. Eismont[5] demonstrated that the greater the degree of cervical stenosis with a specific cervical spine injury, the greater the neurological deficit. Matsuura found that it was not just the central canal diameter but the shape of the canal that is important. The greater the compression ratio, the greater the chance of neurological deficit with a spine injury. Edwards[4] demonstrated that the patient with cervical canal stenosis is more likely to require surgery with a cervical disc herniation and less likely to be able to get well nonoperatively. Radicular pain is more common in smaller canals.

In the Epstein[6] study, there were 20 patients out of 200 admissions to an acute spinal cord injury unit that had no fracture or dislocation, but had complete neurological deficit. Among these cases were various diagnoses of cervical spondylosis, congenital stenosis, etc., but the study points to the fact that permanent neurological deficit can occur with spinal stenosis. The incidence of permanent tetraplegia in spinal column injury has varied from 4% to 70% of pediatric neck injuries, depending on the sample studied. Others have hypothesized on the etiology of quadriplegia without fracture dislocation to be a combination of injury to microvascular blood supply, longitudinal traction on the cord, acute disc prolapse, and/or compromise of the vertebral spinal arterial system. A common disorder in these cases is a central cord infarct. The incidence of permanent cord injury in football is most rare.

Factors in Decision Making in Transient Quadriparesis and Spinal Canal Stenosis

There are numerous decision-making factors in these cases. Among them are severity of the episode, extent of neurological deficit, severity of the symptoms, age, Torg ratio, player position, and neck size. The numerous methods of assessing cervical canal size bear consideration. Regardless of the canal diameter, there is certainly greater danger to someone who suffers a more severe neurological injury with the episode. A person who has had symptoms of myelopathy lasting over 6 months is obviously at greater risk for return of those symptoms than someone who had the episodes for 5 seconds. Each case will be a variation of severity of symptoms, type of neurological deficit, extent of neurological deficit, and longevity of the symptoms. There can be no set standard for measuring each case. The hemiparetic symptoms are different from unilateral arm dysesthesia. The important considerations are history and physical examination. You must document very, very carefully, through the history and physical, exactly what happened. The neurological examination must be immaculate in order to identify and quantify the deficit present.

The severity of the episode is important. We have found the rating system in Table 1 to be helpful in assessing the severity of the episode. Any existing neurological deficit due to a cord neurapraxia should be justification for exclusion from play in any case. As a general guideline, a combined extent/time rating less than 4 is a mild episode, a 4 to 7 a moderate episode, and 8 to 10 a severe episode. When combined with canal size, the severity of the episode can lead to some guidelines for recurrence (Table 2).

The Return-to-Play Decision

Armed with the information from the history of the player's injury, his initial physical exam, radiographic studies, additional tests, and knowledge of the major risk factors (extent, time, and narrowing), the team physician can formulate a reasonable recommendation. Each case is unique, but, in general, up to six additive risk points for all three factors would be considered minimum risk for return-to-play; 6 to 10, moderate; and 10 to 15, severe. For example, a brief episode with a 4-mm canal may absolutely preclude future play. The rating scale

TABLE 1. Rating Severity of Neurological Deficit

Rating	Extent of Deficit
1.	Unilateral arm numbness or dysesthesia, loss of strength
2.	Bilateral upper extremity loss of motor and sensory function
3.	Hemi arm and leg and trunk loss of motor and sensory function
4.	Transitory quadriparesis
5.	Transitory quadriplegia
Rating	**Time**
1.	Less than 5 minutes
2.	Less than 1 hour
3.	Less than 24 hours
4.	Less than 1 week
5.	Greater than 1 week

TABLE 2. Canal Narrowing Rating

Rating	Central Canal Diameter
1.	Greater than 12 mm
2.	Between 10 and 12 mm
3.	10 mm
4.	10 to 8 mm
5.	Less than 8 mm

is only a guideline. Clinically, we use the rating scale, Torg ratios, extenuating factors such as level of play, and risk vs. benefit to the patient, although the risk vs. benefit ratio is often an unquantifiable factor.

Reinjury is *always* a risk when the player returns to the collision environment of the football field. Albright[1,2] showed that, at the high school level, the reinjury rate after all neck injuries, one-third of which had extremity or neurologic symptoms, was 17.2%. The twice-injured players at all levels of play had an 87% chance of future injury. After a time-lost injury, the recurrent injury rate was 42% in the first season back, 62% in the next season, and 67% in future seasons. Therefore, there is a significant recurrent injury rate regardless of the type of injury received, and it is higher with the time-lost neck injury.

Prevention and Treatment

Prevention and treatment of these neck injuries go hand in hand, as most of the injuries are self-limited and most of the players can return to the sport. In addition to the shoulder pad modifications mentioned previously, we emphasize chest-out posturing and thoracic outlet obstruction exercises. It is well documented that using the head for contact in football produces dangerous mechanisms for cervical injury (Case II). This aspect of the sport should be condemned and "trained out" of the younger players. After total recovery from the pain, stiffness, and tenderness of the initial injury, maximum strength should be regained before allowing the player to return to action. Probably the greatest testament to conditioning is the ability of professional football players to deliver or receive high-impact blows as they do without injury.

Chest-out posturing produces three effects:

1. It opens the intervertebral foramina to its maximum size. Pushing the chest out brings the head back over the body and produces a straightening, or less extension, in the cervical spine. Flexion in the cervical spine, while tightening the nerve roots slightly, does increase the size of the intervertebral foramina. Extension closes the foramina and decreases the central canal's diameter.

2. It reduces the effect of the weight of the head. The lever arm effect of the weight of the head on the cervical spine is eliminated as the head is brought back over the body with the chest-out posture. This is important in relieving neck strain and decreasing the force exerted on the spine by the weight of the head.

3. It opens the thoracic outlet. By changing the alignment of the scalene muscles and the clavicle relative to the neck, the thoracic outlet is open with chest-out posturing. A stoop-shoulder, head-forward posture adds to thoracic outlet obstruction and will cause the symptoms of brachial plexus irritation to persist. Many heavily muscled athletes have adopted a round-shoulder, head-forward posture. When they sustain an injury to a nerve or the brachial plexus, symptoms will persist because of their inability to produce proper chest and head alignment. All strengthening of weak muscles as a result of a brachial plexus and/or nerve

CASE II. *A, B,* This head compression resulted from a head-first tackle. There is a 7-mm total overhang on the ring of C-1 on C-2. This represents a Jefferson fracture with a partial tear of the transverse ligament. These findings, shown in the CT scan, demonstrate the fracture.

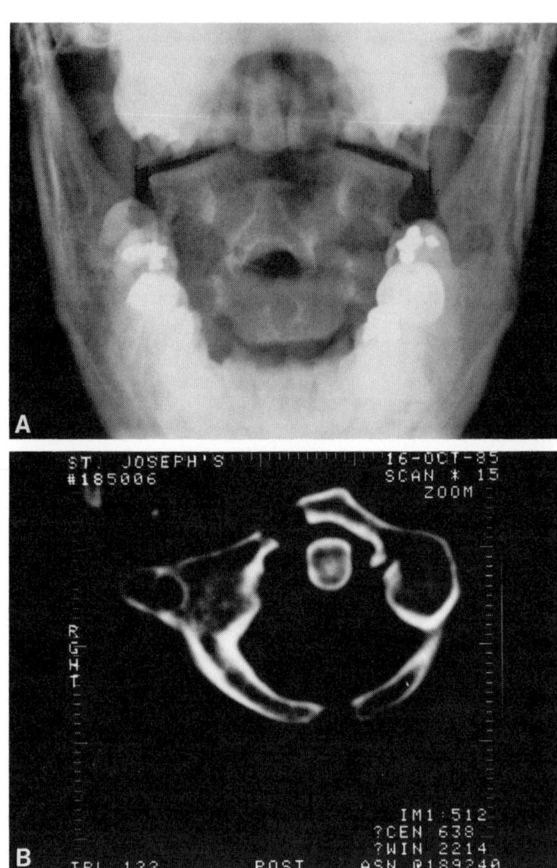

root injury should be conducted while emphasizing a chest-out posture. Weight lifting and strengthening with round-shoulder, head-forward posture can produce increased irritation. In addition to the posture-correcting chest-out exercises, the arm-strengthening exercises are also done with the chest-out posture.

Neck strengthening is important. Neck and radicular pain will cause muscle weakness and dysfunction in the muscles that support the head. Neck muscles in neck injuries should be given the same emphasis as quadriceps strengthening for knee injuries. However, the process must be done carefully. Resistive neck exercises are begun very slowly so the compressive load on the cervical spine does not produce pain. Neck isometrics should be done with the head in the midline only, and resisting forces should be applied perpendicularly to the head from every direction. Very slowly, the head can be taken out of the midline after there is no pain whatsoever, but extremes of head flexion, either anteriorly or posteriorly, or laterally against resistance, are seldom indicated for adequate neck strengthening. Our emphasis has been on midline isometric strengthening and stretching through a full range of motion.

Stretching exercises are critically important to allow the cervical spine a protective flexibility and range of motion. Cervical stiffness is produced by nerve, ligament, or disc injury. The reactive stiffness can produce chronic contractures and a loss of range of motion if not corrected. Chronic contractures are a great enemy of a pain-free neck, in that if a contracture exists, sudden motion at a moment of contact through that restricted range of motion will reproduce the injury and severe pain. Relieve those contractures and restore a protective range of motion with a program of cervical stretching and range of motion exercises. Use the motion in painless ranges initially, then slowly into the painful areas. Extension is usually the most painful exercise but cannot be neglected. Dorsal slides and passive neck stretches are important. Remember that chest-out posturing should be used during the exercises.

The key at this phase of rehabilitation is the return of neck strength and suppleness, with accompanying return of shoulder and upper extremity function. We believe that the reinjury rate is substantially decreased by following these guidelines (Case III).

CASE III. The postoperative x-ray of an anterior cervical fusion in a professional football player. The postoperative cervical fusion at a low cervical level is felt to represent a mild risk of future injury. The higher the fusion in the cervical spine, the greater the risk. A Torg ratio of 0.8 or less is felt to be significantly indicative of cervical stenosis. The exact limits of normality in the general population in relation to symptoms are not well defined. The case is a professional football offensive lineman who suffered a significant cord contusion with residual neurological symptoms and findings. Each of his levels was 11 mm or less. The same offensive lineman had 11 mm central canal diameter, but an abnormal AP compression ratio of 0.5, normal being considered 0.6. The compression ratio may be a more sensitive indicator of spinal stenosis than the central canal diameter or the Torg ratio. This professional defensive back suffered a small unilateral disc herniation that healed well with nonoperative care. He had no symptoms of myelopathy or cord contusion. The abnormal Torg ratios did not correlate well with the amount of reduction of central canal diameter.

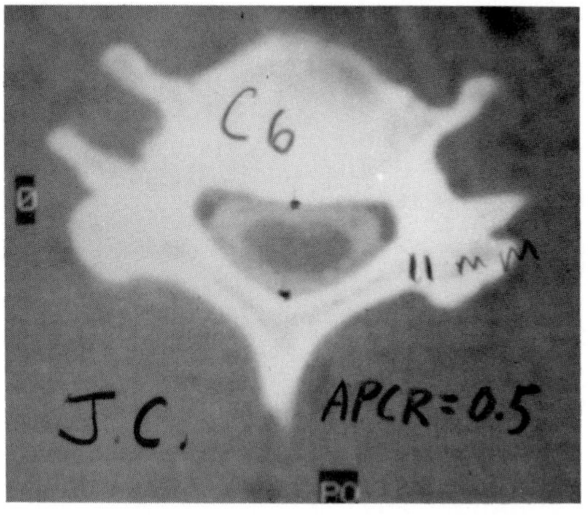

SUMMARY

Cervical spine injuries in football players are common and, at times, a frustrating dilemma for the team physician. With careful evaluation of the patient, the search for residual symptoms, tests as necessary, evaluation of the cervical canal, and proper rehabilitation, safety to the player can be optimized and proper decisions made.

REFERENCES

1. Albright JP, Moses JM, Feldick HG, et al: Non-fatal cervical spine injuries in interscholastic football. JAMA 236:1243–1245, 1976.
2. Albright JP, Van Gilder J, El-Khoury G, et al: Head and neck injuries in sports. In Scott NW, Nisonson B, Nicholas JA (eds): Principles of Sports Medicine. Baltimore, Williams & Wilkins, 1984.
3. Albright JP, McCauley E, Martin RK, et al: Head and neck injuries in college football: An eight-year analysis. Am J Sports Med 13:147–152, 1985.
4. Edwards W, LaRocca H: The developmental segmental sagittal diameter of the cervical spinal canal in patients with cervical spondylosis. Spine 8:20, 1983.
5. Eismont FJ, Clifford S, Goldberg M, Green B: Cervical sagittal spinal canal size in spine injury. Spine 9:633–666, 1984.
6. Epstein J, Carras R, Hyman R, Costa S: Cervical myelopathy caused be developmental stenosis of the spinal canal. J Neurosurg 51:362–367, 1972.
7. Matsuura P, Waters R, Adkins RH, et al: Comparison of computerized tomography parameters of the cervical spine in normal control subjects and spinal cord injured patients. J Bone Joint Surg 71A: 183–188, 1989.
8. Odor JM, Watkins RG, Dillin WH, et al: Incidence of cervical spinal stenosis in professional and rookie football players. Am J Sports Med (Accepted for publication, 1990).
9. Ogino K, Tada K, Okada K, et al: Canal diameter, anterioposterior compression ratio and spondolytic myelopathy of the cervical spine. Spine 8:1–15, 1983.
10. Torg JS: Epidemiology, pathomechanics, and prevention of athletic injuries to cervical spine. Med Sci Sports Exerc 17:295–303, 1985.
11. Torg JS, Das M: Trampoline-related quadriplegia: Review of the literature and reflections on the American Academy of Pediatrics' position statement. Pediatrics 74:804–812, 1984.
12. Torg JS, Vegso JJ, Sennet B, Das M: National football head and neck injury registry: 1971 through 1984. JAMA 254:3439–3443, 1985.
13. Torg JS, Truex R Jr, Quedenfeld TC, et al: National football head and neck injury registry: Report and conclusions 1978. JAMA 241:1477–1479, 1979.
14. Torg JS, Quedenfeld TC, Burstein A, et al: National football head and neck injury registry: Report on cervical quadriplegia: 1971–1975. Am J Sports Med 7:127–132, 1979.

Chapter 18

AEROBIC SPORTS ACTIVITIES AND THE SPINE

Barton L. Sachs, MD

Aerobic exercises are those that increase one's ability to take in and deliver oxygen to all body tissues. To positively affect the condition of one's cardiovascular system, an aerobic exercise must be performed continuously over a sustained period, usually a minimum of 20 minutes.

For the purpose of this chapter, the term "aerobic exercise" is broadly defined as a sport that promotes cardiovascular fitness. This discussion will review the specific musculoskeletal and spinal aspects of (1) diagnostic injury categories, (2) equipment utilization, and (3) rehabilitation relating to aerobic exercise.

CLASSIFICATION OF AEROBIC SPORTS ACTIVITIES

Aerobic sports activities can be classified into noncontact activities, such as swimming, rowing, cycling, and cross-country skiing, or the impact form of aerobic sports. Impact sports are subdivided into high-impact activities, such as jogging, running, and high-impact aerobic dance, or low-impact activities, such as exercise walking and low-impact aerobic dance. The importance of the categorization of exercise activities allows the physician to consider the most likely diagnosis and the most appropriate treatment/rehabilitation program.

PREVALENCE OF INJURIES IN AEROBIC ACTIVITIES

A review by Rothenberger[3] surveyed 726 aerobic dancers. This study attempted to document the prevalence, types and severity of injuries experienced in this sample of dancers. It was found that 49% of the subjects reported a history of at least one injury related to aerobic dancing. Of these, 12.9% occurred as injuries to the lower back, which was the second highest total, preceded only by injuries to the shin. Other than this review, there is very little reported in the scientific literature concerning injuries from aerobic sports activities.

DIAGNOSTIC CATEGORIES

The diagnostic categories of spinal injuries in aerobic exercise are either bone and soft tissue injuries, which anatomically emanate from the spine, or injuries from other associated nonspinal areas of the body. For example, the nonspecific patient complaint of lower back pain from marathon running may actually be secondary to an underlying piriformis syndrome rather than an intrinsic problem found in the spine.

Spinal fractures produced from participation in aerobic exercise fall into the categories of stress fractures, spondylolysis, transverse process fractures, and the vertebral body compression fracture. Impact-loading sports activities produce more fractures. When the body is subjected to repetitive biomechanical loading in a gravitational environment (running, jogging, exercise walking, or high-impact aerobic dance), the possibility of some form of vertebral fracture must be considered.

In order to diagnose a spine fracture, appropriate radiographic studies should be obtained. These include standard radiographs of the spine in the AP, lateral, or oblique views, or sometimes scintigraphic evaluation with a radioisotope for contrast.

If the diagnosis of a fracture is determined, appropriate attention should include at least some form of immobilization. For the lumbar spine, this ranges from the use of a soft corset to a molded thoracolumbar spinal orthosis. For the cervical compression fracture, either a soft collar or rigid Philadelphia or Minerva collar is recommended.

In the specific diagnosis of spondylolisthesis with the acute development of pain, it is important to determine whether the listhesis is of acute or chronic nature. In the case of an acute problem, a rigid orthosis should be utilized. For patients with long-standing chronic listhesis, the treatment may vary but should include activity modification, symptom diffusion with medication and modalities, a possible short course of immobilization, and rehabilitation.

Spine-related Soft Tissue Injuries

The categories of soft tissue injuries include strains, sprains, and contusions. Each of these categories either directly emanates from the spine or is associated with a nonspinal specific anatomical structure. The spinal-specific problems may involve a paraspinal muscular strain syndrome, a paraspinal ligamentous sprain syndrome, or a paraspinal muscular contusion syndrome. A single episode of repetitive over-indulgence may account for the development of any one of these conditions.

Soft tissue-specific spinal disorders also include the discogenic syndromes. These problems include prolapsed or herniated spinal discs or internal disc derangement with an annular tear, with gradual desiccation of the nuclear contents. The discogenic syndromes may develop secondary to a single and forced rotational twist or from a repetitive wear-and-tear phenomenon applied to the spine, such as occurs in the long distance runner.

The nonspinal-specific soft tissue injuries include conditions such as hip capsular tightness, the piriformis syndrome, the iliotibial band syndrome, and the pronated or supinated foot syndromes. When any of these conditions exists in an individual engaged in activities such as jogging, running, aerobic dance, exercise walking, or cross-country skiing, it can account for the common symptom of lower back pain. Because of the intimate relationship of each syndrome to back pain, it is necessary to assess the associated underlying condition; treatment directed to the specific underlying problem will, in turn, allow improvement of the symptom complex, which may involve vague back or neck pain.

Predisposing Etiologic Factors

When assessing injuries in aerobic athletes, the physician should be concerned with underlying predisposing etiologic factors. Those factors may include problems such as osteoporosis in the amenorrheic female, or improper conditioning at any age level, or improper exercise warm-up, or overtraining versus a specific overstress episode, or inappropriate equipment usage. If any of these conditions exists, the physician must draw the athlete's attention to the predisposing factor as part of the treatment process. That means that the amenorrheic female should receive appropriate medical treatment, whereas the runner using worn-out shoes should be counseled to obtain the appropriate equipment.

Disequilibrium

The spine-related soft tissue injuries produced by aerobic exercise usually develop when there is a loss of balanced equilibrium between the physiologic training level and the biomechanical stress to which the individual is subjected. That means that the physician must determine the factors that have produced the disequilibrium state and try to effect a return to equilibration through counseling, treatment, training, and rehabilitation.

TREATMENT AND REHABILITATION

Treatment of the spine-injured aerobic athlete should involve a progressive return to complete participation in the sport. The phased continuum starts with immediate attention to elimination of the patient's painful symptoms. Immediate provision of comfort is attained with initial ice massage, appropriate splinting (with a molded or commercial orthosis or body cast), the use of nonsteroidal anti-inflammatory medication, the elective decision to utilize short-term narcotic analgesic medication, the elective decision to utilize muscle-relaxation medication, the modification of strenuous physical activity (with limited short-term absolute bed rest), and the use of early physical therapy modalities such as ultrasound, diathermy, deep heat, electrical stimulation, or a neuroprobe.

The second phase of treatment/rehabilitation involves progressive stretching of tight or spastic muscles, joints, or ligaments. Stretching should take place in a controlled and phased program specifically outlined by a trained physical therapist or exercise physiologist. In this way, the individual is reconditioning in a manner that is most appropriate for activity return.

The third phase of rehabilitation involves muscular strengthening. It is mandatory to provide a program that involves combined efforts of isometric and isotonic strengthening of muscles utilized for the specific aerobic activity. It is important to include the concept of dynamic balanced equilibrium of all muscle strengths and joint motions. This is best outlined by individuals trained in physical therapy, exercise physiology, kinesiotherapy, or rehabilitation medicine.

The last phase of rehabilitation involves an endurance program that allows the athlete to attain a level of participation in the aerobic sport commensurate with the desired functional level. The outline for endurance training should not be solely left to the athlete. Guidelines and instruction should be provided by the trained person responsible for overseeing the rehabilitation program.

Concurrently, throughout all of the phased levels of rehabilitation, cardiorespiratory function should be maintained. The injured aerobic athlete can continue conditioning in an alternate form of aerobic training activity. The injured runner may maintain conditioning by swimming or using a stationary bicycle; the injured swimmer may continue to walk or run in a lap pool for maintenance.

EQUIPMENT ENVIRONMENT

The management of individuals with spinal injuries from aerobic activity must include equipment evaluation and recommendations. Equipment needs for most aerobic sports are minimal. Common to all types of aerobic activities is the requirement for clothing that is lightweight and nonbinding, to allow for ease of joint and torso mobility. Breathable clothing to allow for loss of body perspiration and appropriate sizing to the individual are also suggested. For outdoor running, cross-country skiing, or bicycling, gloves should be worn to maintain digital warmth and padding.

The most important item of equipment in aerobic sport is the shoe. Much commercial attention has centered on the development of specialized types of shoes for different sports. Requirements that are common to all sports are: (1) shoes should be appropriately sized, (2) they should be new enough to provide appropriate support required for the physical stress, and (3) they should provide appropriate cushion to prevent transmission of undue forces through the lower extremities to the spinal column. It is important to know the age and type of shoe being worn. Running shoes can wear out and fail to provide support or cushion before the soles show excessive wear. Therefore, if possible the physician should examine the shoes.

The last category of equipment requirement involves apparatus that are not worn by the athlete. For aerobic dance activities, this concerns the use of a soft, shock-absorbent type of mat. The cross-country skier needs skis and poles of appropriate length. The bicyclist must have a well-tuned bicycle of proper size with seat and handlebars adjusted to recommended individual specifications.

AEROBIC EXERCISE TRAINING REGIMENS

All aerobic exercise must include proper preparation. Prior to participation, each athlete should undergo appropriate stretching of muscles, including a minimum of 10 minutes of balanced muscular stretching of the torso, hips, hamstrings, quadriceps, triceps surae mechanism, iliotibial band, hip iliopsoas-flexor complex, and the abdominal and paraspinal muscle complex. As the individual commences the aerobic sport, warm-up should take place slowly, working at 40–50% of maximum heart rate and gradually building up to the maximum training heart rate. This heart rate can be determined by the exercise physiologist or physician involved in the care of the patient. After participation in the sport, a cooling-down period of muscle stretching helps prevent muscle tightening and minimizes muscular discomfort while maintaining flexibility.

CONCLUSIONS

Individuals who sustain musculoskeletal or spine-related injuries from participation in aerobic sports activities can be appropriately evaluated, treated, and rehabilitated by the knowledgeable physician. As aerobic sports have become more popular, the level of participation has increased. It is important to have a conceptual understanding of the various sports activities, the categorization of diagnostic entities, an appropriate treatment plan with emphasis toward rehabilitation, and an understanding of equipment needs and training regimens. The basic goal of athletes with spinal injuries is to maintain aerobic conditioning and resume full participation in the aerobic sport. The physician should understand this concept and recommend a safe, planned, and modified program with proper equipment.

REFERENCES

1. Lance K: Low-Impact Aerobics. New York, Crown Publishers, 1988.
2. Nicholas JA, Hershman EB: The Lower Extremity and Spine in Sports Medicine. St. Louis, C.V. Mosby Co., 1986, pp 1171–1229.
3. Rothenberger LA: Prevalence and types of injuries in aerobic dancers. Am J Sports Med 16:403–407, 1988.

Chapter 19

SOFT TISSUE TRAUMA IN EQUESTRIAN PARTICIPATION

Ralph F. Rashbaum, MD

Much attention in equestrian sports has been devoted to osseous injuries to the spinal column, which, by their very nature, are such as to render the victim either seriously injured (in the form of fracture or subluxation with or without neurologic involvement) or a far worse condition of sudden death due to overwhelming spinal cord trauma. It is not the purpose of this article to dwell on these aspects of spinal involvement in equestrian participation, for the reader need only be directed to any number of teaching texts that deal quite well with this subject. Rather this paper is intended to serve as a graphic reminder that there are also soft tissue conditions, precipitated by faulty posture and movements, that can adversely influence participation in this sport so as to make continued riding, whether on a competitive level or for recreation, an impossible task. I hope to achieve this with graphic illustrations representative of correct and faulty posture rather than a wordy discourse on properly seating a horse. For the neophyte rider this should be of measurably more value and importance.

Figures 1, 2, and 3 depict the apparent differences between standing, sitting, and sitting in a saddle as related to the sharing of load. The important feature to note is the sharing of weight on the rider's thighs versus that of a seated posture in a chair where the weight is on the buttocks and sacrum. It is this weight distribution on the muscular medial portion of the thighs that allows for much of the absorption of the concussive forces as the horse begins to walk, trot, or canter.

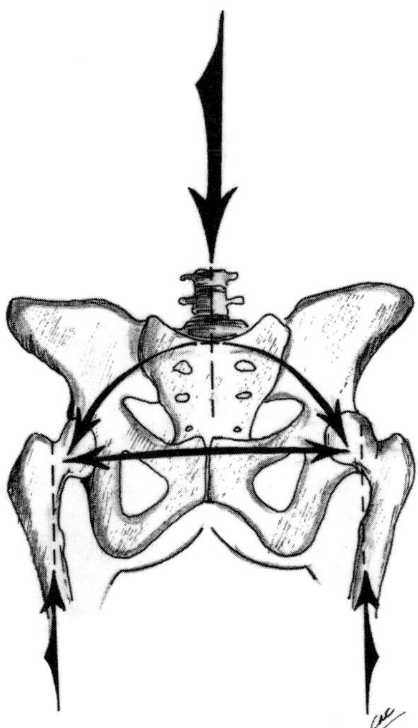

FIGURE 1. Weight distribution while standing.

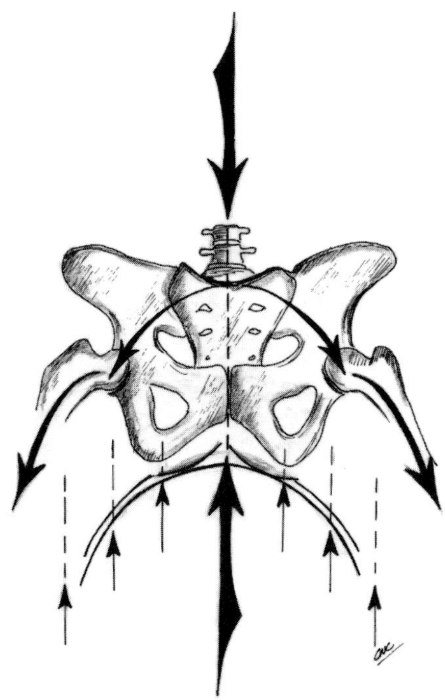

FIGURE 3. Weight distribution while riding.

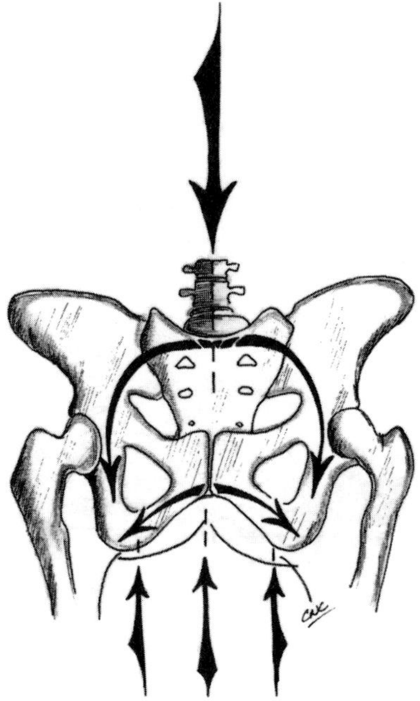

FIGURE 2. Weight distribution while sitting.

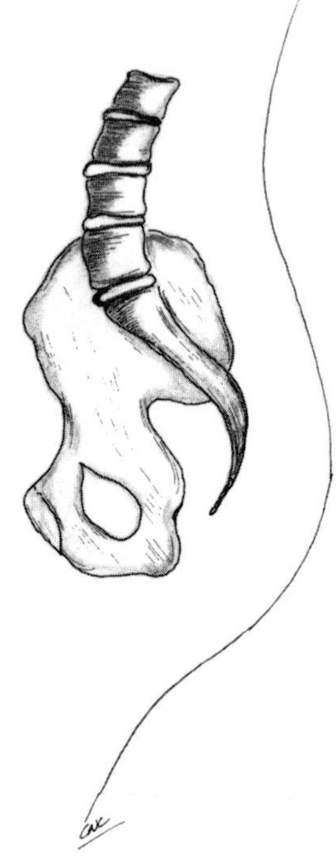

FIGURE 4. Correct lumbar alignment when properly sitting in the saddle

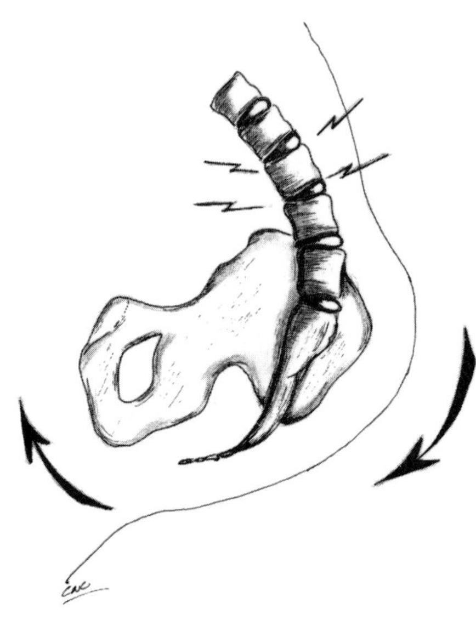

FIGURE 5. The pelvis is rotated clockwise, with the resultant stress being applied to the rider's lower back.

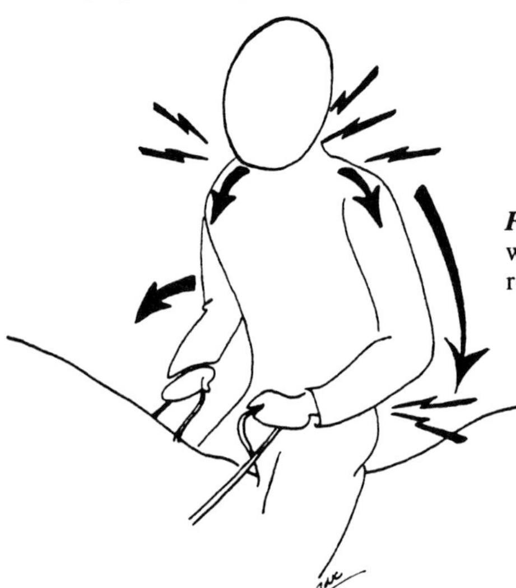

FIGURE 6. Shoulders are forced downward and forward. The upper back is rounded. The neck is placed into extension.

A well-balanced rider, one who is sitting erect in the saddle with the pelvis rolled slightly forward (counterclockwise), does much to diminish the stress applied to the lower back, as seen in Figures 4 and 5.

Improper sitting posture (clockwise rotation of the pelvis) results in compensatory postural changes of the upper back and neck, which, in effect, are an effort to try and "sit a balanced seat." Figure 6 depicts the result of just such

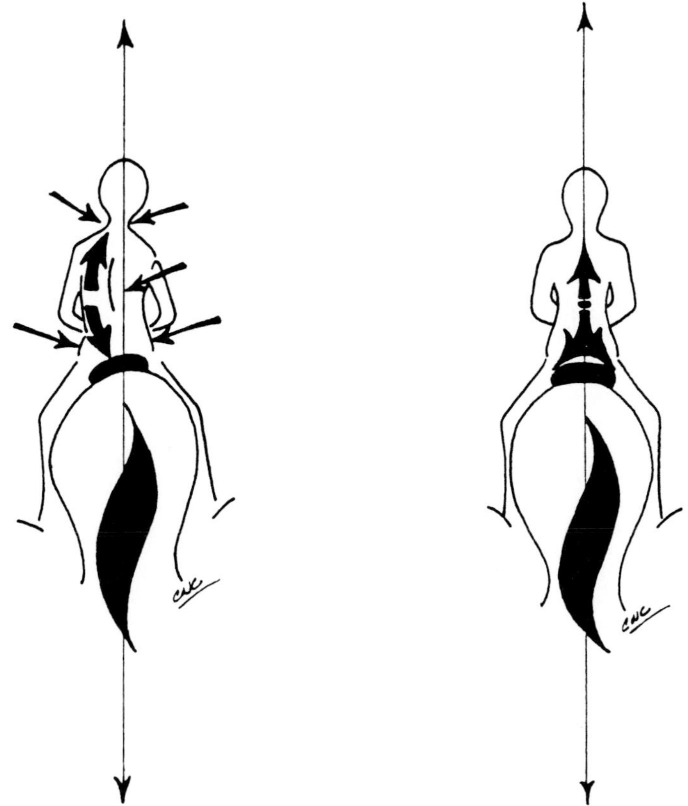

FIGURE 7 *(left).* A common fault is for the rider to sit with the weight on a hip rather than centered on the spine; this causes subtle but continuous stress to the areas indicated. Without being corrected, permanent damage may result over a prolonged period of time. Due to this imbalance, the horse will move away from this pressure, causing the rider to tense the opposite side in order to keep the animal moving in the desired direction.

FIGURE 8 *(right).* Correct position from the rear; weight is evenly distributed.

an attempt as it reflects stress applied to the rider's upper back, neck, and shoulders. This is a position that quickly leads to muscle stress, fatigue, and, without correction, subsequent soft tissue injury.

In Figure 7, a common fault is seen that can lead to postural stresses distributed unequally to the rider's spinal axis as well as the hip. This will ultimately result in a painful ride. The posture will also result in undesired movements of the horse, as he is trained to move away from the rider's leg pressure, which is being inadvertently applied. The overall effect is that the rider must now exert far more counterforce on a continual basis in order to correct this unwanted movement on the part of the horse. Ultimately this will limit the duration of the ride due to rider fatigue. Figure 8 depicts the correct seated posture from behind.

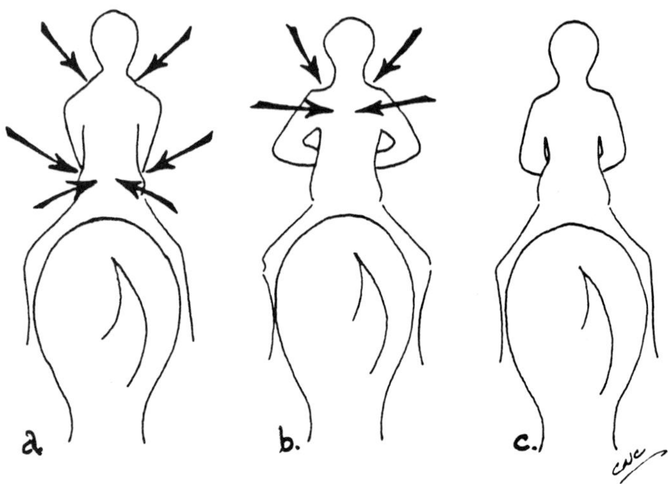

FIGURE 9. *A,* Rider with pinched-in elbows and dropped shoulders tightening the neck, spine, and lower back. The rider becomes rigid and his back receives the shock of movement. Lower back and neck pain result. *B,* Rider wings elbows out—impinging neck and tensing shoulders. Upper body stiffens causing lateral tension and neck stiffness, and the lower body has to support the constantly off-balanced upper body. *C,* Relaxed rider—arms hang naturally, lower back is relaxed, body flows with the movement of the horse. Spinal shock is minimized.

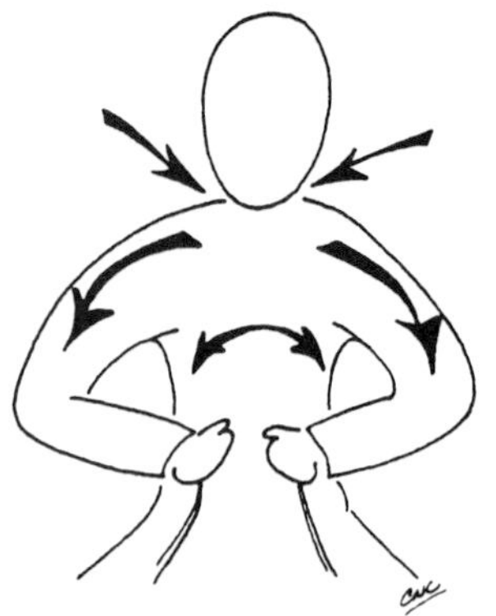

FIGURE 10. The rider has his shoulders rolled forward, causing his chest to be concave, resulting in stiffness in neck area, restricted use of upper back and rigidity in arms and wrists. This creates extra stress on the lower back and waist, as the upper body now must rely on the reins to maintain balance.

Figure 9 shows the effect of positioning of the rider's elbows as it relates to postural stresses imposed on the neck, shoulders, and back. The illustration once again serves to underscore the integral relationship between proper sitting posture and its effects on minimizing postural stresses to the spine. Figure 10 illustrates this problem viewing the rider from the front.

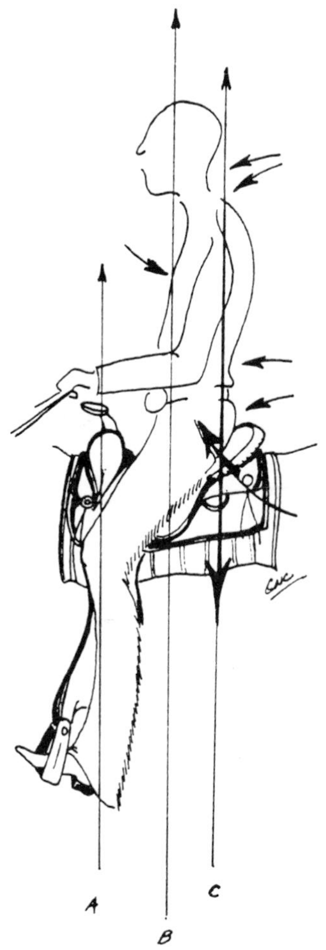

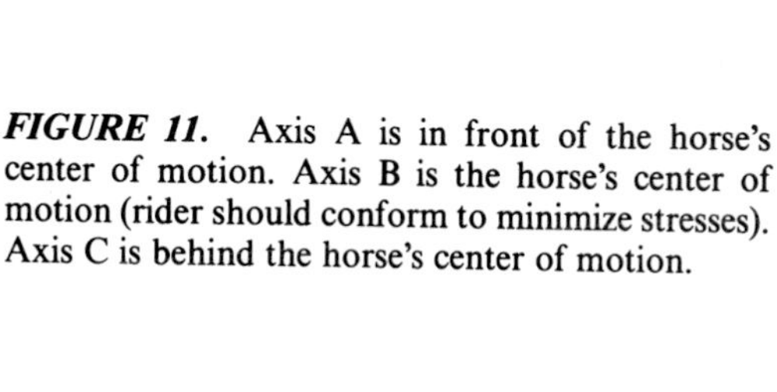

FIGURE 11. Axis A is in front of the horse's center of motion. Axis B is the horse's center of motion (rider should conform to minimize stresses). Axis C is behind the horse's center of motion.

Figure 11 shows a rider who is sitting in three vertical planes. Axis B is the center of motion of the horse and is the plane in which the rider seeks to sit to optimally reduce both the stress applied to his spine as well as to that of the horse. To minimize concussive stresses applied to the rider, his heels should be brought back under his trunk and his pelvis rotated forward (counterclockwise). This will allow the rider's trunk to move forward in the saddle to a point above the center of motion of the horse. This will also necessitate the rider sitting up straight with his shoulders back, so as to bring the upper trunk and head over this point as well. The resultant "balanced posture" is one of minimal muscle stress as well as pelvic flexibility to better absorb concussive shocks associated with the movement of the horse through the animated gaits.

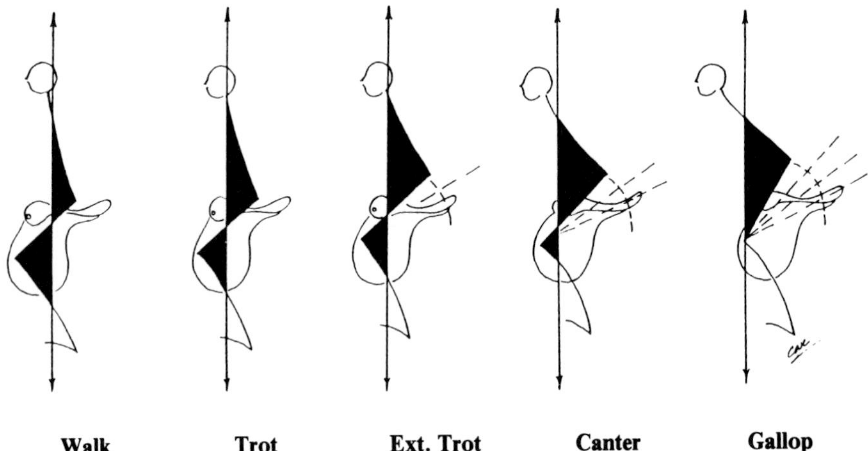

FIGURE 12. Changes that are seen in balance and trunk inclination as the rider goes through the various transitions of gait. There is a proportionate increase in low back stress as the center of gravity of the rider moves forward.

The previous figures have depicted problems associated with mere sitting errors and how they relate to postural stresses on the spine. The following illustrations will deal with problems of the rider's posture relative to the moving horse. In the series of stick figures seen in Figure 12, an attempt is made to show the increased stress in the lower back that would normally arise as the rider's posture accommodates the forward movement of the horse through these animated gaits.

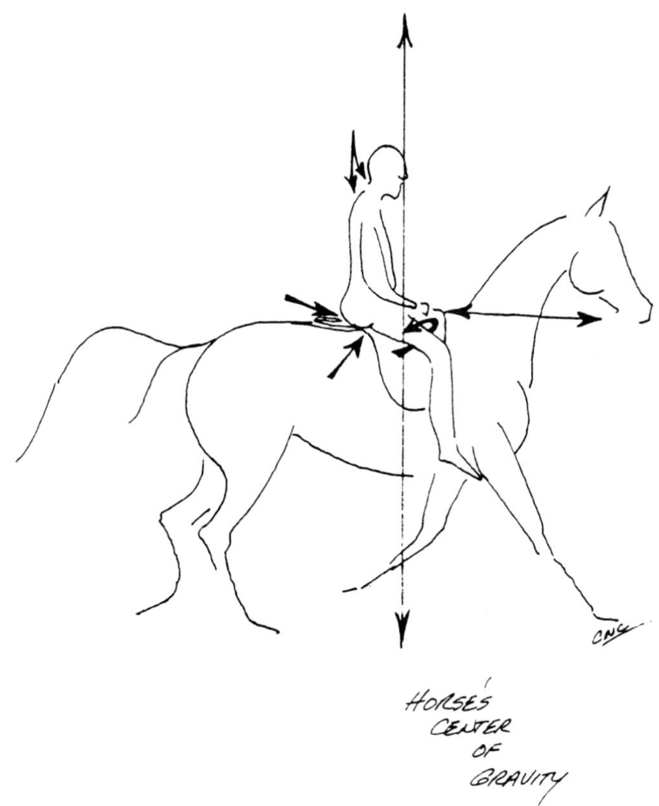

FIGURE 13. Rider moves against the motion of the horse; shocks to spine radiate throughout the body; hips are rolled outward, with the flexed part of the thigh against the saddle. The feet are carried with the toes downward and heel up, causing the support of the calves to be useless. The hands maintain constant tension on the reins for balance. The rider cannot maintain continuity with the center of gravity and natural motion of the horse.

Figure 13 illustrates the trotting horse with the rider seated behind the center of motion of the horse and with little or no attention paid to the position of the rider's legs or heels, or proper positioning of the rider's thighs. It is easy to see how the concussive forces of "posting to the trot" can be transmitted to the rider's pelvis and spine.

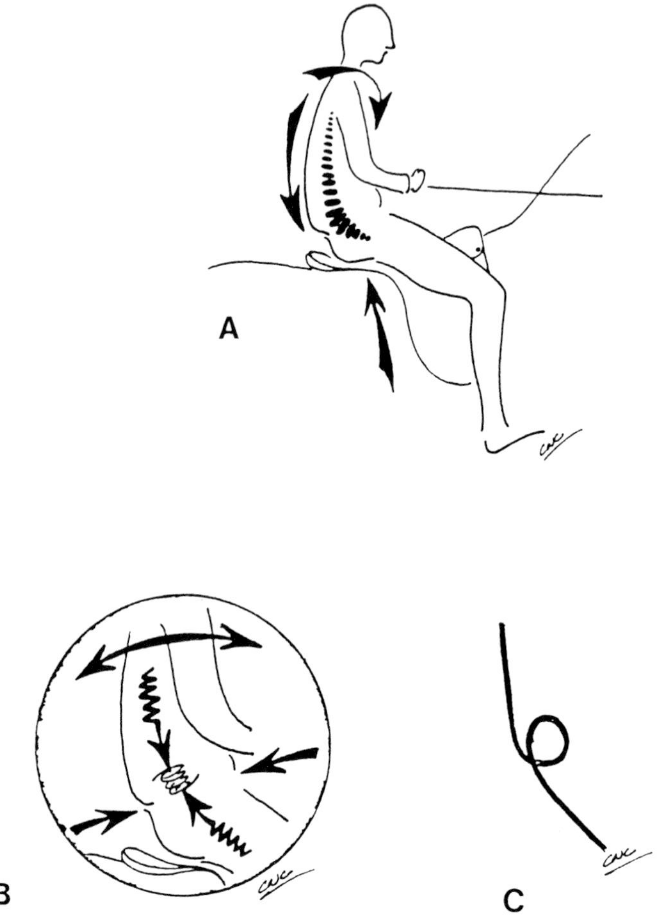

FIGURE 14. *A,* Vertical and forward forces are opposing each other—vertebrae become compressed. *B* and *C,* Pelvis may become the focal point of absorbed shock, like a tension spring.

Figure 14 depicts what might be happening to the spine, likening it to a flexible spring. Figure 15 both explains and depicts the effect of proper sitting posture while riding the trotting horse.

Figure 16 demonstrates the problems associated with progressive displacement of the rider's center of gravity relative to that of the horse's center of motion. It is quite easy to see how the simple act of leaning backwards brings with it a number of attempts to compensate or regain the balance of the rider. The extreme results of such a movement are seen in Figure 16E, with the rider "dashboarding" (legs almost straight ahead instead of straight down) and "balancing on the horse's mouth" by pulling back hard on the reigns.

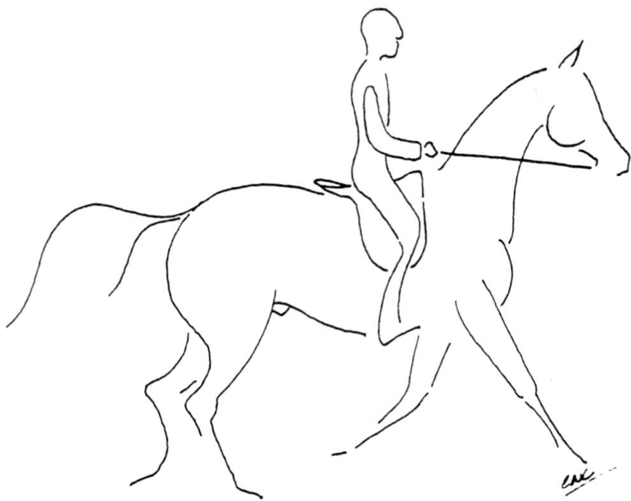

FIGURE 15. Rider naturally in balance; muscles absorb much of the shock of movement; spinal stress is minimized; weight is evenly distributed. The heels are down and thighs are rotated in, which allow for weight to be borne by the thigh muscle and to be distributed to the stirrups. This will allow the hips, knees, and ankles to absorb concussive shocks.

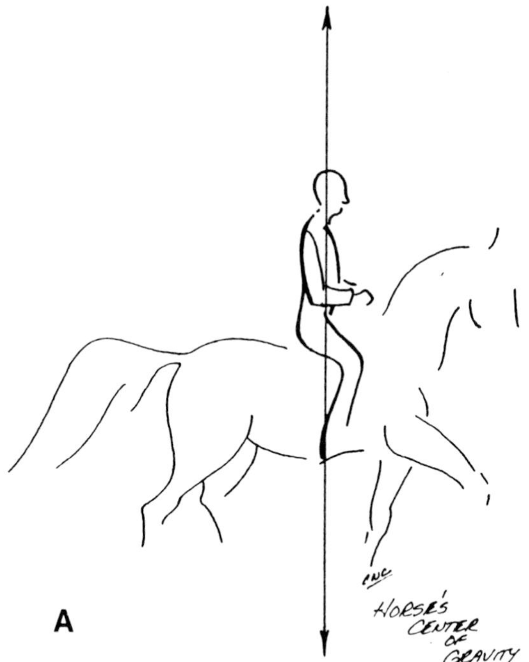

FIGURE 16. *A,* The rider is in proper position—in balance with the horse, relaxed, moving with the center of gravity of the horse. The spine is erect and able to absorb shocks without trauma/stress.

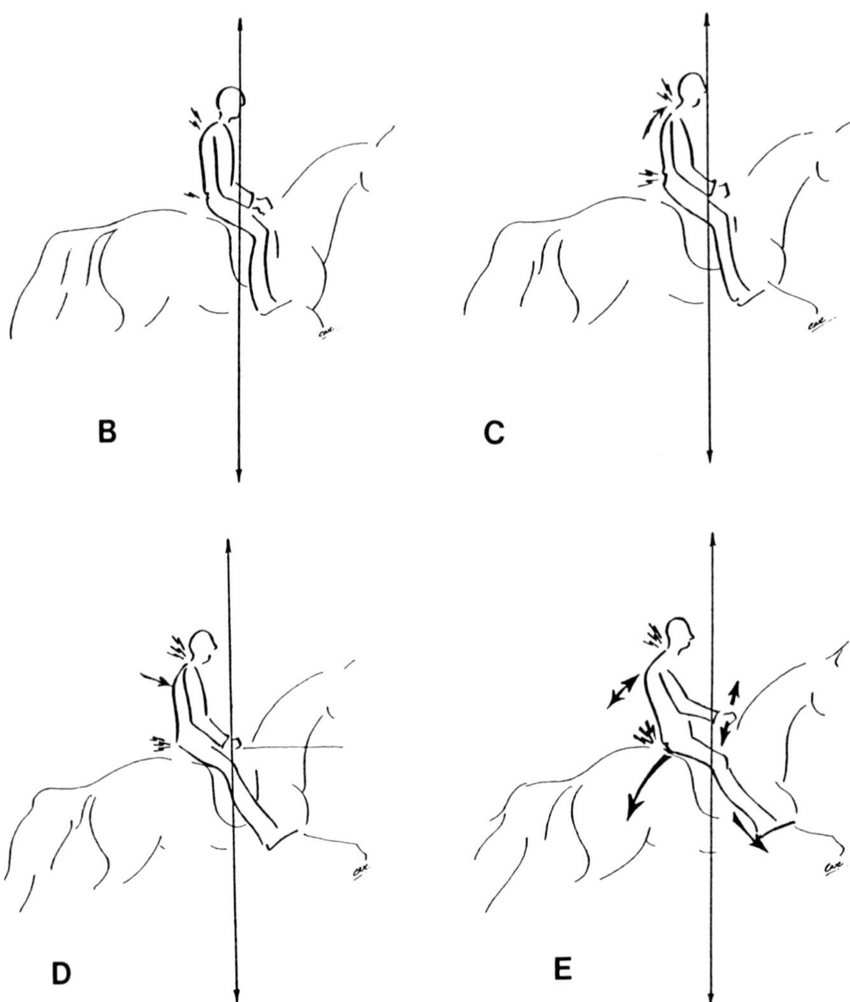

FIGURE 16. *(continued).* *B,* The rider has assumed a "couch potato" posture, rotating his pelvis and rounding neck and shoulder. His weight is behind the motion of the horse. *C,* The rider has further rounded the shoulders and is bracing off his hands and stirrups. The spine is stiffened; shock increases to lower back and hips. *D,* The pelvis is thrust forward and upward in front, increasing tension in the lower back. The rider's weight moves further to the rear, behind the motion of the horse. He inclines his head forward to compensate—arms and wrists stiffen. *E,* The rider is totally behind the horse and the lower back takes vertical and lateral shocks; neck and shoulder impingement results.

Our discussion now brings us to a natural endpoint. We have progressed from the seated posture through walk, trot, and canter, and it is now time to stop the horse. This is graphically depicted in Figure 17. The rider has remained behind the horse's center of motion. To do this, he has both leaned back and rotated this pelvis clockwise. This will force his pelvis and sacrum down into the saddle as the horse slows. The weight of the downward sinking body of the rider

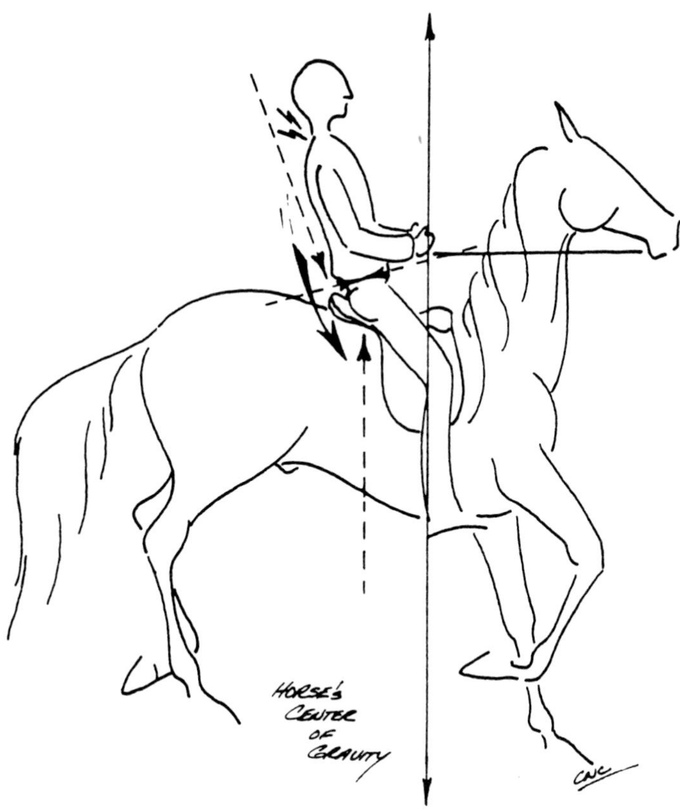

FIGURE 17. The rider is behind the motion of the horse; sacrum and pelvis have been forced downward and forward; weight of downward sinking body meets upward shock from horse.

meets the upward movements of the horse, resulting in "tooth-rattling" concussions transmitted to the rider through his seat. Had the rider been sitting appropriately, this concussive force would have been absorbed by the effective range of movement of the pelvis and hips, as well as by the soft tissues of the rider's legs (thighs, knees, and ankles). In conclusion, it is only when the rider has paid attention to the proper seating postures that stress and strain on the soft tissue structures of the spine and pelvis will be minimized and the resultant ride will be both picture perfect and comfortable.

Acknowledgment. The author would like to thank Craig Christiansen for preparing all the artwork in this chapter.

Chapter 20

LUMBAR INJURIES IN GYMNASTICS

Jeffrey A. Saal, MD

The number of gymnasts has grown tremendously in the past decade. In 1986, more than 130,000 female gymnasts were registered in the U.S., 48,000 in the competitive class.[36] This large number of participants as well as the changes in performance standards probably account for the steady increase in the rate of injury observed in this sport.

Gymnastic injury rates, which have been reported to be twice those of other noncontact sports, approach the rates noted in football and wrestling.[24] Additionally, the injury rate in gymnastics appears to be proportional to the skill and competitive level of the athlete. Injury rates show a steady rise as the level of competition accelerates from high school and club level to the collegiate and elite level.[19,32,41,49] Currently gymnastics trials for women are composed of four events. These events are: balance beam, uneven parallel bars, vault exercises and floor exercises. Men compete in six events: parallel bars, horizontal bars, rings, pommel horse, long horse vault, and floor exercise.

Until 1976, trampoline was also a competitive event, but it was banned in an attempt to reduce catastrophic head and spinal cord injury. Numerous studies have reported that the floor exercise event has the highest injury rate.[11,19] Balance beam and uneven parallel bars are ranked second, and vaulting reportedly is the safest of all the events.[23,41] When analyzing gymnastics-related injury, a number of factors must be considered, namely, the degree of difficulty of the gymnastic routine, proper or improper technique, and adequacy of spotting. Additionally, inappropriately advancing the athlete, overuse, and poor training habits can be contributing factors.

EPIDEMIOLOGY OF INJURY

The lower extremities, the area most frequently injured during gymnastic activities, account for 50–66% of all reported injuries. The trunk and spine account for 12–19% of reported injuries.[11,19,26,41,51,56] The elimination of the trampoline event reduced the injury rate to the head, neck, and lower spine by 19%. Injuries from overuse, which are the most difficult to document and analyze, account for 43% of all injuries.[56,57] Unfortunately, the majority of lumbar injuries fall in this category. Rarely is the lumbar injury the result of a particular traumatic event such as a fall. More commonly the gymnast reports an insidious onset of low back pain that is exacerbated by certain routines. The athlete is rarely able to pinpoint a specific history for the injury or note a time of occurrence.[40]

LUMBAR INJURY TYPES

Precise data are unavailable to clarify the actual incidence of each diagnostic subcategory of lumbar pain affecting the gymnast. However, in one study, female gymnasts participating in competitive events were reported to have an almost fivefold increase in the incidence of spondylolysis when compared to nonathletic females of the same age. Radiographs of 100 competition class gymnasts revealed an 11% incidence of injury compared to the 2.3% incidence of a nonathletic group.[25] However, the incidence of the pars interarticularis defect in the general population has been reported to be as high as 4.2% in one study[43] and 5.8% in another[4] (Fig. 1). Moreover, the rates vary according to race and gender, white males having the highest rates, 6.4%, and black females, the lowest, 1.1%.[4] None of the aforementioned studies demonstrated that the anatomic defect was indeed a symptomatic condition. Fatigue loading of the neural arch while performing back and front walkovers has been hypothesized to be the major cause in the development of the pars lesions. Additionally, dismounts in lumbar extension have been implicated in the condition's etiology.[6]

Although lumbar intervertebral disc herniation has been reported in the pediatric and adolescent population, no epidemiologic data exist for this condition in gymnasts. Repetitive torsional forces coupled with lumbar flexion place excessive mechanical stress upon the posterior annulus fibrosis, predisposing the disc to prolapse.[14] The model of gradual disc prolapse would explain how an overuse mechanism can cause this injury.[3] Repetitive microtrauma weakens the annular fibers initially in the inner zone, gradually spreading radially and leading to nuclear extrusion. In younger gymnasts the high level of nuclear hydration and the concomitant increase in swelling pressure increase the likelihood of nuclear extrusion.[16] Compare this scenario with that of the desiccated adult intervertebral disc.

Posterior disc herniation in the skeletally immature athlete often will be coupled with an apophyseal rim lesion.[13] This lesion may lead to the later development of central canal stenosis. The motion segments at risk for torsional injury lie above the intercristal line, i.e., usually the L4–5 interspace coupled with the L3–4 interspace. The L5–S1 motion segment would seem to be protected from torsion but is exposed to repetitive flexion and axial loading.[3,16]

Intraosseus intervertebral disc herniation presumably caused by axial loading across the disc space has been reported in gymnasts.[40] Jarring dismounts

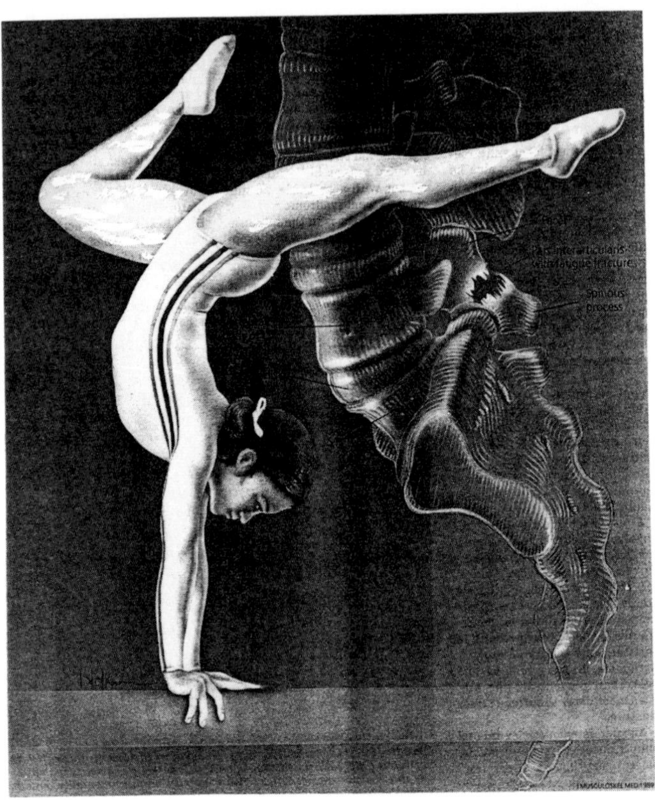

FIGURE 1. During growth, hyperlordosis is increased. Repeated stresses to the hyperlordotic lumbar spine, especially in sports such as gymnastics, can result in failure of the pars interarticularis. Reproduced with permission from The Journal of Musculoskeletal Medicine, February 1989.

may be a logical but as yet unproven cause for this injury type. Schmorl's node formation is caused by intraosseus disc herniation of nuclear material into the relatively soft vertebral endplate.[37] The interruption of the vertebral endplate, which occurs due to disc herniation, will disrupt nutrient flow to the nucleus and lead to premature disc desiccation.[38] This presumably occurs due to the inability of the nucleus to be replenished with hydrophilic proteoglycan moieties, leading to progressive water loss and secondary annular degeneration. Radial annular tears and internal disc disruption without obvious nuclear migration may also occur as a result of a particular injury or from repetitive torsional and axial load microtrauma.

Neural arch fatigue fractures are not the only posterior element injuries that are observed in gymnasts. The apophyseal joints, i.e., facet joints, are consistently placed under mechanical stress loading with gymnastic routines. Repetitive torsional stresses and lumbar extension are likely to cause injury to the articular surface of the facet joints, leading to bouts of synovitis and ultimately to degenerative changes in the articular cartilage.[31] If a motion segment has already suffered structural damage to the disc, the load borne by the facet joints may further predispose them to injury.[10] Occasionally, an athlete may present with lumbar pain with or without radicular referral, and developmental stenosis coupled with multilevel disc degeneration will be noted on imaging studies, i.e., MRI. A possible explanation of this complex situation is that the developmental stenosis and poor disc nutrition are probably the result of a genetic condition that has become symptomatic when stressed by athletic activity.[21]

INJURY PRESENTATION AND WORKUP

The first and most important task when faced with a gymnast suffering from low back pain is to establish a diagnosis. Without an accurate and timely diagnosis, it is virtually impossible to plan a specific treatment and rehabilitation program to enable the patient to return to his or her preinjury competitive level. Localization of the pain generator is paramount in spinal pain diagnostics. Indeed, the structure that appears to be most involved on a CT scan or other imaging study may not be the structure that is generating the disabling pain. Therefore, a careful correlation of the history, mechanism of injury, physical examination, and diagnostic studies is imperative to establish the location of the pain generator(s).[44]

Diagnostic studies that examine only structural changes are unable to establish the cause of persistent pain when used in isolation. This has been demonstrated repeatedly in studies attempting to correlate structural changes seen on lumbar x-rays, myelograms, and CT scans with patients' pain complaints.[5,9] The diagnostician must have the ability to sort through the clinical information derived from the history, the mechanism of injury, a careful physical examination, the electrophysiologic studies (i.e., EMG, SSEP), imaging studies, results of previous treatment, and the social factors surrounding the patient's pain to arrive at a diagnosis. An adequate understanding of spinal biomechanics, referral pain, and potential pain generators is therefore necessary for making an accurate diagnosis.[9]

The diagnosis of lumbar pain syndromes remains a difficult conundrum. Pain syndromes are given many names in an attempt to describe what would most appropriately be designated *nonspecific lumbar pain with and without radicular referral.*[46] The terms used to identify pain syndromes reflect the background, training, specialty, and bias of the examiner. Some commonly utilized terms include: *lumbar sprain, lumbar strain, lumbago, myofascial pain, iliolumbar ligament syndrome, sacroiliac dysfunction, lumbar malalignment,* and *multifidus syndrome.*

Many athletes are diagnosed as having lumbar sprains and strains, technically meaning that they have injuries of the ligaments and muscles. However, there exists no scientific evidence that muscles are a primary cause of back pain. Pain referred to the musculature can arise from any source that enters and is modulated by the dorsal ramus system.[45] Basic scientific findings suggest that ligaments and fascia may be sources of primary pain, but there is no evidence that they cause pain syndromes that persist longer than 4–6 weeks. The soft tissues of the lumbar region must obey the same biologic rules as other areas of the body. For example, hamstring muscle injuries do not create pain syndromes that persist beyond the normal point of healing. Acute injuries of the lumbar spine may indeed involve soft tissue structures but rarely require aggressive rehabilitation. Nonspecific local treatment and time will enable these conditions to become asymptomatic. However, if lumbar pain persists for a period greater than 6 weeks, a search for the underlying structural and biomechanical cause is in order.

Presenting Symptoms and Signs

The athlete who presents with posterior element pain will often report vague low back pain that may radiate to the buttocks and posterior thigh, and occasionally into the calf or ankle when the pain intensifies. The pain will be reported as being worse when standing, improved when sitting, and usually worse if the athlete lies supine with legs extended. On physical examination the pain is provoked by extension maneuvers and maneuvers that couple extension with rotation and axial loading. Moreover, the pain can be further intensified with ipsilateral single-leg standing while carrying out extension maneuvers. During the examination, the patient's posture is often found to be lordotic. Straight leg raising may cause back pain without radicular referral, but hamstring musculature is usually quite flexible in gymnasts, rendering this test useless. However, often poor flexibility of the iliopsoas will be observed, especially on the side with pain involvement.

Local paraspinal tenderness with reproduction of pain may be noted by the experienced examiner familiar with palpation techniques. Localized deep paraspinal muscle spasm can also be observed over the affected joint or neural arch. History and physical examination alone can not differentiate between the gymnast suffering from facet joint synovitis versus pars interarticularis stress fracture, or an exacerbation of a previously sustained pars fatigue fracture. However, spondylolisthesis will be accompanied by a prominence of the affected spinous process coupled with localized paraspinal guarding and hypermobility upon segmental palpation. These signs upon palpation allows spondylolisthesis to be identified on physical examination.

Unless there is accompanying intervertebral canal stenosis or disc herniation, no neurologic deficit will be noted with posterior element injury subtypes. However, lower extremity referral zone pain is not uncommon due to dorsal ramus activation. Additionally, lower extremity paresthesias may occur as a result of excitation of the sensory fibers of the exiting mixed spinal nerve that lay adjacent to the medial edge of the facet joint capsule. If the athlete is suspected of having a neural arch fracture, radiographs that include oblique projections are necessary. If a pars defect is noted, the chronicity cannot be confirmed without obtaining a radionuclide bone scan.[6]

Cases may also be encountered in which the defect is not seen on the radiographs, but in which the examiner's high index of suspicion motivates a bone scan that may demonstrate a discrete area of increased uptake over the pars interarticularis.[40] A bone scan without localized increased uptake, coupled with a radiographic defect, is considered a chronic lesion.[6,40] However, this chronic lesion may still be the cause of the athlete's complaint of pain. Selective injection of the lytic defect and the facet joint at contiguous levels may be necessary to sort out complex and refractory cases.

The gymnast with an intervertebral disc herniation may complain of back and leg pain. However, if the herniation is in the exit zone of the nerve canal or is extraforaminal, the athlete may only experience leg pain without back pain. Gymnasts will often state that the pain is only experienced while attempting to stretch for an event, and that they are asymptomatic while performing routines. The leg pain is usually worse after practice sessions and cool down. On physical assessment, the athlete will often display a loss of lumbar lordosis coupled with a pelvic obliquity and a list. A dramatic list may be noted during forward flexion and when accompanied by provocation of the leg pain. Straight leg raising will often display marked asymmetry in the young athlete with only minimal complaints of pain. They may describe the pain as *pulling* or they may describe paresthesias of the foot while performing the maneuver. A neurologic deficit may be present without the young athlete realizing it. Overall, young athletes tolerate pain associated with disc herniation quite well and complain less in the presence of more obvious physical signs than their adult counterparts. An athlete with an intraosseus disc herniation rarely presents as a patient with acute symptoms. The insidious onset of low back pain usually prompts the athlete to seek medical attention.[37] The finding of a Schmorl's node on routine radiographs may then be noted. Obviously, this radiographic finding does not reveal the age of the lesion nor does it reveal whether the lesion is indeed the cause of the pain. Localized increased uptake on a radionuclide bone scan may yield a clue as to the age of the endplate lesion. Discography is the only means to confirm the presence of pain generation of this type of lesion.[58] However, this is never necessary in athletes with vague nondisabling low back pain.

On the other hand, individuals with disabling low back pain who cannot sit even for a few minutes, and therefore cannot attend school or go to work, are another issue. These patients are usually in their 20s or 30s and have had extensive workups that have all been declared normal. However, their extreme debility continues. Such patients may be diagnosed as having internal disc disruption, a condition that can only be confirmed by discography.[7] In the diagnostic evaluation, the patient's history and physical examination must correlate with the structural evaluations noted on imaging studies. Additionally, electrophysiologic studies and selective block procedures may be necessary to sort out complex cases.

REHABILITATION OF LUMBAR INJURIES

The goal of rehabilitation must be to return the athlete to the highest level of performance possible. Fortunately the majority of injuries can be successfully treated nonoperatively.[46]

A rehabilitation program can be divided into two phases: a pain control phase and a training phase.[45] The pain control phase may include a variety of passive modalities, for example, flexion or extension exercises, lumbar mobilization, traction, and selective injection procedures. However, the key element of the rehabilitation program is the training phase, which emphasizes back school, functional movement training, and specific, dynamic muscular lumbar stabilization exercises.

THE TREATMENT PROGRAM: THE PAIN CONTROL PHASE

Pain control treatment should be instituted as early and efficiently as possible. It is important not to get stuck in the pain control phase, but rather to advance as rapidly as possible to the training phase of treatment. The initial stage of pain control, back first-aid, treats the pain and teaches the patient to control pain and muscle spasm. The treatment includes the application of ice,[12] resting in a position of comfort, and basic instruction in body mechanics to facilitate pain-free movement while performing normal daily activities. The use of medications can then be kept to a minimum. Dependent upon the type of injury sustained, anterior structures (the discovertebral joints) or posterior structures (the facet joints and neural arch) will determine the position and comfort. Athletes with acute uncomplicated anular tears, with or without small focal protrusions, will find pain relief in extension. Athletes with posterior element pain will find pain relief in slight flexion. During this initial phase, rest may also be specifically prescribed. It may only need to be used to control pain in the early days following the injury. The athlete must be given exact instructions regarding their activity level. The instructions must be communicated to the coach as well.

Pain relieving modalities such as transcutaneous nerve stimulation (TENS)[17] and pulsed alternating electrical muscle stimulation coupled with ice can also be useful to reduce the acute pain.[17,27] Extension exercises are valuable to reduce pain in discogenic injury subsets.[33] The principle of extension exercises may very well be explained by a reduction in neural tension rather than by nuclear migration as initially proposed.[48] When extension exercises cause centralization of low back pain without exacerbating or peripheralizing the lower extremity, i.e., radicular pain, they can be utilized. Peripheralization of the pain, i.e., an increase in radicular referral pain into the buttock or lower extremity, is a contraindication to the use of extension exercises and may indicate the presence of significant stenosis, posterior element disease, or disc herniation in the subarticular, foraminal, or extraforaminal zones. The correction of a list is necessary before beginning extension exercises. If the exercises are attempted while the patient is still listed, exacerbation of pain may occur that might lead to an erroneous decision to abandon the extension exercises. The overuse of extension exercises can lead to facet pain, which may delay the treatment program.

Flexion exercises are most useful for patients suffering from facet pain or symptomatic neural compromise from a stenotic canal. Flexion has been noted to cause a reduction in articular weight-bearing stress to the facet joints.[2] Flexion exercises have an additional benefit of stretching the dorsolumbar fascia.[15] Flexion must be used cautiously owing to the rises in intradiscal pressure that result and the heightened stress that is placed upon the posterior annulus. Flexion exercise in the seated position is most precarious due to the acute rise in intradiscal pressure that will result. In addition, lumbar flexion exercises performed with the legs fully extended creates the greatest degree of flexion upon the lower spine segments and will predispose the posterior annulus to the receipt of forces that can disrupt the integrity of these segments. Therefore, flexion exercises, if they are to be done, should be in spine-safe positions. These positions will unload the spinal segment but still allow a flexion stretch to occur. However, the data do not clearly support the absolute necessity for bracing to achieve successful fracture healing.

The use of mobilization techniques can be extraordinarily useful to attain articular as well as soft tissue range of motion.[54] Stiffened segments should be mobilized and tight soft tissues should be adequately stretched. Ultrasound application can facilitate soft tissue extensibility in order to allow adequate articular as well as soft tissue mobilization to occur.[28] Caution must be taken with the use of ultrasound in the presence of an acute radiculopathy. Possible post-treatment exacerbation of radicular symptoms, which may be related to neural swelling, may occur. Mobilization treatment is appropriate for the thoracolumbar junctional segments, which can often become hypomobile and indeed be a pain generator in their own right, often masquerading as a lumbar pain syndrome.[34] This will frequently be encountered in the gymnastic population, presumably due to the excessive lumbar lordosis transferring mechanical stress to the junctional segments. Over vigorous mobilization can be harmful in all types of injuries and should be carefully graded and timed during the treatment program.

The gymnast will often display signs of lumbar segmental hypermobility, and therefore mobilization treatment should be approached cautiously.

Although many studies report subjective symptom improvement, there is no scientific evidence to support the contention that any of the traction techniques actually facilitate nuclear migration. There is also no direct correlation with disc contour changes before and after traction.[22]

One of the most powerful tools in the pain control phase is the use of selective injections. The list of selective injections includes epidural cortisone injections from the translumbar or sacral approach, intra-articular facet injections, and lumbar selective nerve root blocks. These procedures can also be used for precise diagnostic localization of spinal pain generators.

The use of an epidural cortisone injection in the face of a disabling lumbar radiculopathy caused by disc injury or stenosis can provide dramatic relief.[8,59] The rationale for using corticosteroid anti-inflammatory agents is well established.[20] Epidural cortisone is most beneficial for patients with more leg pain than back pain, and for those who manifest dural tension signs on physical examination. Intra-articular lumbar facet injections under fluoroscopic guidance place corticosteroids into inflamed facet capsules.[30] Actual injection of spondylitic defects has also been found to give symptomatic relief, probably due to the spreading of the medication onto an inflamed exiting nerve root subjacent to the lytic defect. These techniques are especially useful in gymnastics-related posterior element pain syndromes. Lumbar selective nerve root block instills medication around an inflamed nerve root that is principally entrapped within the foramen or is entrapped by a large lateral disc fragment that has migrated foraminally.[53]

Acupuncture is a useful adjunct in the treatment of a variety of painful lumbar disorders in athletes. It has been reported that trigger points are found in predictable locations and that they correspond to well-established acupuncture points.[39] Dry needling a trigger point is just as effective as injecting the trigger point with local anesthetic solution alone, saline alone, or local anesthetic solution plus corticosteroid.[18,19] Endorphin release following acupuncture treatment has also been scientifically demonstrated.[50,52,55] Naloxone can block endorphin release and can blunt acupuncture analgesia.[35] There are numerous well-controlled scientific studies that demonstrate the usefulness of acupuncture in the relief of pain.[42] Acupuncture may break a pain cycle, thereby facilitating an active exercise program. It must be kept in mind that acupuncture, as well as the other injection procedures described above, are purely facilitators of treatment and should be considered as adjunctive therapy only. These techniques decrease the activity of inflammatory foci[47] and thereby speed the progression of treatment in the training phase.

THE TREATMENT PROGRAM: THE TRAINING PHASE

After having successfully completed the pain control phase of the rehabilitation program, the athlete should begin the training phase. The key element in the training phase is to attain the adequate musculoligamentous control of lumbar spine forces to eliminate repetitive injury to the intervertebral discs, facet joints, and related structures. Without progressing beyond the pain control phase, the athlete may be at risk of a repeat injury, further limiting his or her activity. It is crucially important to try to identify why gymnasts were injured and what risk factors for further injury they face. Analyzing their dismount techniques and floor routines is an important element of treatment and prevention. They gymnast must be made aware of proper spinal positioning and muscle bracing to avoid injury.

Stabilizing Concepts

Repetitive flexion and torsional stress to the lumbar intervertebral discs and facet joints will lead to advanced degenerative changes.[14,16] In addition, gradual disc prolapse secondary to fatiguing of the annular fibers is also important for understanding repetitive microtrauma to the lumbar segments.[3] Stabilization involves elimination of this repetitive microtrauma to the lumbar motion segments, thereby limiting the injury and allowing healing to occur. It can also potentially alter the natural history of degenerative processes.

Muscle fusion is essentially the use of the musculature to brace the spine and protect the motion segments against repetitive microtrauma and excessively high single occurrence loads. The abdominal mechanism, which couples the midline ligament as well as the dorso-lumbar fascia, combined with a slight reduction in lumbar lordosis, can eliminate shear stress to the lumbar intervertebral segments. The abdominal musculature has the unique ability to flex the lumbar spine with its action upon the superficial portion of the dorsolumbar spine and the superficial portion of the dorsolumbar fascia, and to extend the lumbar spine by its action upon the deep portions of the fascia that form the alar interspinal ligaments. This coupled action allows the abdominal muscles to corset the lumbar region when used in concert with the latissimus dorsi, which also acts upon the dorsolumbar fascia. The lowering of the center of gravity with slight knee flexion facilitated by adequately strong quadriceps musculature is an important part of the formula for bracing the spine.

Due to the changes in axial rotation that are possible at the intervertebral segments at different degrees of lordosis, control of lordosis in flexion/extension is extremely important. Knowledge of these mechanisms can lead to an understanding of the balanced muscular function and flexibility that leads to the control of stresses applied to the lumbar intervertebral segments. Reducing lumbar lordosis will decrease facet loading but also limit the amount of torque delivered to the disc.

The concept of the muscle fusion involves the co-contraction of the abdominal muscles to maintain a corseting effect to the lumbar spine, using the midline ligament and thoracolumbar fascia, coupled with proper pelvic positioning, to accomplish the task. The use of the spinal extensor muscles to reduce translational stress to the intervertebral segments is important during activity as well as for balancing shear stress to the intervertebral segments. The multifidus muscle appears to be the most active in this regard.

In order to apply the muscle fusion, adequate flexibility and spinal range of motion must be attained. Some interesting work presented by Adams et al. regarding diurnal variations and stresses on the lumbar spine reports changes in lumbar disc and ligament extensibility as the day progresses.[1] These changes are based upon the creep of soft tissue structures, leading to an increased range of motion. Adams et al. point out that bending and lifting activities performed early in the morning, when undertaken by nonextensible ligamentous and annulus fibers, will cause the disc to accumulate fatigue damage more easily than similar activities performed later in the day. This observation suggests a need for flexibility of the structures to eliminate this repetitive fatigue stress to the intervertebral joint. We should also think of the muscles that attach to the pelvis as guy wires that can effectively change the position and symmetry of the pelvis. Considering that the pelvis is the platform on which the lumbar spine rests, pelvic positioning is the key to postural control of the lumbar spine. Therefore, adequate flexibility of hamstring, quadriceps, iliopsoas, gastrocsoleus, hip rotator, and iliotibial band (ITB) muscles is important. There is also a need for flexible neural elements as well. Gymnasts will often have excellent hamstring flexibility but poor iliopsoas flexibility. Improving flexibility of the hip flexors can reduce the lumbar lordosis and thereby reduce lumbar segmental torque.

Stabilization exercise is designed to develop isolated and co-contraction muscle patterns in order to stabilize the lumbar spine in its neutral position. Neutral position is defined for each individual. Neutral position of the spine does not necessarily mean zero degrees of lordosis, but rather the most comfortable position for the individual. It is more appropriately referred to as the position of optimal function (POOF). The gymnast is taught to incorporate stabilization training into the athletic routines. This is most useful during dismount techniques. Obviously, athletes must be able to perform their gymnastic routines in the extremes of motion. However, if neutral spine positioning can be used in daily activities and during dismount, the cumulative forces upon the lumbar spine can be greatly reduced. Additionally, limitation of excessive practicing of the particular routines that subject the spine to the limits of extension will help reduce recurrent injuries.

During sports-specific training programs, the athlete progresses through a basic level of exercises and continues through an advanced level of training, finally undertaking the sports-specific training.[45,46] The sports-specific training begins with hands-on, one-on-one mat work, proceeding from isolated to compound movements. The use of videotaped exercise sessions and videotaped performances of specific athletic techniques is a valuable coaching and training aid. The principles of athletic spine training can be applied to virtually all sports. It is important to work carefully with individual coaches before designing any training programs. Figure 2 illustrates a few examples of dynamic lumbar stabilization exercises.

PREVENTION OF LUMBAR INJURIES

Numerous factors have been implicated in the cause of gymnastics injuries. The equipment and mats do not appear to play a significant role in the development of most lumbar injuries, considering that these injuries are associated with overuse phenomena. Coaching techniques and the intensity of practice sessions probably play greater roles in injury prevention than any other factors. The poor postural habits that young gymnasts learn in practice create the injuries of tomorrow. Proper coaching of dynamic lumbar stabilization techniques while stretching and while dismounting should have a dramatic effect upon injury reduction.

CONCLUSION

Gymnastics-related lumbar spine injuries are frequently encountered. With the rise in the number of participants in the sport, these injuries can be expected to increase. A methodology for diagnosis, treatment, and prevention of these injuries has been presented that has been developed over many years of sports medicine experience with spinal injuries. Diagnosis must be timely and precise. Treatment must incorporate dynamic muscular stabilization exercises to prevent repetitive forces from injuring the spine.

San Francisco Spine Institute Patient Exercise Program — Stabilization

Bridging

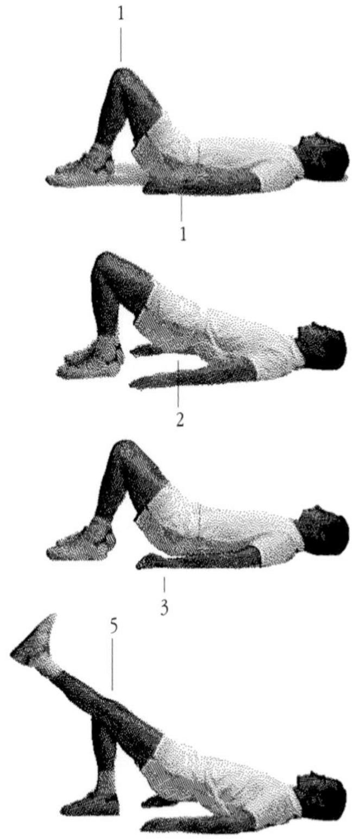

Purpose: To strengthen your abdominal, buttocks and low back muscles.

1. Lie on your back with knees bent.
2. Raise your hips and back from the floor. Hold this neutral bridge position.
3. Lower yourself to within one inch off the floor. Repeat the exercise.

With Leg Extension

4. Perform steps 1 and 2 above.
5. From the neutral bridge position, slowly straighten your left leg from the knee. Hold this position. Lower your left leg. Then extend your right leg.

Caution: This exercise will train you to stabilize your spine properly. It will enable you to be active without placing undue stresses on your spine. Stabilization requires strength, flexibility and coordination.

The exercise must be performed maintaining your spine's neutral position as identified by your trainer. This position is unique to your spine and posture.

This exercise sheet is not designed to replace a trainer's instruction. If you experience an increase and/or persistence in low back pain, leg pain or tingling while performing this exercise, stop. Consult with your physician or trainer.

Training Notes:

San Francisco Spine Institute Patient Exercise Program

Stabilization

Quadriped Arm and Leg

Purpose: To strengthen your abdominal, buttocks and back muscles.

1. Get down on your hands and knees. Tighten your stomach and buttocks muscles.
2. Raise your arms alternately.
3. Raise your legs alternately.
4. Alternately raise your opposite arms and legs.

Caution: This exercise will train you to stabilize your spine properly. It will enable you to be active without placing undue stresses on your spine. Stabilization requires strength, flexibility and coordination.
The exercise must be performed maintaining your spine's neutral position as identified by your trainer. This position is unique to your spine and posture.
This exercise sheet is not designed to replace a trainer's instruction. If you experience an increase and/or persistence in low back pain, leg pain or tingling while performing this exercise, stop. Consult with your physician or trainer.

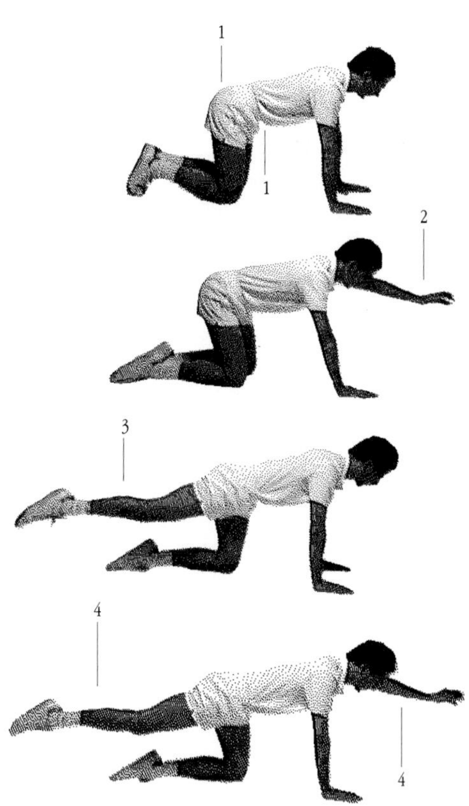

Training Notes:

 San Francisco Spine Institute Patient Exercise Program | Stabilization

Forward Lunge

Purpose: To strengthen your thigh and buttocks muscles.

1. Stand with your feet, shoulder width apart, knees slightly bent.
2. Lunge forward with your left leg. Your right knee should almost touch the floor. Return to your original standing position. Repeat the exercise with the opposite leg.

Caution: This exercise will train you to stabilize your spine properly. It will enable you to be active without placing undue stresses on your spine. Stabilization requires strength, flexibility and coordination.

The exercise must be performed maintaining your spine's neutral position as identified by your trainer. This position is unique to your spine and posture.

This exercise sheet is not designed to replace a trainer's instruction. If you experience an increase and/or persistence in low back pain, leg pain or tingling while performing this exercise, stop. Consult with your physician or trainer.

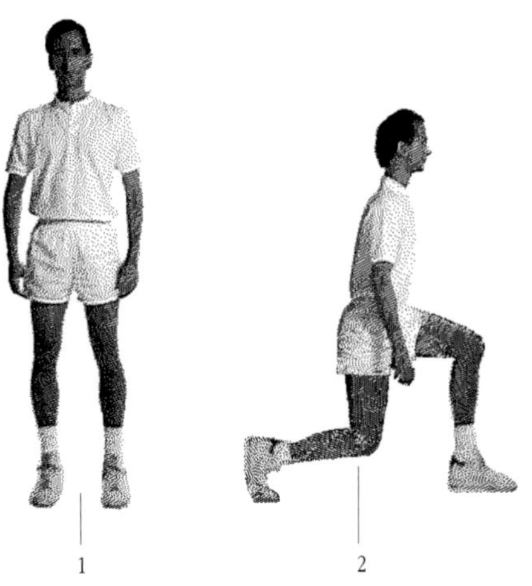

Training Notes:

REFERENCES

1. Adams MA, Dolan P, Hutton WC: Diurnal variations in the stresses on the lumbar spine. Spine 12:130–137, 1987.
2. Adams MA, Hutton WC: The mechanical function of the lumbar apophyseal joints. Spine 8:327–330, 1983.
3. Adams MA, Hutton WC: Gradual disc prolapse. Spine 10:524–531, 1985.
4. Baker DR, McHollic W: Spondyloschisis and spondylolisthesis in children. J Bone Joint Surg 32A:933, 1956.
5. Barton PN: The significance of anatomical defects of the lower spine. Index Medicus 17:37, 1948.
6. Ciullo JV, Jackson DW: Pars interarticularis stress reaction, spondylolysis, and spondylolisthesis in gymnasts. Clin Sports Med 4:000, 1985.
7. Crock HV: Internal disc disruption: A challenge of disc prolapse fifty years on. Spine 11:650–653, 1986.
8. Derby R: Diagnostic block procedures: Use in pain location. Spine: State Art Rev 1:47–65, 1986.
9. Diveley RL, Oglevie LL: Preemployment examination of the low back. JAMA 160:556, 1956.
10. Dunlop RB, Adams MA, Hutton WC: Disc space narrowing and the lumbar facet joints. J Bone Joint Surg 66:706–710, 1987.
11. Eisenbery I, Allen WC: Injuries in a women's varsity athletic program. Phys Sportsmed 6:112–120, 1978.
12. Eldred E, Lindsky DE, Buchwald JS: The effect of cooling on mammalian muscle spindles. Exp Neurol 2:144–157, 1960.
13. Epstein JA, Epstein NE, Marc J, et al: Lumbar intervertebral disk herniation in teenage children: Recognition and management of associated anomalies. Spine 9:427–432, 1984.
14. Farfan HF: Effects of torsion on the intervertebral joints. Can J Surg 12:336–341, 1969.
15. Farfan HF: Muscular mechanism of the lumbar spine and the position of power and efficiency. Orthop Clin North Am 6:135–144, 1975.
16. Farfan HF, Cossette JW, Robertson GH, et al: The effects of torsion on the lumbar intervertebral joints: The role of torsion in the production of disc degeneration. J Bone Joint Surg 52A:468–497, 1970.
17. Fox EJ, Melzack R: Transcutaneous electrical stimulation and acupuncture: Comparison of treatment for low-back pain. Pain 2:141–148, 1976.
18. Frost FA, Jessen B, Siggaard-Andersen J: A control, double-blind comparison of mepivacaine injection versus saline injection for myofascial pain. Lancet 8:499–500, 1980.
19. Garrick JG, Requa RK: Epidemiology of women's gymnastics injuries. Am J Sports Med 8:261–264, 1980.
20. Ghosh P: Influence of drugs, hormones, and other agents on the metabolism of the disc and the sequelae of its degeneration. In Ghosh P (ed): The Biology of the Disc. Boca Raton, FL, CRC Press, 1988.
21. Gibson MT, Szypryt EP, Buckley JH, et al: Magnetic resonance imaging. J Bone Joint Surg 69B:699–703, 1987.
22. Gillstrom P, Ericson K, Hindmarsh T: Autotraction in lumbar disc herniation: A myelographic study before and after treatment. Arch Orthop Trauma Surg 104:207–210, 1985.
23. Haycock CE, Gillette JV: Susceptibility of women athletes to injury: Myths vs. reality. JAMA 236:163–165, 1976.
24. Jackson DS, Furman WK, Berson BL: Patterns of injuries in college athletes: A retrospective study of injuries sustained in intercollegiate athletics in two colleges over a two-year period. Mount Sinai J Med 47:423–426, 1980.
25. Jackson DW, Wiltse LL, Cirincione RJ: Spondylolysis in the female gymnast. Clin Orthop 117:68, 1976.
26. Kirby RL, Simms FC, Symington VJ, et al: Flexibility and musculoskeletal symptomatology in female gymnasts and age-matched controls. Am J Sports Med 9:160–164, 1981.
27. Lampe GN, Mannheimer JS: Clinical Transcutaneous Electrical Nerve Stimulation. Philadelphia, F.A. Davis, 1984.
28. Lehman JF, DeLateur BJ: Therapeutic heat. In Lehman JF (ed): Therapeutic Heat and Cold. Baltimore, Williams & Wilkins, 1982.
29. Lewit K: The needle effect in the relief of myofascial pain. Pain 6:83–90, 1979.
30. Lippitt AB: The facet joint and its role in spine pain: Management with facet joint injections. Spine 9:746–750, 1984.
31. Liu YK, Goel VK, Dejong A, et al: Torsional fatigue of the lumbar intervertebral joints. Spine 10:894–900, 1985.

32. Lowry CB, Leveau BF: A retrospective study of gymnastics injuries to competitors and noncompetitors in private clubs. Am J Sports Med 10:237–239, 1982.
33. MacKenzie R: Mechanical Disorders and Treatment of Lumbar Spine Disorders. New Zealand, Spinal Publications, 1981.
34. Maigne R: Low back pain of thoracolumbar origin. Arch Phys Med Rehabil 61:389–395, 1980.
35. Mayer DJ, Price DD, Rafii A: Antagonism of acupuncture analgesia in man by the narcotic antagonist naloxone. Brain Res 121:368–372, 1977.
36. McAuley E, Hudash G, Shields K, et al: Injuries in women's gymnastics: The state of the art. Am J Sports Med 15:558–565, 1987.
37. McCall IW, Park WM, O'Brien JP, et al: Acute traumatic intraosseous disc herniation. Spine 10:134–137, 1985.
38. McFadden KD, Taylor JR: End-plate lesions of the lumbar spine. Spine 14:867–869, 1989.
39. Melzack R, Stilwell DM, Fox EJ: Trigger points and acupuncture points for pain: Correlations and implications. Pain 3:3–23, 1977.
40. Micheli LJ: Back injuries in gymnastics. Clin Sports Med 4:000, 1985.
41. Pettrone FA, Ricciardelli E: Gymnastic injuries: The Virginia experience 1982–1983. Am J Sports Med 15:59–62, 1987.
42. Reichmanis M, Becker RO: Relief of experimentally-induced pain by stimulation at acupuncture loci: A review. Compendia Medicus East West 5:281–288, 1977.
43. Roche MB, Rowe GG: Incidence of separate neural arch and coincident bone variations. J Bone Joint Surg 34A:491, 1952.
44. Saal JA: Diagnostic studies of industrial low-back injuries. Topics in Acute Care and Trauma Rehabilitation 2:31–49, 1988.
45. Saal JA: Rehabilitation of football players with lumbar spine injury (Part 1 and 2). Phys Sportmed 16:61–67 (Pt 1), 117–125 (Pt 2), 1988.
46. Saal JA, Saal JS: Nonoperative treatment of herniated lumbar intervertebral disc with radiculopathy: An outcome study. Spine 14:431–437, 1989.
47. Saal JS: High levels of inflammatory enzyme activity in lumbar disc herniations: Analysis of phospholipase A2 activity. International Society for the Study of the Lumbar Spine Annual Conference, 1989.
48. Schnebel BF, Chowning J, Davidson R, et al: A digitizing technique for the study of movement of intradiscal dye in response to flexion and extension of the lumbar spine. International Society for the Study of the Lumbar Spine, 1987.
49. Silvij S, Nocini S: Clinical and radiological aspects of gymnast's shoulder. J Sports Med Phys Fit 22:49–53, 1982.
50. Sjolund BH, Eriksson MBE: Endorphins and Analgesia Produced by Peripheral Conditioning Stimulation. New York, Raven Press, 1979.
51. Snook GA: Injuries in women's gymnastics: A 5-year study. Am J Sports Med 7:242–244, 1979.
52. Takagi H: Critical review of pain relieving procedures including acupuncture: Advances in pharmacology and therapeutics II CNS pharmacology. Neuropeptides 1:79–92, 1982.
53. Takeshi T, Kouzaburou F, Eisuke K: Selective lumbosacral radiculography and block. Spine 5:68–78, 1980.
54. Van Hoesen LS: Mobilization and manipulation techniques for the lumbar spine. In Grieve (ed): Modern Manual Therapy of the Vertebral Column. Edinburgh, Churchill Livingstone, 1986.
55. Watkins LR, Mayer DJ: Organization of endogenous opiate and nonopiate pain control systems. Science 216:1185–1192, 1982.
56. Weiker GG: Club gymnastics. Clin Sports Med 4:39–43, 1985.
57. Weiker GG: Injuries in club gymnastics. Phys Sportsmed 13:63–66, 1985.
58. Weinstein J, Claverie W, Gibson S: The pain of discography. Spine 13:1344–1348, 1988.
59. White AH: Injection techniques for the diagnosis and treatment of low back pain. Orthop Clin North Am 14:553–567, 1983.

Chapter 21

THE SPINE AND GOLF

Valerie K. VanderLaan, PA-C
and Robert W. Gaines, Jr., MD, FACS

EPIDEMIOLOGY

Low back pain in golfers is a relatively common complaint. It has been reported that less than 10% of sports-related injuries involve the spine. However, touring golf professionals have exhibited a 29% incidence of acute or chronic lower back complaints throughout their careers.[16] More recently, Duda has reported that 90% of all tour injuries have been to the cervical or lumbar spine.[7] Realizing that in a good drive the ball leaves the head of the club at approximately 136 mph, that the swinging club can travel up to 110 mph in velocity, and that the swing only lasts approximately 2 seconds, it is easy to appreciate the strength and power necessary for a successful shot. Injuries can be related to overuse, improper swing mechanics, poor overall conditioning,[14] or a combination of these factors. Pre-existing spine problems may be primary or aggravating factors.

McCarroll and Gioe[11] mailed questionnaires to 500 professional golfers of the Tournament Players Association and Ladies Professional Golf Association. The average ages of these golfers were 30 and 24 for men and women, respectively. Average years on tour were 18 and 9, respectively. Throughout their careers, 103 men and 87 women reported symptoms. The low back and left wrist were most commonly injured. From 10 to 30% of touring professionals play injured at any given time.[11]

While age and pre-existing structural disorders affect golfers individually, obvious differences in overall conditioning and swing mechanics between "professional" golfers and the "weekend" golfer permit the vast majority of golfer's spinal injuries to be separated by these two simple factors. The better golfer is generally more flexible and stronger, the weekend golfer is generally stiffer and less agile. The better golfer's rhythmic swing minimizes muscular effort, disc and facet loading, and muscle tears, whereas weekend golfers subject their backs to higher loads, greater muscular efforts, higher disc pressures, and they have less endurance. Thus, acute back injuries occur much more commonly in the weekend player and are generally muscle strains or muscle-tendon junction problems. Spondylolisthesis, disc disease, or spinal stenosis may occur in either group, and may produce more chronic problems.

In the senior golfer, loss of strength, loss of flexibility, and loss of coordination, as well as excessive weight and collagen brittleness, can take their toll on the spine. Muscle exercises to maintain strength, golf lessons to maintain a rhythmic swing, and a good warm-up can aid in prevention of serious injuries. Only rarely do structural changes limit participation.

In summary, conditioning, age, skeletal and disc abnormalities, and swing mechanics are the factors that determine the risk and patterns of injury in the spines of golfers.

BIOMECHANICS OF THE GOLF SWING

The spinal column is the axis around which the upper and lower extremities move during the golf swing. During a rhythmic swing, there is movement of a relatively small degree of all of the motion segments in the thoracolumbar spine. None of the motion segments, however, reaches the extreme of motion.

The illustrations on the following pages detail spinal kinesiology during the six separate phases of the golf swing:

1. **Address (Fig. 1)**

   Spinal contours are close to standing posture. The entire torso leans forward, pivoted at the hip joints. Spinal extensors and hip extensors are tonically active to maintain in the upright posture and limit further flexion. Pressure in lumbar discs is mildly increased compared to the pressure in the upright standing posture.
2. **Take-away (Fig. 2)**

   Pelvis rotates clockwise (when viewed from the top down, looking from the back forward). The spine also starts to rotate clockwise.

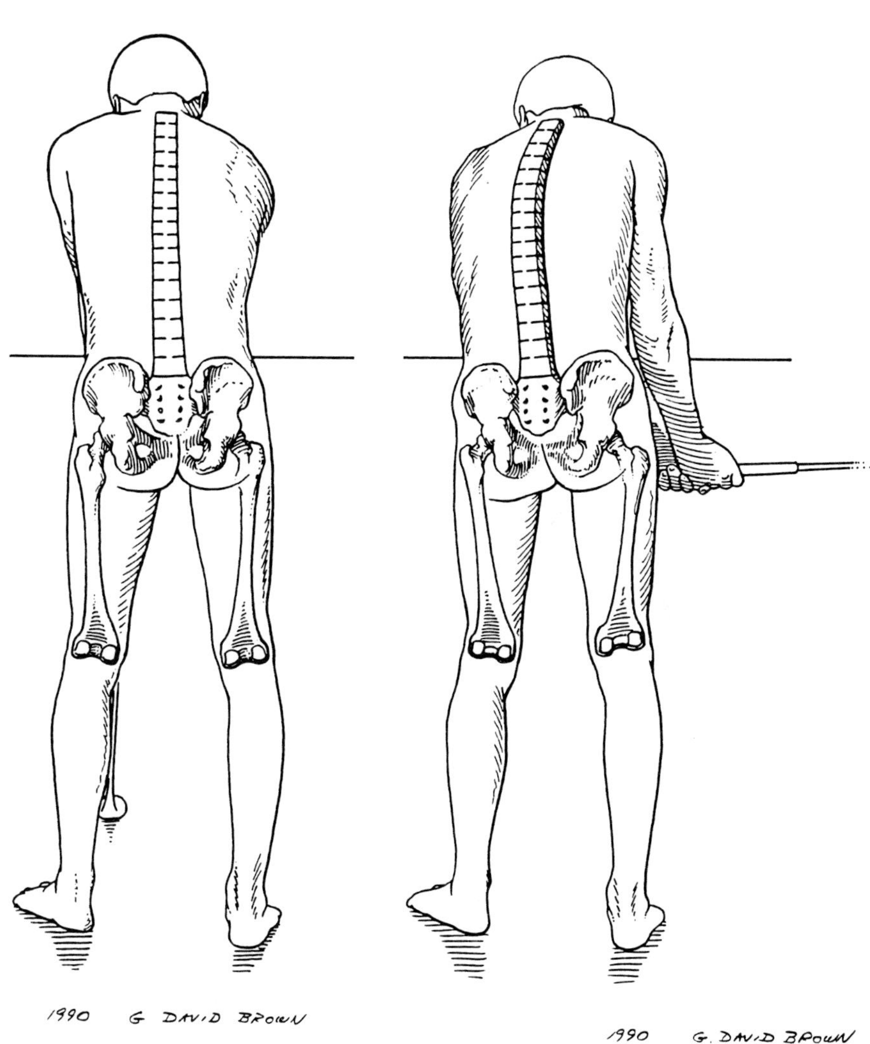

FIGURE 1. The address.

FIGURE 2. Take-away.

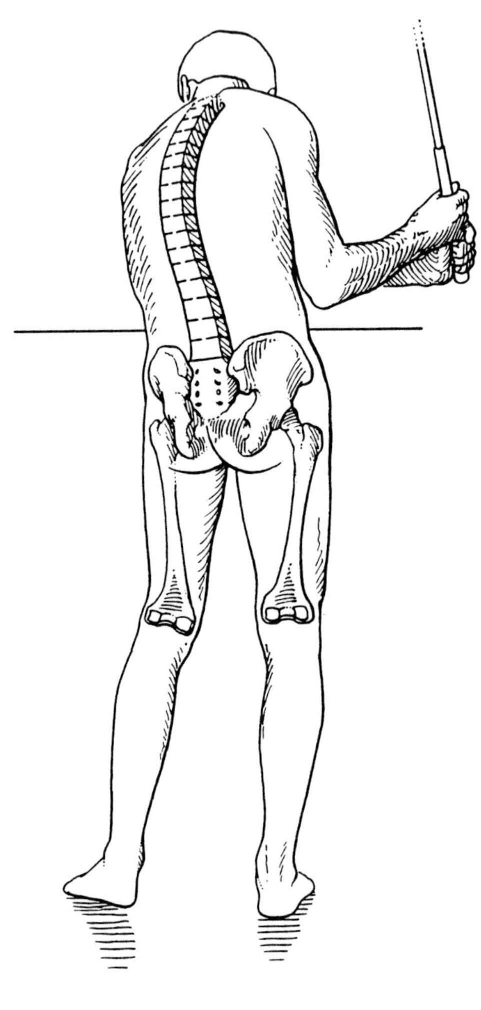

FIGURE 3. At the top.

3. At the Top (Fig. 3)

The shoulders are rotated 45 to 90 degrees posteriorly, and the pelvis is rotated clockwise 15 to 45 degrees. The clockwise rotation of each spinal motion segment is maximal at this phase. Disc pressures are increased by co-contraction of the spinal extensors and the abdominals, which stabilize and move the spine.

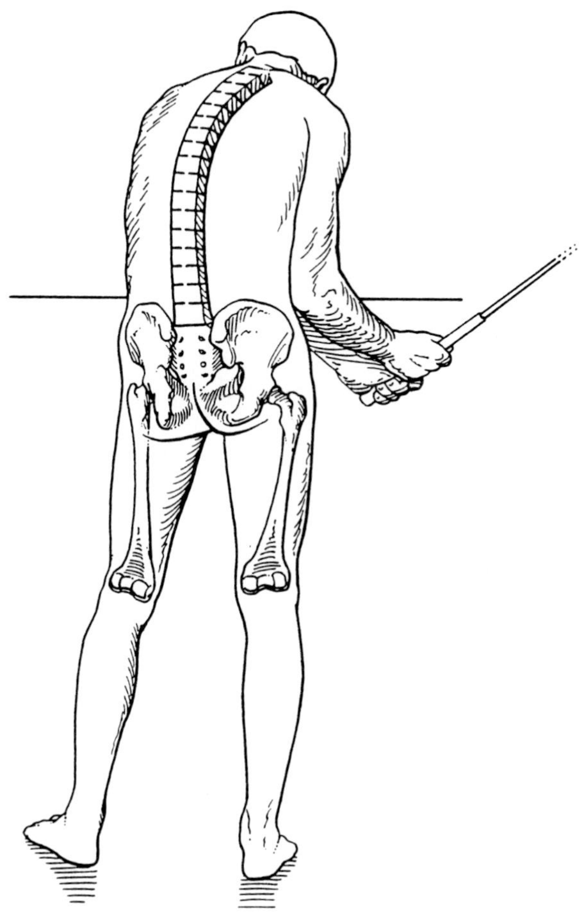

FIGURE 4. Downswing.

4. Downswing (Fig. 4)

Counterclockwise rotation of all spinal motion segments begins. Knee and hip joint movements, and leg and hip muscles derotate the pelvis back toward the "address" position. Active muscle recruitment of spinal and abdominal muscles increases disc and facet pressures.

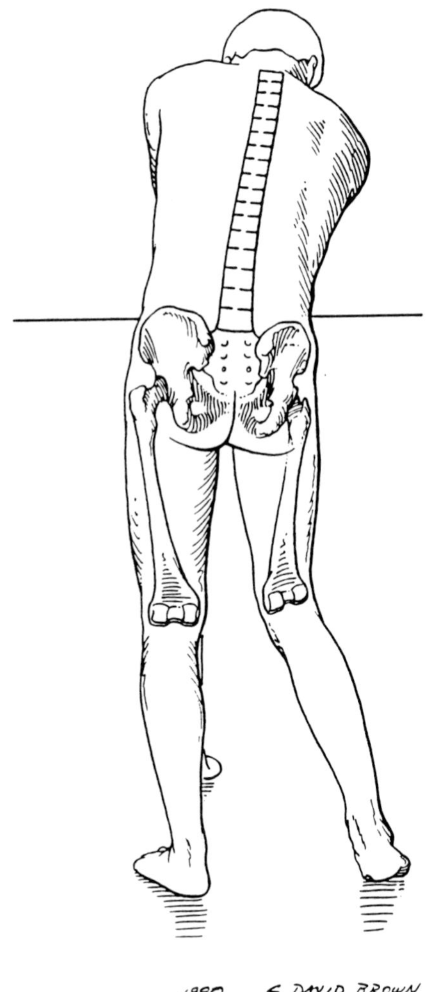

FIGURE 5. At impact.

5. At Impact (Fig. 5)

Spinal motion segments and the pelvis return toward the “address” position. Disc pressures and muscular contraction forces are maximal. Since the ball is so light, there is very little additional impact loading in the spine due to striking the ball (unlike baseball).

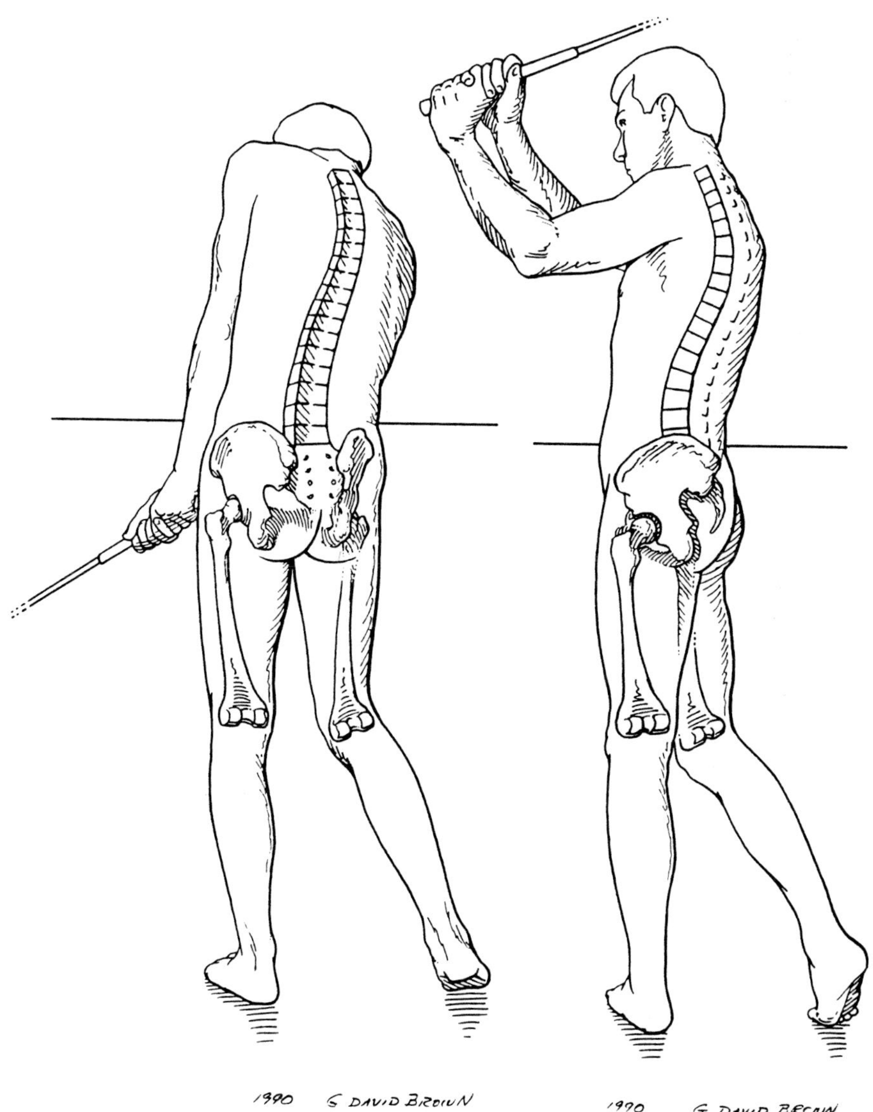

FIGURE 6. Follow-through.

FIGURE 7. Finish.

6. Follow-through and Finish (Figs. 6 and 7)

Continuing counterclockwise, rotation of the pelvis and all spinal motion segments occurs to the maximum range. The pelvis and the chest face the path of the ball at the finish. Pelvic rotation occurs as a consequence of rotations in the knee and hip joints. Gradual decreases in muscular effort and disc pressures occur back to the baseline level necessary to maintain the upright posture, while decelerating the trunk and upper extremities.

COMMON ACUTE SPINAL INJURIES IN GOLFERS AND THEIR RECOGNITION

Vulnerable tissues in the spine of golfers include:

1. Muscle bellies
2. Muscle and tendon attachments
3. Disc
4. Spinous processes and lamina

Muscle Belly Injuries. These occur from particularly violent swings or sudden stops during the downswing (hitting a root or a rock), or overuse from playing too many holes. Tenderness in the spinal muscles confirms the diagnosis.

Muscle and Tendon Attachment Injuries. These may arise from minimal or excessive use, swing abnormalities, or accidents. Tenderness at attachment sites along the spine, iliac crest, or ribs confirms the diagnosis.

Disc Injuries. Disc injuries can occur from swing accidents but generally are not directly related to a rhythmic swing. Golf can aggravate a pre-existing lesion, however. A positive deep-tenderness test and/or a positive straight leg raising test are physical findings associated with disc disease.

Laminal and Spinous Processes Impingement Injuries. Since impingement of spinal structures can only occur by maximal hyperextension of spinal segments, this problem is very unusual in golfers unless they have a very marked spinal hyperextension at the finish, or a striking reverse pivot during the take-away. Pain with hyperextension and interlaminar tenderness confirms the diagnosis.

PRE-EXISTING SPINAL ABNORMALITIES (CHRONIC SPINAL PROBLEMS)

Conditioning and good swing mechanics minimize risk of acute back injury. However, in conditioned or unconditioned golfers, underlying disease states may predispose to acute or chronic problems. Usually these conditions are self-limiting. However, disc disease, spondylolysis, spondylolisthesis, and spinal stenosis can occur in golfers as they do in the rest of the population. If extensive treatment becomes necessary for a golfer, it is almost always due to one of these structural problems.

Disc Disease

As aging proceeds, degenerative disc disease develops. Normal disc function is directly related to the elasticity of the annulus fibrosus and the stress distribution characteristics of a normal nucleus pulposus. Torsional loading of the disc space, fundamental to golf, is best handled by the younger, more responsive disc. Water content of a healthy disc is 88% at the time of birth and decreases with aging, reaching 40–60% by age 70.[13] This decrease in disc hydration (desiccation), combined with crystallization of the collagen fibrils in the annulus, leads to weakening and breakdown of disc architecture.

Symptomatic lumbar disc disease is relatively common among golfers. While disc injuries can occur during play, they usually present before or after a round. If a disc injury occurs during a golf swing, it is generally due to a swing accident. Most disc injuries occur in the L4–5 or L5–S1 level, as in the general population.[16] The sudden onset of low back pain with or without radicular symptoms suggests disc rupture. The high torsional and compressive loads that occur during golf readily explain the aggravation of symptoms that occasionally occurs among golfers with pre-existing disc disease.

The diagnosis is suggested by a positive deep tenderness test and/or a positive straight leg raising test over the involved disc. It can be confirmed by plain x-rays and a CT or MRI scan. Expedient and accurate diagnosis and management are essential to returning the golfer to the course.

Spondylolysis and Spondylolisthesis

Spondylolysis results from repeated stress to the pars interarticularis during lumbar hyperextension.[13] The golfer who first notices back pain after playing or practicing, but continues to play, may be placing extraordinary stress on the pars, with the end result being cortical fatigue and fracture.[16] While most spondylolysis is acquired, those athletes with a genetic predisposition for this condition are at risk for more significant injury during athletic activity. It then becomes important to assess whether this condition is acute or chronic for initial treatment and future management.

Golfers found to have bilateral spondylolysis on plain radiographs are at risk of developing spondylolisthesis as disc degeneration occurs. These athletes may present with paraspinous spasm and/or radicular symptoms during or after activity.[16] Cessation of athletic play is occasionally recommended for symptomatic spondylolisthesis of grade II or greater. Surgical stabilization may be warranted for chronic instability and continued or increased pain. The older golfer who presents with spondylolysis or spondylolisthesis in conjunction with back pain must be carefully evaluated in order to rule out disc herniations, recess stenosis, or spinal stenosis.[13] Diagnosis is similar to disc disease and confirmed by x-ray and MRI or CT scan.

Spinal Stenosis and Degenerative Facet Disease

Golfers over age 60 may show symptoms related to facet degeneration or spinal stenosis. Golfers with stenosis present with pain or radicular symptoms that are increased by hyperextension of the spine and relieved by flexion. Occasionally surgical decompression may be required to alleviate thecal sac and/or nerve root tension.

Degenerative facet disease may be delineated by pain relief following facet injections with local anesthetic. If this type of pain seems to be mechanically induced, facet rhizotomy may alleviate all or most of the symptoms temporarily. Once again, spinal fusion may be the ultimate outcome.[13]

TREATMENT

The diagnosis and treatment of most back problems can be based on a careful history and physical examination. Plain x-rays, MRI, CT scanning, myelography, and/or discography are only necessary if response to treatment is delayed. Once the diagnosis has been made, initial treatment of most problems of short duration can include rest, swing alterations, and mechanical modalities such as massage, ice, or heat.

Massage and chiropractic manipulation often help to reduce spasm and may even promote better mobility. Acupuncture can also be used to reduce pain. Gravity inversion can relieve spasm and spinal pressure in very resistant cases. This procedure requires a golfer to hang suspended either upside down or right side up in a traction-type device to reduce loads on the facets and disc spaces. As with any ancillary treatment, gravity inversion can worsen a golfer's symptoms if it is not applied gently. Also, the cardiovascular detriments of gravity inversion must be minimized or avoided. Anti-inflammatory agents, anti-spasmodics, and analgesics can be used if there is incomplete response to mechanical treatment.

Surgical management can take many forms and should not be considered until all conservative means have failed. Rhizotomy, chymopapain, percutaneous discectomy, simple laminectomy/discectomy, and spinal fusion should never be a mainstay in treating athletic injuries. However, golfers occasionally need these procedures, as do other athletes, if their symptoms fail to respond to conservative management.

After adequate pain relief has been achieved, by either conservative or operative treatment, an exercise program aimed at trunk and abdominal strengthening should be initiated. Exercises geared toward increasing spinal flexibility are essential to returning a golfer to the game. Aerobic and cardiovascular conditioning as well should enable the player to increase his or her endurance and power both on and off the course.

PREVENTION AND CONDITIONING

The initiation of an early exercise regimen is most important to both the amateur and tour professional in the prevention of golf injuries. The acute onset of lower back pain during play should not be the catalyst for exercise. Those programs aimed at increasing abdominal tone and lower back strength are the mainstay of athletic conditioning in this sport. Flexibility is another key component of prevention. Adequate stretching prior to exercise will inevitably aid in increased flexibility. Prone press-ups, hamstring stretching, and lateral side-bending are all excellent warm-up exercises for increasing a golfer's flexibility.[4]

Exercises to strengthen abdominal tone include abdominal isometrics, sit-ups performed supine on a rubber ball, and abdominal curls. These maneuvers increase abdominal and trunk control, both of which are key when handling transfer of power upward through the body during impact and follow-through.

The most crucial factor in injury prevention concerns modification of the swing. The editors of *Golf Magazine* have proposed the "no strain swing" in an effort to minimize lower back pain resulting from repeated spine hyperextension during aggressive play.[8] This swing is comprised of three components: (1) relaxed posture at address, (2) a three-quarters back-swing, and (3) increased hand action and a shorter finish. Keeping the head still and rounding the back at address will also serve to reduce lower back tension. Narrowing the putting stance will decrease postural strain as well.

The reverse-swing exercise[12] is advocated for increasing flexibility on the principle that the golfer must balance muscle pull by performing the opposite of the normal swing mechanism. This is done by taking swings, or upper extremity and pelvic rotations in the opposite direction repeatedly during warm-up and exercise.

Although activity modification needs emphasis, other factors inherent to the game itself are equally important. Wearing spikeless shoes and avoiding bouncing golf carts can reduce chronic pain during play.[13] Flexing the knees while lifting a golf bag, avoiding unilateral carrying or lifting, switching shoulders while carrying a golf bag, and taking care to keep the knees flexed when bending over should be part of any rehabilitative education program.[3]

Lastly, "self-awareness" and education about injury prevention are vital. Teaching the golfer to modify his swing, thereby reducing stress and torsional forces on the spine, will not only aid in injury reduction but enhance the golfer's game and overall physical fitness.

CONCLUSION

Most acute low back problems that plague the golfing athlete are due to the golf swing itself. The key to prevention of these injuries is abdominal and trunk strengthening, as well as a knowledge and application of proper swing mechanics so that the muscular effort and pressures generated in the spine are smooth and gradual, and that peak loads are avoided.

Injuries that become chronic and do not respond to conservative treatment or swing changes generally relate to the common spinal problems seen in the general population, i.e., spondylolisthesis, spondylolysis, disc disease in its various forms, or spinal stenosis. Thorough work-up and conservative or operative treatment of golfer's back problems generally result in prompt response to treatment, and return to the course.

Proper preparation for injury-free golf involves a recognition of a player's level of conditioning, lessons from a professional to minimize injury through proper swing mechanics, and proper diagnosis and treatment of injuries if they occur. If these guidelines are followed, golf should be a sport that can be played for a lifetime with very few lay-offs due to spinal disability.

Acknowledgment. The authors would like to thank golf pro Willard Crenshaw for his assistance in preparing this chapter by demonstrating and discussing the mechanics of a golf swing.

REFERENCES

1. Berry IW: Enemy number one. Golf Magazine March:34–39, 1984.
2. Blanstein JL: Injuries in Sport, 1973.
3. Carney R: Back savers: Stay off the disabled list with these five easy tips. Golf Digest 46–49, 1986.
4. Carney R: Oh, my aching lower back. Golf Digest 146–149, 1987.
5. Chasuat D: Golf injuries. Medicine du Sport (Paris) 61(5):253–255, 1987.
6. Dannenberg AL, et al: Leisure time activity in the Framingham Offspring Study. Am J Epidemiol 129:76–86, 1989.
7. Duda M: Golfers use exercise to get back in the swing. Phys Sportsmed 17(8):109–113, 1989.
8. Editors of Golf Magazine: The no-strain swing. Golf Magazine 40–43, 1984.
9. Kerian RK, et al: Golf injuries. Sportsmed Digest 5(7):6–7, 1983.
10. McCarroll JR: Golf. In Schneider RC, Kennedy JC, Plant ML: Sports Injuries: Mechanisms, Prevention and Treatment. Baltimore, Williams & Wilkins, 1985.
11. McCarroll JR, Gioe TJ: Professional golfers and the price they pay. Phys Sportsmed 10(7):64–70, 1982.
12. McCleery P: Bad back: How to avoid an old hang-up. Golf Digest March:58–65, 1984.
13. Nicholas JA, Hershman EB: The diagnosis and treatment of injuries of the spine in athletes. In Nicholas JA, Hershman EB: The Lower Extremity and Spine in Sports Medicine. St. Louis, C.V. Mosby, 1986, pp 1204–1226.
14. Schulenberg CAR: Medical aspects and curiosities of golf. Practitioner 217:625–628, 1976.
15. Shulz R, Curnow C: Peak performance and age among super athletes: Track and field, swimming, baseball, tennis and golf. J Geratology 43(5):113–120, 1988.
16. Spencer CW, Jackson DW: Back injuries in athletes. In Jordan Bd, Tsairis P, Warren RF: Sports Neurology. Rockville, MD, Aspen Publishers, 1989, pp 159–177.
17. Vinger PF, Hoerner EF (eds): Sports Injuries: The Unthwarted Epidemic. Littleton, MA, PSG Publishing, 1981.

PART III

EVALUATION AND TREATMENT OF SPINAL INJURIES IN THE ATHLETE

Chapter 22

RADIOGRAPHIC EVALUATION OF THORACOLUMBAR SPORTS-RELATED INJURIES

Philip R. Shalen, MD

The increasing importance of fitness in North America has resulted in individuals of all ages participating in athletics. Acute, chronic, and/or repetitive stresses upon the spinal elements hasten the occurrence of thoracolumbar pain syndromes. Although most of the associated injuries and their clinical presentations are self-limited, some are acutely severe, or persistent and chronic, and may have radiographic equivalents that are conducive to treatment.

The diagnostic radiologist's contribution to evaluating sports-related spinal injuries is to use the appropriate imaging modality for outlining normal and pathologic anatomy and to assist the referring physician in establishing criteria for surgical vs. nonsurgical disease. One objective is to enable the competitive athlete to return expeditiously to his sport with a decreased risk of aggravating the previous injury.

Clinical experience determines the radiologist's ability to accurately and noninvasively diagnose spinal disease. Radiologists must cooperate in devising sensible and affordable diagnostic approaches for evaluating sports-related spinal injuries.[14] The purpose of this chapter is to:

1. Outline the most common mechanical etiologies of thoracolumbar back pain.

2. Explain the roles of conventional radiography, including tomography, as well as nuclear radiology, water-soluble myelography, unenhanced and intrathecally enhanced computed tomography (myelo-CT), magnetic resonance imaging (MRI), discography, and CT-discography (discocat).

3. Discuss diagnostic approaches for evaluation of thoracolumbar spine pain in athletes.

ETIOLOGIES OF THORACOLUMBAR PAIN IN ATHLETES

The most common etiologies are:

1. Acute mechanical disorders (e.g., muscle and ligament strain, HNP, fracture).

2. Chronic mechanical disorders and those secondary to repetitive stress (e.g., stress fracture, disc disruption, Scheuermann's disease, "kissing" spines, and leg-length discrepancies).[6,7,15]

3. Nonmechanical disorders that simulate categories 1 and 2 above (e.g., neoplasm, disc-space infection, paraspinal muscle mass, aortoiliac aneurysm).

ACUTE MECHANICAL DISORDERS

Muscle and Ligament Strain

Muscle and ligament strain are among the most common sports-related injuries in either well-conditioned or sedentary adolescents and adults.[15] These are usually self-limited processes and are rarely evaluated radiographically. Muscle injuries can be imaged with MRI but are not a common indication for this examination.[13]

Herniated Nucleus Pulposus

Most patients with clinically suspected herniated nucleus pulposus (HNP) will have a conventional lumbosacral spine survey to exclude spondylolysis and spondylolisthesis, post-traumatic changes (including compression fractures and subluxations), and gross congenital deformities. Approximately 10% of patients who have persistent pain for more than 3 months will have a disc injury requiring further radiographic evaluation (Algorithm I).[14,16] The decision tree of this algorithm starts with either unenhanced CT or MRI. Both can be sensitive, specific, and highly accurate. Many referring practitioners are comfortable with the availability, accuracy, and reasonable cost of CT. Magnetic resonance imaging, if readily available, is attractive because:

1. Visualization of the conus medullaris is routine.
2. Unsuspected intrathecal neoplasms may be detected (Fig. 1).
3. MRI can ascertain whether discs are dehydrated (degenerated).
4. MRI is not an x-ray procedure with associated radiation.
5. With surface coil technology, MRI can frequently and effectively image obese patients.

If MRI with T1- (short TR, short TE) and T2- (long TR, long TE) weighted images (T1W1 and T2W1) is the initial examination, consideration of surgical intervention may be warranted after demonstration of a clinically correlating HNP and after failure of continued conservative care. If the MRI is negative for HNP, then a myelo-CT is obtained (usually as an outpatient). This procedure may be performed after conventional water-soluble myelography or as a low-dose myelo-CT (i.e., lumbar puncture with a 25–27 g needle, with intrathecal

Algorithm I

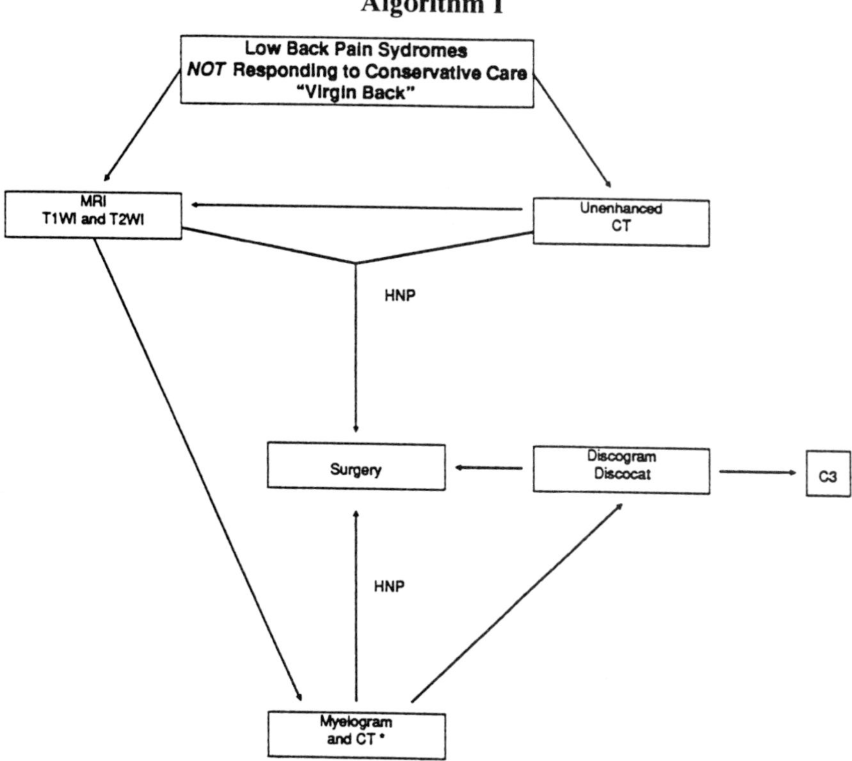

* CT after myelography may not be necessary if unenhanced CT was the initial exam. However, the myelo/CT may be easier to interpret, especially in obese patients.

administration of 3–5 cc of contrast). The myelo-CT avoids the diagnostic pitfalls associated with conventional myelography by visualizing the following:

1. The "insensitive" ventral epidural space at L5–S1.
2. Neuroforaminal and lateral recess stenoses.
3. Far-lateral HNP.
4. Pars defects.
5. Facet disease.
6. Differentiates the extradural defects of spurs from discs.

A small free fragment, facet-joint arthropathy, a pars defect, and bone metastases are more obvious on CT. If the myelo-CT is negative, a lumbar discogram and discocat may yield information unobtainable by other examinations (i.e., eliciting concordant discogenic pain and demonstration of annular disruptions that are suboptimally visualized on conventional CT or MRI). If this examination is also negative, the existence of surgical disease seems remote.

If the initial unenhanced CT is negative, then unenhanced MRI with T1W1 and T2W1 should be performed. The algorithm then proceeds with myelo-CT and lumbar discography/discocat, as described previously.

The radiographic findings associated with adult HNP have been extensively described and are beyond the scope of this review. However, the rare disc protrusions in older children and teenagers may be quite different in appearance,

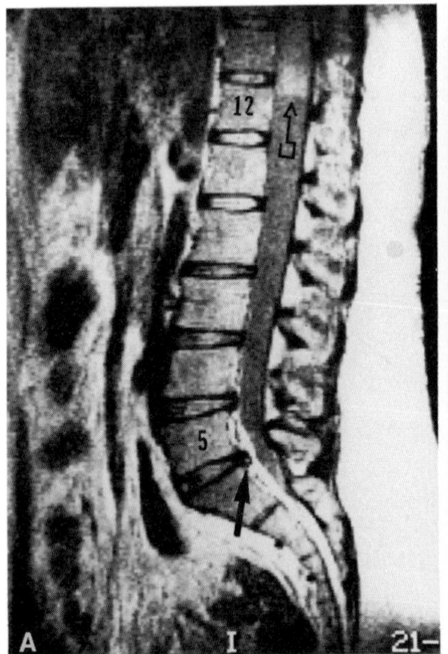

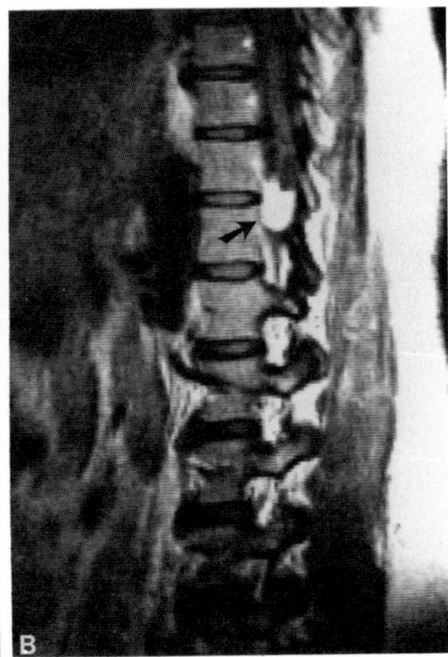

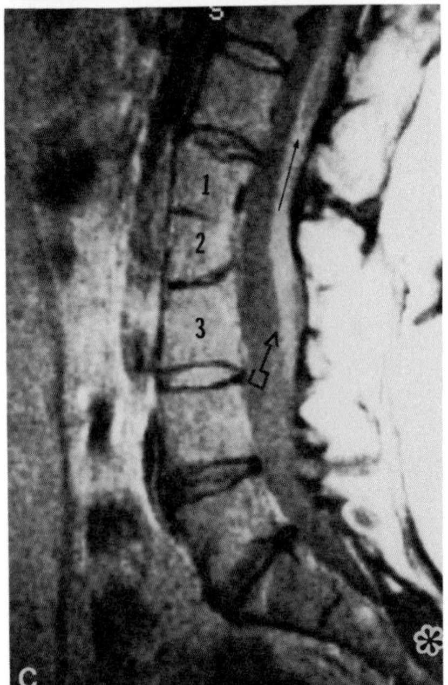

FIGURE 1. Patient with lumbar radicular syndrome. *A,* Disc protrusion at L5–S1 (closed arrow). Abnormal increased signal from central canal at T11–12 level (open arrow). *B,* Extramedullary schwannoma: homogeneous enhancement after intravenous gadolinium DTPA (arrow). *C,* Syrinx: This patient had back pain after being injured at work. Low conus (closed arrow), fusiform "mass" (syrinx) (open arrow) congenital L1–3 fusion, and sacral meningocele (✻).

symptoms, and pathophysiology.[3,11,15] Their disc lesions may be multiple; associated with large, avulsed apophyseal fragments; and present with severe low back pain, with or without radiculopathy (Fig. 2).

Thoracic disc herniations are rare, usually small, partially calcified, and may present with symptoms suggestive of a spinal cord tumor.[1] The most expeditious

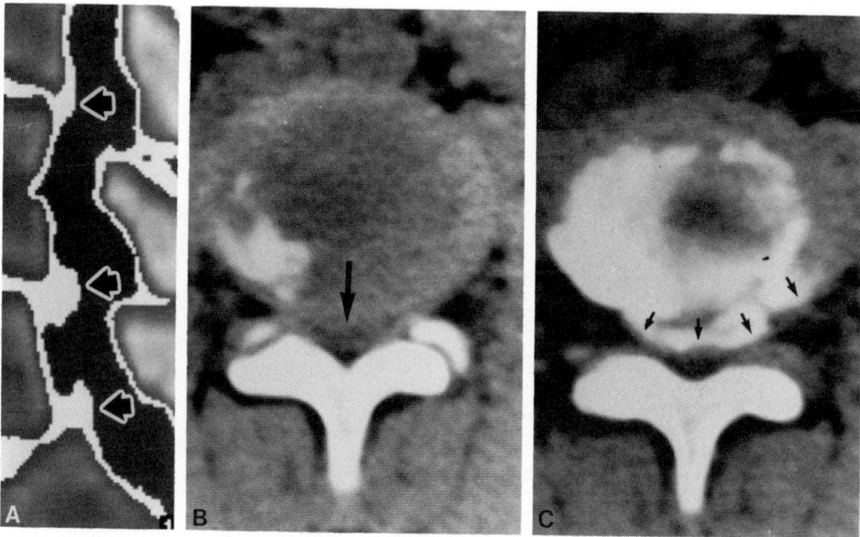

FIGURE 2. A 13-year-old patient with back pain. *A,* Multilevel protrusions on sagitally reformatted CT (arrows). *B,* Adult-type protrusion at L4–L5 (arrow). *C,* Adolescent-type endplate avulsion-protrusion (arrows) at L5–S1.

diagnostic screening study for the thoracic spine is MRI (Fig. 3). HNP, hematoma, and abscess (extra-axial lesions) are distinguishable from hydrosyringomyelia, neoplasm, hemorrhage, and arteriovenous malformations (intra-axial lesions) (Fig. 4). Further specificity may be possible with a limited CT thoracic myelogram (Fig. 5). If MRI is contraindicated or not well-tolerated, then conventional water-soluble thoracic myelography followed by a limited CT thoracic myelogram could be performed (Fig. 6).

Spinal Fractures

Injured athletes with thoracolumbar spine fractures do not always present with profound neurologic deficits. Consequentially, the initial radiographic examination, although simple in scope, must be of the highest possible quality. In the emergency situation, I prefer an initial two-view spine examination (AP and lateral, cross-table, if trauma is severe). If these are negative for fracture and/or subluxation, careful flexion and extension views are obtained when possible to demonstrate any latent instability.

Further evaluation with CT or pluridirectional, thin-section tomography is indicated if (1) a fracture is seen on plain films or (2) the patient's clinical condition precludes adequate plain films, but the mechanism of injury makes fracture a reasonable probability.

Computed Tomography. CT is an excellent examination under these circumstances because (1) minimum patient manipulation is necessary, (2) compression fractures and subluxations may be visualized on digital radiographic localized images (Fig. 7), (3) the patient can be intubated and chemically paralyzed, and all life-support systems are compatible with performance of the exam *(this is not the case with MRI),* (4) bony and soft tissue anatomy is discernible in minute detail, and (5) the exam can be performed after myelography

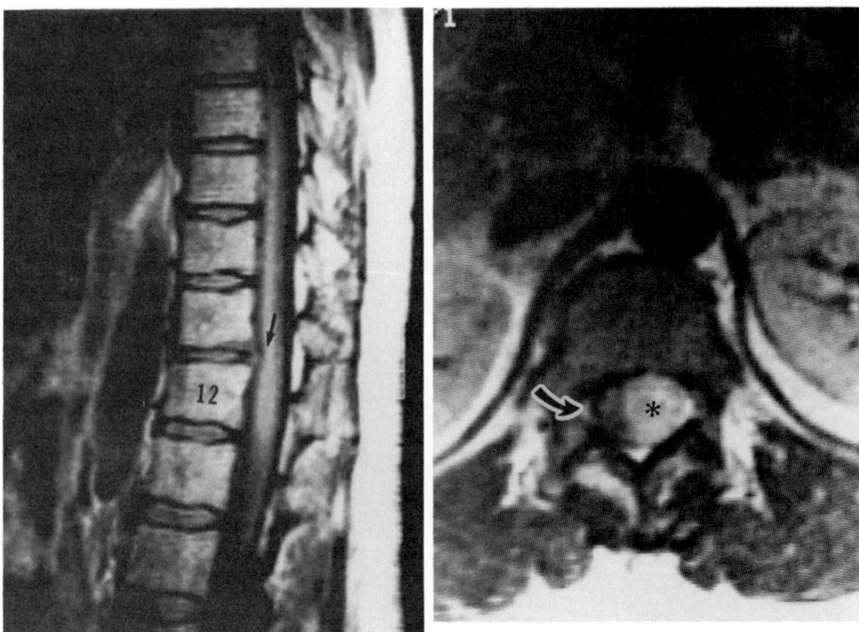

FIGURE 3 (left). A T11–12 protrusion with ventral spinal cord compression (arrow).

FIGURE 4 (right). Meningioma: T2WI showing large, hyperintense extramedullary mass (✱) displacing the lower thoracic spinal cord (arrow) to the right.

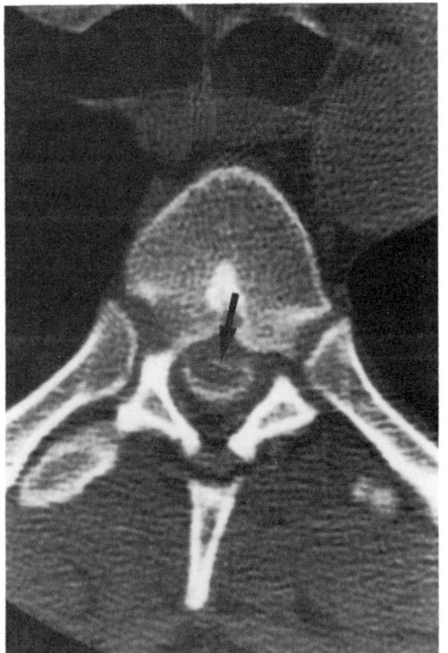

FIGURE 5. CT thoracic myelogram; ventral spinal cord compression (arrow).

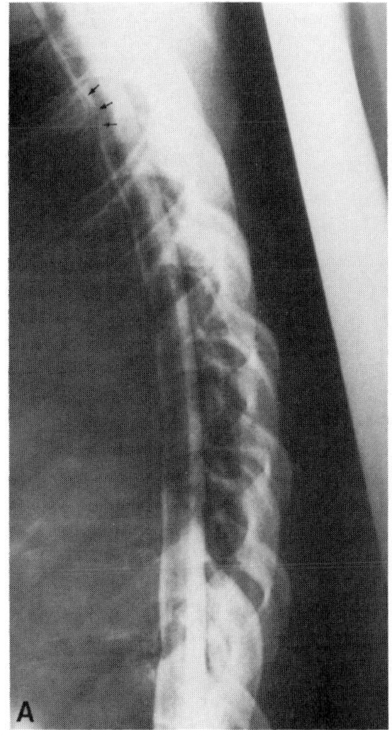

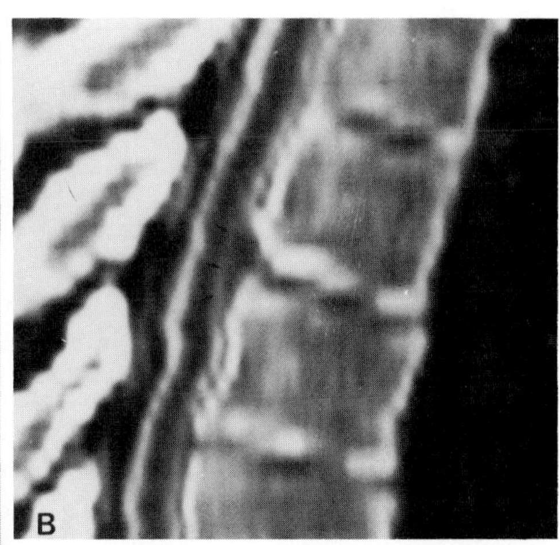

***FIGURE 6** (above).* Thoracic HNP on *A,* decubitus lateral (arrows) and *B,* sagittal reformation (arrows) after CT myelography.

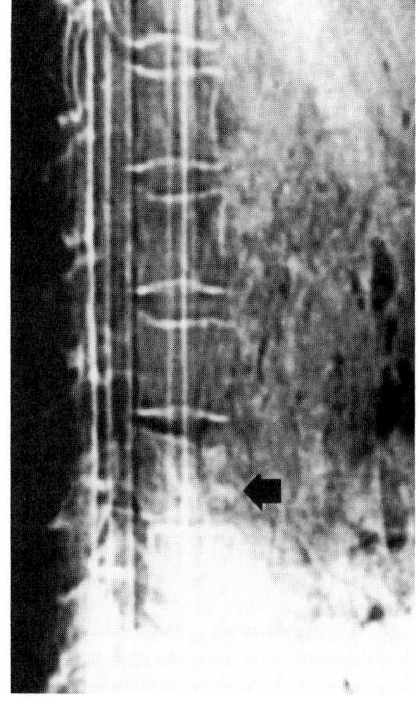

***FIGURE 7** (right).* Digital lateral localizer image: lumbar fracture (arrow) visualized despite artifacts from trauma board.

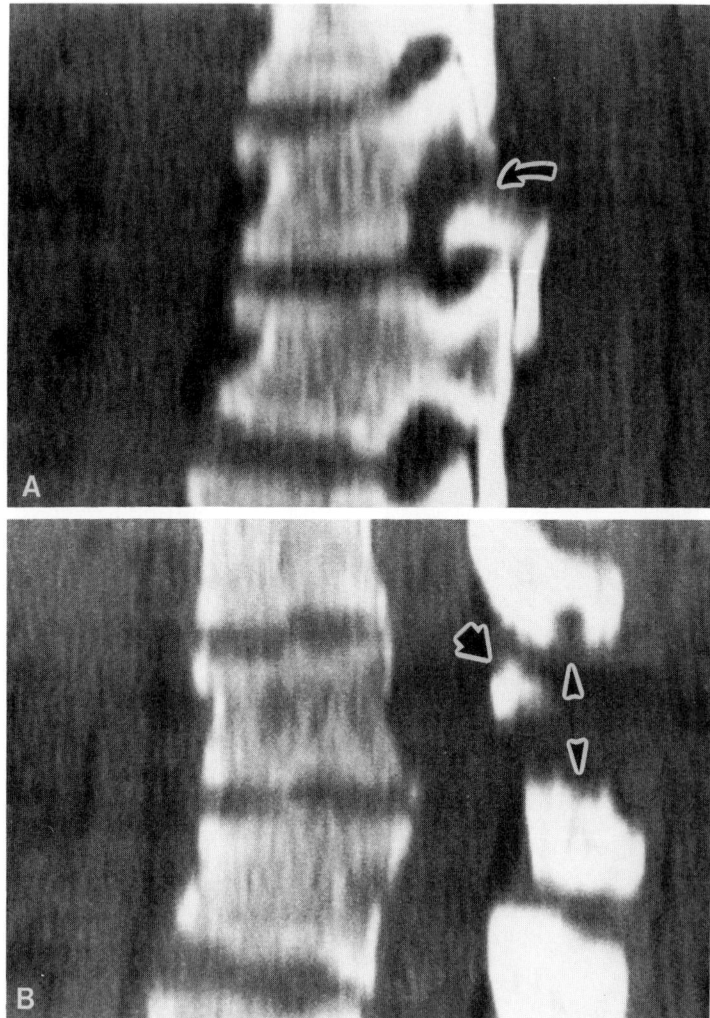

FIGURE 8. *A*, Parasagittal and *B*, midline sagittal CT reformations. Acute pars (arrow in *A*) and spinous process fractures (arrow in *B*) are present. Note widening of interspinous space (arrowheads).

to evaluate a high-grade or total block, or to increase the CT's sensitivity. CT technique should include 4–5 mm overlapped transaxial or thinner contiguous sections through suspicious regions, using high-resolution bone and soft tissue algorithms. The slices are overlapped to allow better quality sagittal and coronal reformations (Fig. 8).

Tomography. Thin-section, pluridirectional tomography is a superb examination for demonstrating spinal fractures (Fig. 9). However, its use has decreased markedly with the nearly universal availability of thin-section, high resolution CT. The relative disadvantages of conventional x-ray tomography include (1) higher radiation dose; (2) poor visualization of intra- and extraspinal

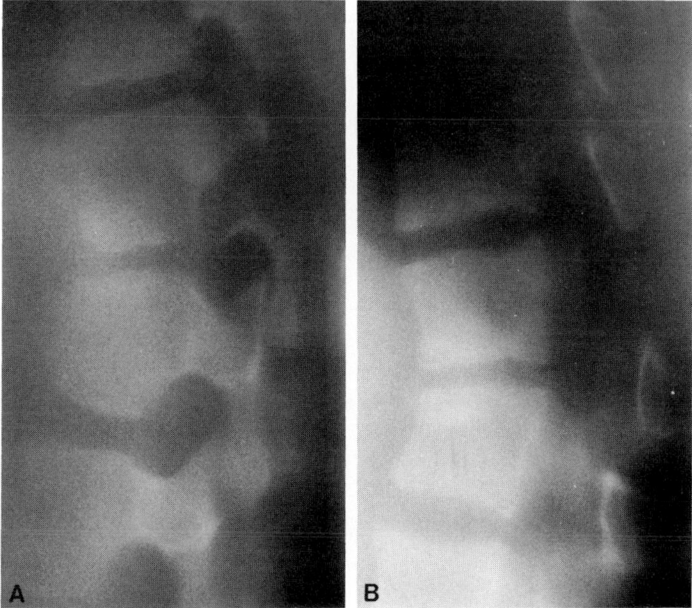

FIGURE 9. *A,* Parasagittal and *B,* midline sagittal pleuridirectional tomographic images correspond to Figure 8 *A, B.*

soft tissues; (3) having to move the patient into the recumbent and decubitus positions; and (4) the inability to perform multiplanar reconstructions.

CHRONIC MECHANICAL DISORDERS

Stress Fractures

Pars disruptions in adults are generally thought to represent unrecognized stress fractures that occurred in childhood or early adolescence.[8] Rothman defined four stages in the natural history of spondylolysis:[11]

I. Acute fracture
II. Healing fracture
III. Unhealed fracture
IV. Healed fracture.

Spondylolisthesis, disc degeneration, HNP, neuroforaminal stenosis, and hypertrophy of the contralateral pars, pedicle, and lamina may be associated anatomical findings. Clinical symptoms may include low back pain initially, and radiculopathy ultimately.

Radiologic imaging techniques and findings will vary with Rothman's stages I–IV. Until spondylolysis occurs, repetitive micro- (stress) fractures may be radiographically invisible. These prespondylitic pars stress fractures may be detectable on radionuclide scans.[5,8,9,10,12] A subacute or healing (Stage II) fracture should be discernible on lumbar spine radiographs, CT, and radionuclide scans. An unhealed (Stage III) fracture is visible on plain films and CT. A bone scan is likely to be negative, unless there are degenerative pseudarthroses. The evaluation can be confusing with mixed-stage disease, e.g., with a unilateral stage III and a

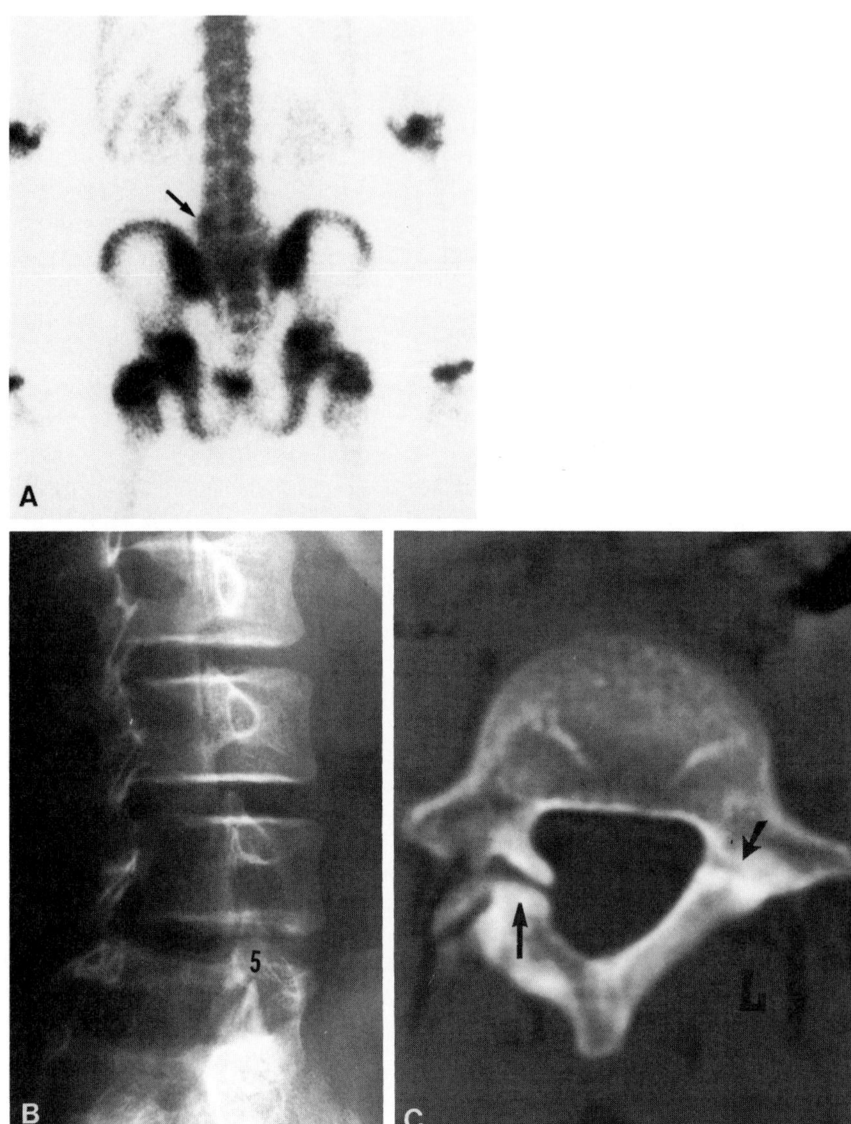

FIGURE 10. Young gymnast with chronic low back pain. *A,* Radionuclide bone scan: increased activity at L5 on the left (arrow). *B,* Oblique lumbar spine: "normal" L5 pars interarticularis on the left. *C,* Transaxial CT at L5: Stage II and Stage III fractures on left (curved arrow) and right (straight arrow), respectively.

contralateral stage I or II (Fig. 10), or if there is compensatory hypertrophy of the intact posterior elements, then the radionuclide scan could be positive on the radiographically unfractured side. Finally, Stage IV (healed) lesions may not be recognized as such. Thickening of the pars or hockey-stick deformities on CT sagittal reformations are highly suggestive.[11]

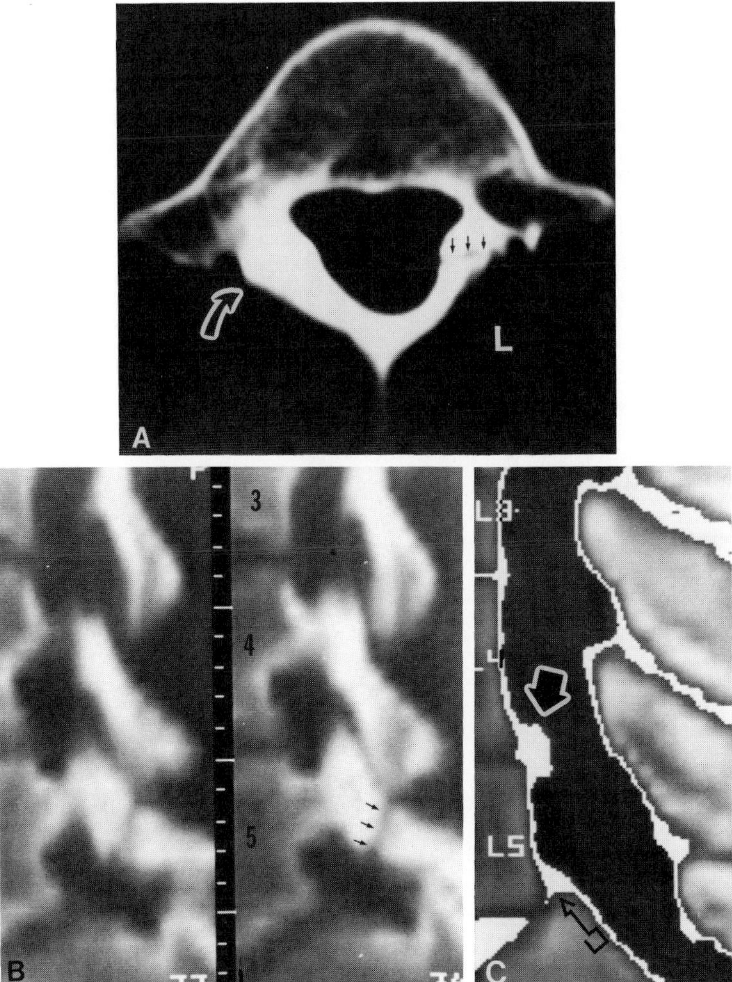

FIGURE 11. *A,* Transaxial CT at L5: Stage IV and Stage III fractures on right (curved arrow) and left (small arrows), respectively. *B,* Sagittal reformat through L3–L5 left-sided pars interarticularis. Note L5 pars fracture (small arrows). *C,* Highlighted midline sagittal reformat: There is a Grade I spondylolisthesis at L5–S1 (open arrow), and a disc protrusion at L4–5 (closed arrow).

CT is usually the single best examination for delineating pars fractures, spondylolisthesis, associated disc herniation, air vacuum disc, neuroforaminal stenosis, and posterior element hypertrophy (Fig. 11). MRI will visualize the larger, distracted fractures and help to differentiate pseudo-bulges, secondary to spondylolisthesis, from frank disc ruptures. The decreased signal associated with dehydrated or degenerated discs is only seen on MRI (Fig. 12).

Disc Disruption

The etiology of athletically induced low back pain may remain obscure, despite extensive diagnostic testing. As suggested in Algorithm I, it is at this point

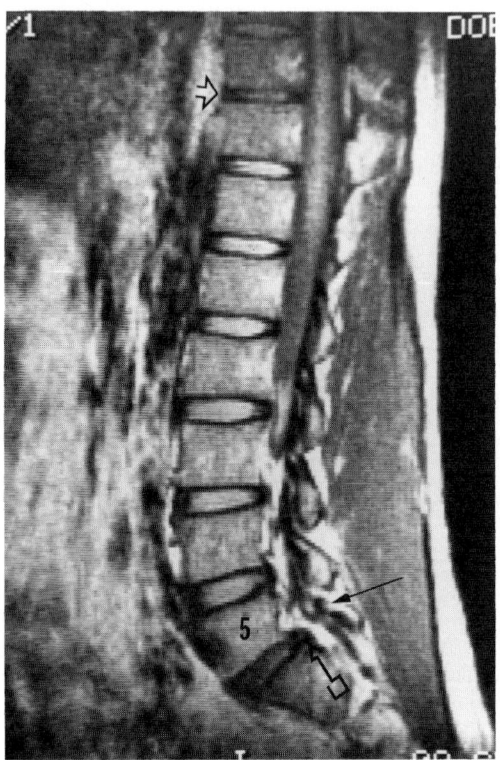

FIGURE 12. Sagittal MRI: Pars defect (closed arrow), Grade I spondylolisthesis with posterior L5–S1 protrusion (open arrow). Decreased signal from the narrowed (degenerated) T10–11 disc space.

that discography and CT-discography might be considered. After intradiscal contrast injection, there may be *exact* reproduction of the patient's clinical symptoms, i.e., a concordant pain response. A different therapeutic approach may then be warranted.[7,13,15]

Scheuermann's Disease

Scheuermann's disease represents vertebral endplate stress fractures seen in young children and adolescents. A higher incidence has been described in competitive swimmers specializing in the butterfly stroke and in weight lifters[6] (Fig. 13).

Affected patients may have low back pain, kyphoscoliosis, irregular and poorly formed thoracolumbar vertebral endplates, and intravertebral disc herniations (Schmorl's nodes, limbus vertebrae). Pathologically, there is avascular necrosis of secondary ossification centers of vertebral endplates. Although there is usually no evidence of an identifiable traumatic event, the mechanism of injury may be comparable to the chronic stress and microfractures thought to cause spondylolysis.[2]

The radiographic diagnosis is not complicated. All of the pathologic findings are seen with frontal and lateral projections of the spine, CT with sagittal reconstructions, and multiplanar MRI.

Leg-length Discrepancies

Leg-length discrepancies of 1 cm or more can result in a functional scoliosis and pain in the sacroiliac joints and along the course of the sciatic nerve at the

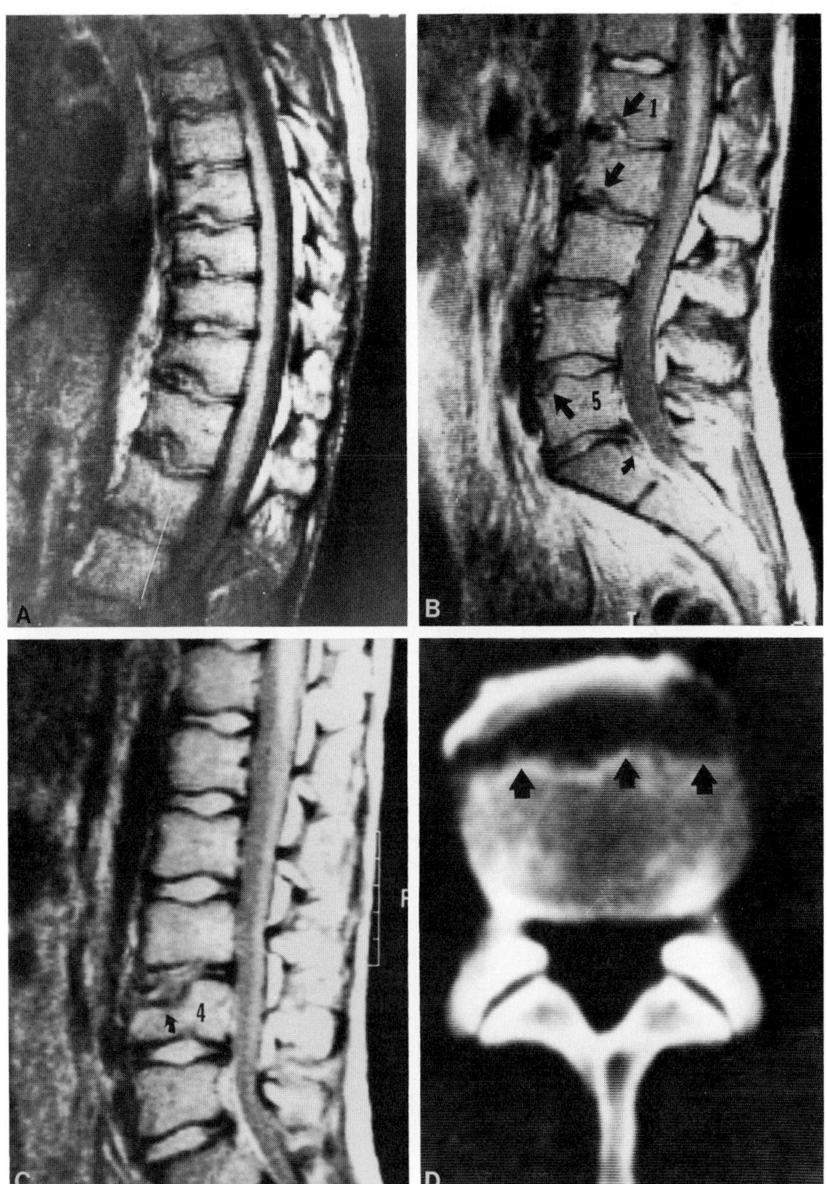

FIGURE 13. *A,* An 18-year-old swimmer with chronic back pain: Scheuermann's disease with multilevel Schmorl's nodes. *B,* A 27-year-old weight lifter with acute and chronic back pain. An L5–S1 HNP (curved arrow) and multiple Schmorl's nodes (straight arrows) are visible. Note L1–2 through L5–S1 degenerative disc signals. *C, D,* Anterior Schmorl's node and limbus vertebra at L4 on MRI (curved arrow in *C*) and transaxial CT (arrows in *D*).

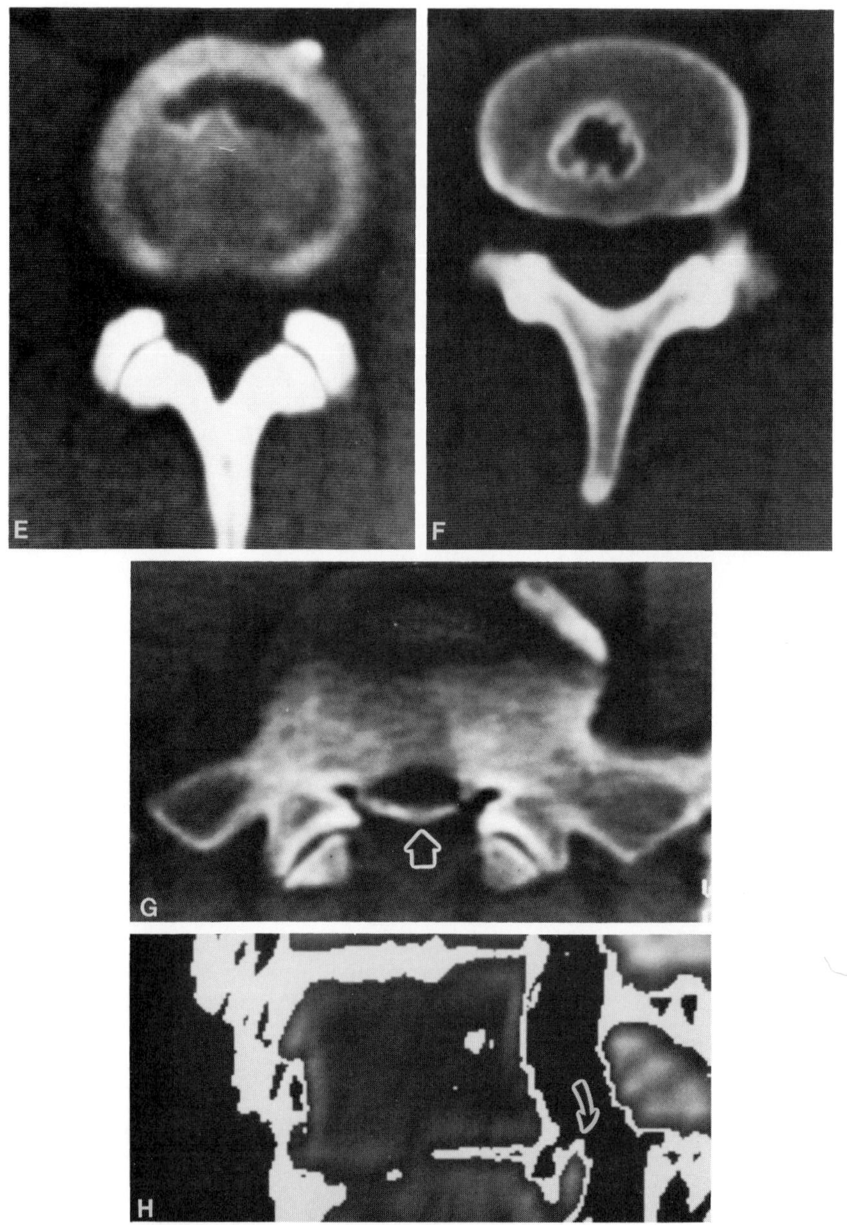

FIGURE 13 (continued). *E, F,* Schmorl's nodes involving anterior and central portions of the endplate. *G, H,* Transaxial (arrow in *G*) and sagittally (curved arrow in *H*) reformatted images of a posterior Schmorl's node and posterior limbus vertebrae (uncommon).

sciatic notch ipsilateral to the smaller extremity. The diagnosis can be made by measuring the distance between the medial malleoli and the anterior superior iliac spines. The dull, aching pain may be relieved by a heal lift.[6,7]

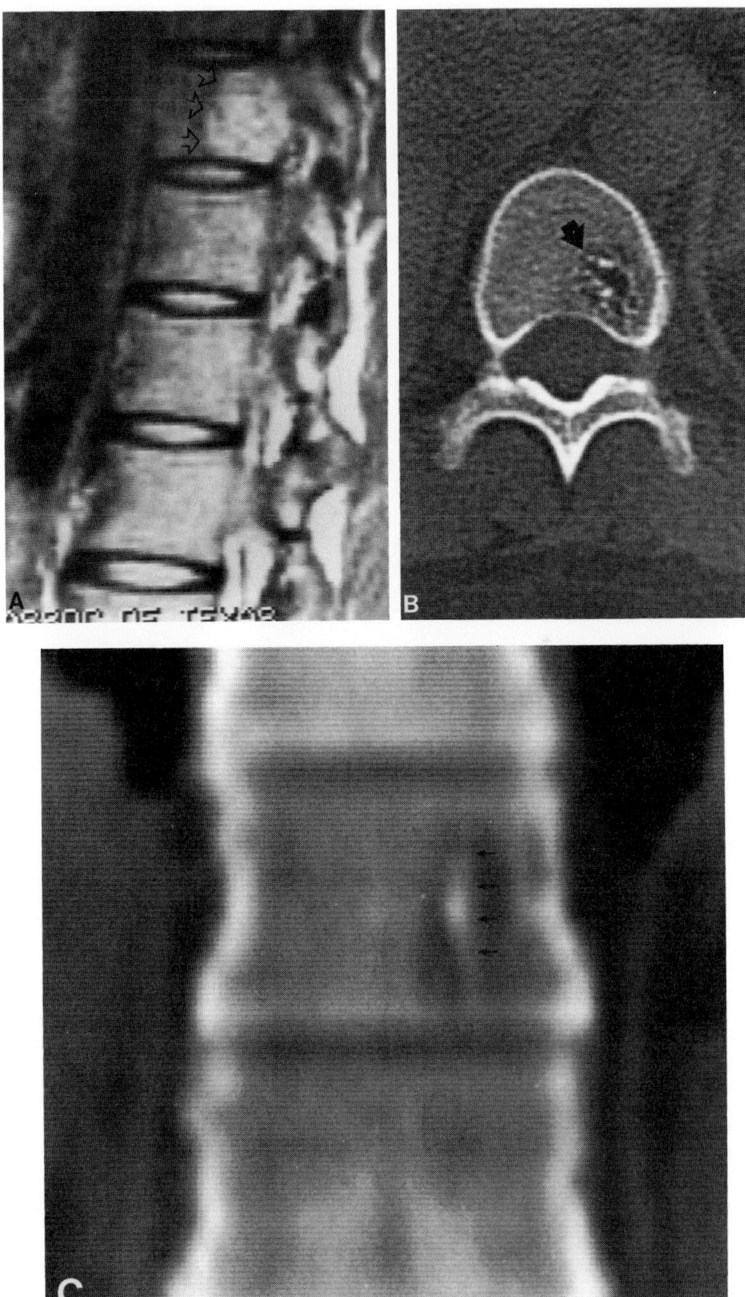

FIGURE 14. *A,* T10 hemangioma on sagittal MRI: well-circumscribed, nearly homogenous increased signal emanating from the vertebral body centrum (open arrows). *B, C,* Transaxial (arrow in *B*) and coronal (small arrows in *C*) CT reformation of L3: sharp demarcation and bony spiculation is characteristic of a vertebral hemangioma.

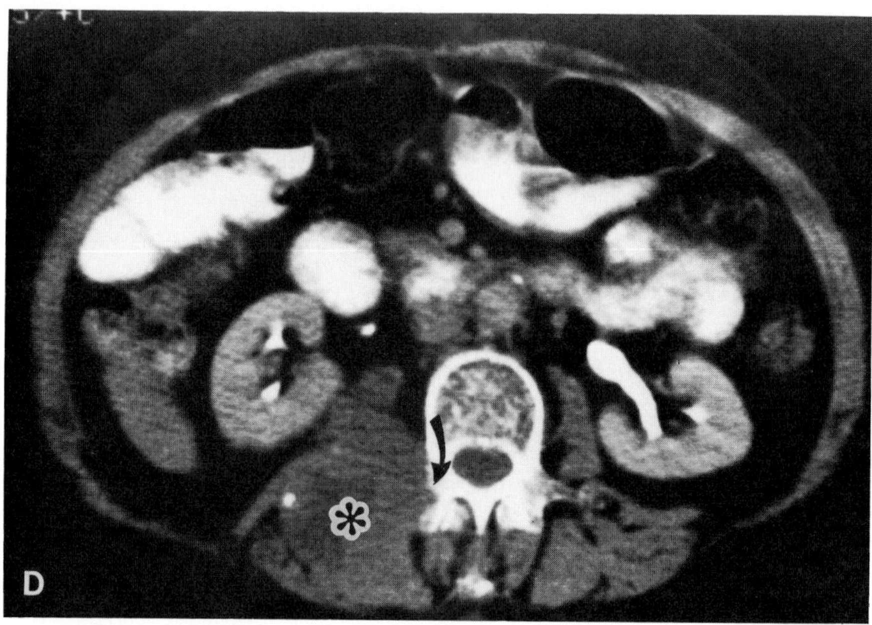

FIGURE 14. (continued). D, Back pain patient with transverse process destruction (curved arrow) secondary to a large, quadratus lumborum neoplasm (*).

Interspinal Osteoarthrosis and Lumbar Interspinous Process Bursitis (referred to as "kissing spines")

This mechanical cause of low back pain is seen after repetitive hyperextension maneuvers, resulting in interspinous tissue injury and localized bursitis. Diagnosis is made by history and physical examination, as there are no radiographic equivalents.

NONMECHANICAL SPINAL DISORDERS SIMULATING ATHLETIC INJURY

A variety of intra- and paraspinal disease processes may result in low back and radicular syndromes precipitated during physical exertion. These abnormalities are rare in young people, but readily diagnosable with modern imaging techniques. Benign and malignant neoplasms may involve the paraspinal musculature and bone (Fig. 14). Direct compression (invasion) of nerves and pathologic fractures are discernible (Fig. 15). Disc space infections, osteomyelitis, paraspinal and intraspinal extradural abscesses, and hemorrhages (Fig. 16) can result in severe, acute low back pain clinically indistinguishable from other more common entities. Discitis may result in narrowing of the intervertebral disc space, irregularity, demineralization, and lysis of the contiguous vertebral endplates and vertebral centra (osteomyelitis). An epidural empyema may result.

Aortoiliac aneurysms and dissections may cause back pain and radicular syndromes, but are not usually seriously considered in the differential diagnosis of low back pain syndromes in athletes.

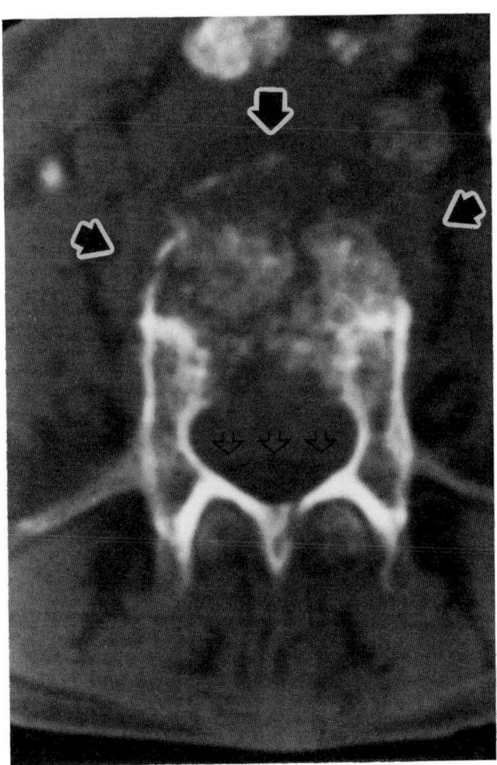

FIGURE 15. Vertebral body metastasis, pathologic fracture, and a large intra- (open arrows) and paraspinal (closed arrows) mass.

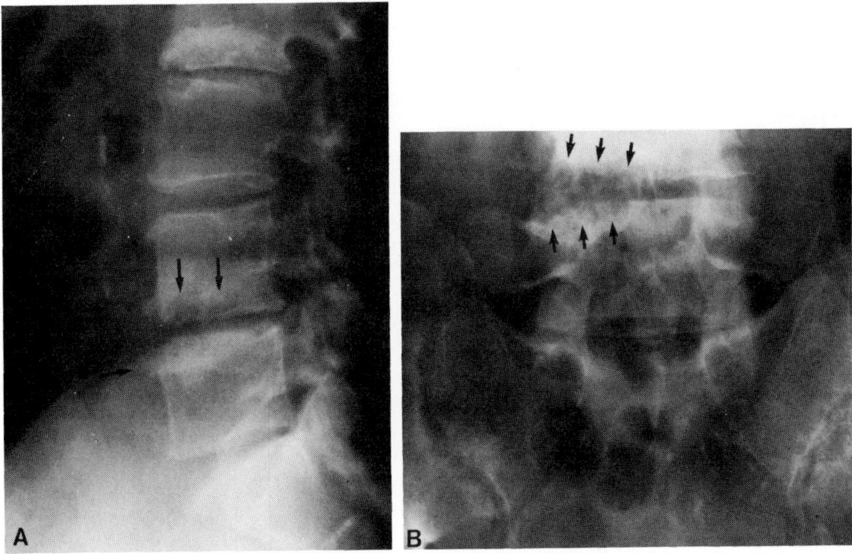

FIGURE 16. *A, B,* AP/lateral radiographs: focal endplate destruction (arrows) and mixed lytic-blastic reactive changes are characteristic of discitis and vertebral body osteomyelitis.

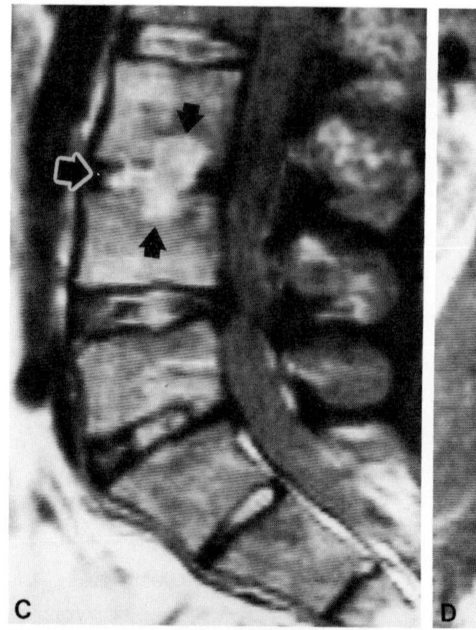

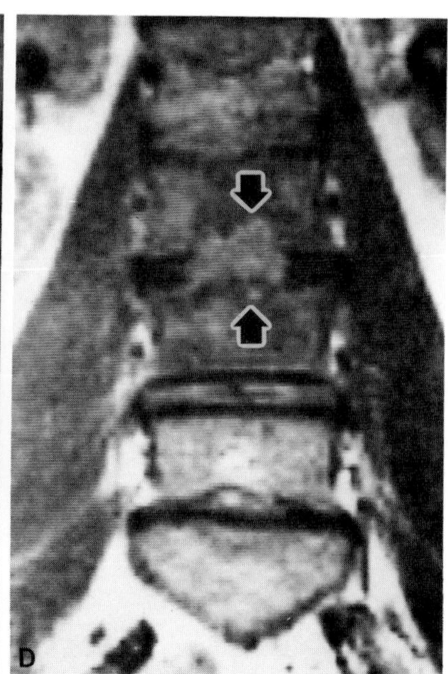

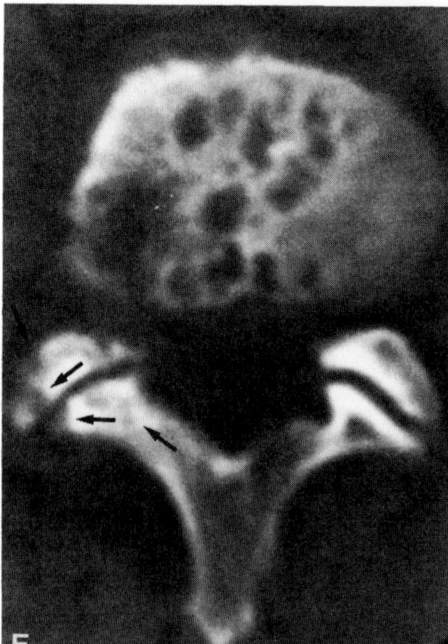

FIGURE 16. *(continued). C, D,* Sagittal and coronal MRI: abnormal increased signal from disc space and vertebral body (arrows) and focal endplate destruction consistent with infection. *E,* Transaxial CT image: destructive inflammatory changes of endplate, facet elements, and facet joint (arrows).

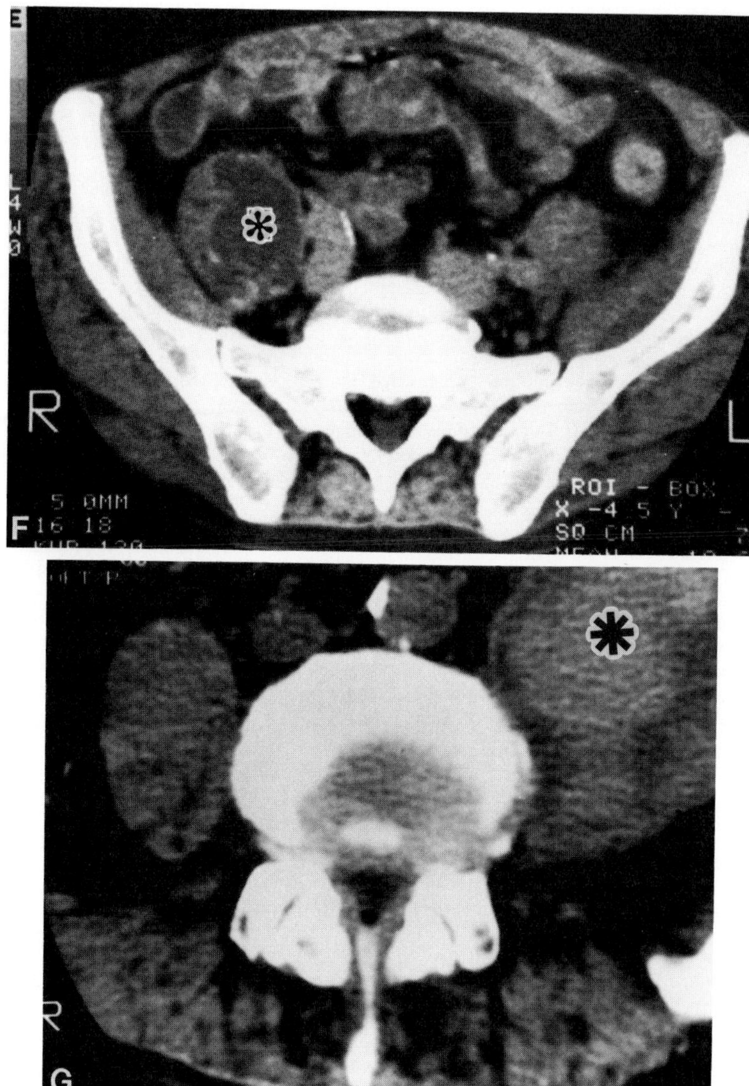

FIGURE 16 (continued). *F,* Right psoas abscess (✱). *G,* Left psoas hematoma (✱)

CONCLUSION

Most sports-related injuries involving the thoracolumbar spine are self-limited and do not require medical intervention. Occasionally, disabling syndromes occur that, when appropriately diagnosed and treated, further injury may be prevented and more rapid return of the athlete to training and competition may be allowed. The radiologist may contribute significantly to this process.

Acknowledgments: Special thanks to Denise Williams and Kass Jackson for preparation of the manuscript and to Michael Lorfing for photographic reproductions.

REFERENCES

1. Cacayorin ED, Hochhauser L, Petro GR: Lumbar and thoracic spine pain in the athlete: Radiographic evaluation. Clin Sports Med 6:767–783, 1987.
2. Edeiken J, Hodes PJ: Roentgen Diagnosis of Diseases of Bone. Baltimore, Williams & Wilkins, 1967.
3. Ehni G, Schneider SJ: Posterior lumbar vertebral rim fracture and associated disc protrusion in adolescence. J Neurosurg 68:912–916, 1988.
4. Fleckenstein JL, Weatherall PT, Parkey RW, et al: Sports-related muscle injuries: Evaluation with MR imaging. Radiology 172:793–798, 1989.
5. Jackson DW, Wiltse LL, Dingeman RD, Hayes M: Stress reactions involving the pars interarticularis in young athletes. Am J Sports Med 9:304–312, 1981.
6. Keene JS, Drummond DS: Mechanical back pain in the athlete. Comp Ther 11:7–14, 1985.
7. Keene JS: Low back pain in the athlete. Sports-Induced Back Pain 74:209–217, 1983.
8. Letts M, Smallman T, Afanasiev R, Gouw G: Fracture of the pars interarticularis in adolescent athletes: A clinical biomechanical analysis. J Pediatr Orthop 6:40–46, 1986.
9. Papanicolaou N, Wilkinson RH, Emans JB: Bone scintigraphy and radiography in young athletes with low back pain. Am J Radiol 145:1039–1044, 1985.
10. Pennell RG, Maurer AH, Bonakdarpour A: Stress injuries of the pars interarticularis: Radiologic classification and indications for scintigraphy. Am J Radiol 145:763–766, 1985.
11. Rothman SL: Computed tomography of the spine in older children and teenagers. Clin Sports Med 5:247–270, 1986.
12. Rupani HD, Holder LE, Espinola DA, Engin SI: Three-phase radionuclide bone imaging in sports medicine. Radiology 156:187–196, 1985.
13. Sachs BL: Discography as a diagnostic modality for use in low back pain. Spine State Art Rev 3:49–55, 1989.
14. Shalen PR: Radiologic techniques for diagnosis of lumbar disc degeneration. Spine State Art Rev 3:27–48, 1989.
15. Spencer CW III, Jackson DW: Back injuries in the athlete. Clin Sports Med 2:191–215, 1983.
16. Thomas JC Jr: Plain roentgenograms of the spine in the injured athlete. Injuries to the Spine 5:353–371, 1986.

Chapter 23

NONSURGICAL TREATMENT OF SPORTS-RELATED SPINE INJURIES

INTRODUCTION

Fortunately, most low back injuries sustained by athletes can be successfully treated conservatively. The methods of conservative treatment available for athletes are the same as for others with low back pain. However, when treating injured athletes, special consideration needs to be given to the importance of athletic activity to them and the physical demands they will face upon returning to their chosen athletic endeavors.

The purpose of this chapter is to discuss different conservative methods available to treat athletes with low back injuries, including rest or reduced activity, various modalities, manipulation, acupuncture, injections, and psychological intervention. Several of these methods may be combined as the patient progresses through a rehabilitation program.

I. Modalities

DONNA D. OHNMEISS, MS

The majority of low back pain experienced by athletes is related to problems of strained muscles or ligaments, which are often associated with the great demands athletes place on their spines, especially when the load is combined with a twisting motion. Discussed below are some of the more common modalities used to treat athletic low back injuries.

Rest

Rest from activity provides a period when no or only minimal stress is placed on injured tissue, thereby providing a more favorable healing environment. Although some advocate a period of bed rest lasting up to several weeks, Deyo reported favorable results with just 2 days bed rest for low back pain.[3] Prolonged bed rest can be detrimental. It is associated with rapid deossification of weight-bearing bones and loss of muscle strength and bulk,[2] the reason being that these tissues are only maintained by putting some degree of stress on them. During bed rest the structures are not stressed and thus no rebuilding occurs. Also, prolonged bed rest may be detrimental to the disc, since the disc depends on diffusion induced by motion for its nutrition.[6,23,24] Stanish points out that in recreational athletes there may be a danger of prescribing rest, in that once a person leaves activity due to a painful injury, he or she may have fear of reinjury and be less likely to return to sports.[20]

Compliance with several days of strict bed rest may be rather poor, especially among motivated athletes in training. Athletes resting from their usually demanding training can still engage in other activities, so long as they do not aggravate their pain. Swimming or hydrotherapy may be particularly beneficial very early in the rehabilitation process, since the buoyant force of the water greatly decreases the loads placed on the spine.

Some authors recommended bed rest for patients with a herniated disc, usually in the range of 5 to 14 days before returning to reduced activity, although no rationale for this has been presented.[16] Recently, very favorable results have been reported among low back pain patients in the treatment of herniated nucleus pulposus (HNP) by avoiding prescription of bed rest and promoting activity.[19]

Cryotherapy

The initial physiologic responses to cold have been reported to be vasoconstriction, decreased nerve conduction velocity, decreased blood flow and decreased capillary permeability, and an increased pain threshold.[5,12,13] The pain-controlling mechanism is thought to occur by either or both producing counter-irritant signals (and thus blocking the pain signals) and also be reducing muscle spasm and thereby reducing pain. Because of these properties, ice (in the form of ice packs, massage, or spray-on cooling agents) is commonly applied several times a day during the first 24 to 48 hours of injury to provide pain control and reduce edema and bruising. The mechanism of cold applied to the skin to reach deep injuries in spinal musculature has not been clearly determined.

Among authors,[9,18,22] the recommended duration of application of ice varies from 8 to 20 minutes. Several authors have reported that ice applied for more than 20 to 30 minutes results in intermittent cycles of vasodilation and vasoconstriction. Sometimes referred to as the "hunting reaction," this is thought to be a protective mechanism to help maintain a safe temperature of the skin and other tissues.[12,18] Prolonged application of ice can result in superficial tissue damage or frostbite, and therefore it should not be applied for more than 20 minutes in a single session.[12] Ice massage is less likely to produce damage, since the ice is being moved over the skin rather than a continuous application. Spray-on cooling agents should be used with care, since they rapidly cause great decreases in skin temperature, thus increasing risk of damage. Also, cooling reduces elasticity of collagen, and therefore vigorous activity should be avoided immediately following ice application to avoid further injury.[18] Slow, smooth stretching movements are preferred following cryotherapy.

Heat

The physiologic effects of applying heat are increased blood flow, increased capillary permeability, decreased pain, and decreased muscle spasm.[5,12] These can be beneficial responses in the healing process. Also, application of heat has been found to increase the extensibility of collagen tissue.[11] Because of these properties, heat should be applied prior to stretching exercises.

There are several methods of delivering heat to an injured back. These can be classified into surface or superficial heating that directly affects the skin temperature, such as hydrocollator packs, heat lamps or pads, or other conductive methods that deliver heat to muscles and other structures by having it pass through the skin, or deep heating methods, such as shortwave diathermy, microwave, and ultrasound, that directly increase the temperature of the muscles and have less effect on skin temperature.[18] Of the deep heating systems, ultrasound seems to be the most popular and will be discussed subsequently.

Heat should not be applied for at least the first 48 hours following injury or perhaps longer if significant signs of edema are noted. The application of heat should not be so great that the athlete feels uncomfortably warm. During the initial heat application, the patient should be closely monitored. Fair-skinned patients may be particularly sensitive to heat. If the patient reports discomfort or burning sensations, the heat treatment should be stopped and the intensity, duration, or both reduced during the next session.

If the athlete is undergoing some form of thermotherapy, use of analgesic cream should be eliminated or reduced, because the injured area has been made more sensitive by heat treatment.

Ultrasound

Ultrasound is a vibration occurring at frequencies too high to be detected by the human ear. These sound waves can provide deeper penetration than other forms of heat application.[5,12] Consequently, in patients with injury to deep spinal musculature, ultrasound may be better able to reach the injured tissue than other forms of conductive heat. It produces increased cell membrane permeability, increased extensibility of connective tissue, and muscle relaxation. It is not clearly understood if these effects are only of a thermal nature or if these changes are produced by some other biological or mechanical action, such as micromassage produced by the vibrating sound waves.

Ultrasound is contraindicated in patients with advanced heart disease, tumors, or pregnancy. Also, it should not be used over the spinal cord, spinous process, or any bony prominence.[17,18,21] It has been recommended not to use ultrasound or other means of deep heating tissue in an area where disc herniation or nerve entrapment is present or suspected.[12] Heat causes tissues to enlarge, which may worsen a situation where nerve compression is already located in a confined space.

In the course of treatment, ultrasound should be used to alleviate pain localized in a small area, acute muscle spasm, or deep tissue injury. Conductive, superficial methods are to be used for general pain relief and to warm and elongate tissues prior to stretching exercises.

Transcutaneous Electrical Nerve Stimulation (TENS)

The idea of treating pain with electrical stimulation is an old one, but generally it fell into disfavor until the publication of the gate-control theory. In general, this theory suggests that pain sensations can be inhibited by input from other sensory fibers. It has been hypothesized that TENS produces these pain-blocking signals. Also, electrical stimulation has been associated with an enhanced release of endorphins, which aid in pain reduction.[7,10] TENS varies greatly in terms of the pulse frequency, pulse width, and waveform. Well-defined standards concerning appropriate combinations of these variables, as well as duration of treatment, have not yet been established. As is true of many conservative treatments, there have been no well-designed comparative studies evaluating the effectiveness of TENS in the treatment of low back pain; however, many feel that this is a useful treatment for many patients. One advantage of the TENS unit is that the athlete can easily wear it while participating in physical activities.

There are few contraindications for using TENS. This treatment should not be used by patients with a cardiac pacemaker, during pregnancy, or when masking pain during vigorous activity may result in further injury.[7] Some patients experience skin irritation from the electrodes or gel.

Braces and Corsets

The use of spinal braces or corsets has been demonstrated to increase intra-abdominal pressure, reduce intradiscal pressure, and increase skin temperature.[4,15] For years weight lifters and others have used abdominal supports to help reduce the chance of injury when lifting very heavy loads. Some authors feel that the brace provides support and reduces the load on spinal structures. Braces have been reported to be beneficial in several studies dealing with sports participation and spinal deformity or injury to bony structures.

Micheli reported on the use of a modified Boston brace system to reduce lordosis in treating young athletes with spondylolisthesis, discogenic pain, apophyseal fracture, and mechanical pain.[14] The braces were modified to allow the youths to participate as much as possible in their sport. Among the 31 athletes, 28 reported a return to full activity with little or no residual pain. The only patients who did not return to activity were 3 of 6 who had discogenic pain.

Wilson and Lindseth reported on using the Milwaukee brace in athletes with kyphosis.[25] The brace was worn 23 hours a day. The athlete was allowed to practice and compete in swimming meets during the time the brace was off (except for the butterfly stroke, which produces hyperlordosis). The authors also felt that being allowed to remain active in swimming had a positive psychological effect.

Benson et al. reported very favorably about using the Milwaukee brace to treat young athletic patients with scoliosis or Scheuermann's kyphosis, and whose curve patterns were amenable to bracing.[1] The authors strongly advocate allowing the patient to be as physically active as possible, including participation in competitive sports. This allows the patient to maintain better overall fitness and has psychological advantages.

Most authors recommend antilordotic bracing along with activity modifications for athletes who have stress fractures of the posterior elements.[8,14,16]

Bracing may be beneficial in the treatment of nonbony injuries as well. Early in the rehabilitation process, a brace or corset produces restricted movement and thus prevents overstretching of healing tissues. Grew and Deane reported that wearing a corset retains heat.[4] This may aid in keeping collagen tissues warm and more extensible, also serving to reduce the chance of tissue damage during stretching exercises.

DISCUSSION

Although the outlook for recovery from low back pain in athletes is good, bouts of low back pain should not be ignored. They should be considered a warning of potential recurrent problems. Merely getting over the painful episode should be considered as only a first step, rather than the last step, in the rehabilitation process. The use of pain-controlling agents should be employed only on a short-term basis while the patient is involved in physical rehabilitation and conditioning. Otherwise, these agents may mask pain, and the injury causing the pain may be ignored, resulting in recurrent or more serious injury.

During the period of rest and reduced activity following a low back injury, the athlete and those involved with his or her training should take advantage of this opportunity to try to identify the cause of the injury and modify activity accordingly. If the athlete returns to the same activity level as he or she had before the injury, the injury may recur. Many injuries are due to weakness or lack of flexibility. Injury is associated with having less strength, endurance, or flexibility than the activity demands; injury is likely to recur unless modifications are made. This evaluation should include assessing muscle strength and endurance, muscle balance, flexibility, and warm-up and stretching techniques (for more information on these topics, see chapters 1–3), as well as body mechanics, shoes, and the training surface. Following assessment, the athlete should gradually return to activity, incorporating the necessary modification identified during the assessment. Often the athlete may benefit from participation in swimming or hydrotherapy early in the rehabilitation program, since this allows the patient to be active but with buoyant forces reducing stresses on healing tissue.

II. Manipulation

JOHN J. TRIANO, DC
THOMAS E. HYDE, DC

The sports physician encounters a large number of musculoskeletal injuries, with as much as a 20% incidence affecting the neck and back.[1,2] The main outcome of interest to the athlete and his or her coach is to avoid significant compromise in performance for a prolonged recovery time before returning to play. Back injury can be one of the more demanding and exasperating of disorders for the physician to follow. Even with minimal objective findings, it carries the potential for permanently disabling the patient's performance and ending a productive career. There is increasing interest in claims by top athletes that regular and specific manipulation by chiropractors and manipulating physicians assists in optimizing their performance.[3,4] Manipulation is used along with other manual methods to relieve muscles that are painful or in spasm, to restore movement to stiffened joints, and to correct subluxed joints. This section will attempt to briefly explain the theoretical basis for these claims and to review some of the available clinical and scientific information. Examples of how the procedures are incorporated in managing the athletic musculoskeletal injury will be presented.

APPROPRIATENESS OF CARE

The greatest obstacle hampering research of the efficacy and efficiency of manipulation is the absence of a sound scientific diagnosis of the lesion present in the majority of back and neck pain cases.[5] The result is an ongoing controversy as to the appropriate care that should be applied. Indications from clinically derived data[6] lead to wide-ranging treatment variations found in common practice. Persistence of widely differing viewpoints about appropriate standards of care exists because of the uncertainty that comes from the untested theories behind assorted practices. Recognition of this state has been articulated as the professional uncertainty hypothesis, which lends some perspective to this current sociomedical climate.[7] The conditions under discussion are common to clinical practice, and the alternative forms of treatment that are available for such disorders may be comparably appropriate or inappropriate.

Although many of the applications for manipulation remain to be substantiated on a research basis, their utility is often strongly asserted by both the athletes and their clinicians. In the current milieu there is little justification for withholding these procedures. In cases where contraindications are absent, a trial therapy of manipulation often seems to be helpful in identifying those who are likely to respond. Many hold that athletes are kept playing and long periods of convalescence are reduced. Table 1 lists the outcomes from nine of the more recent studies of manipulation. Seven of them suggest greater therapeutic benefit from manual procedures than for alternative treatments.

Although no direct studies on athletic populations are available, descriptive reports on frequency and duration of care for spinal disorders in the general population have been made. The evidence[17] indicates that patients seen by health care providers trained in manipulation have the same clinical and sociological characteristics as those who seek nonmanipulative care. Severity of injury being similar, the natural history and course of the condition will also be the same. A cumulative total of 4,917 patients were followed in three descriptive studies.[18–20]

TABLE 1. Outcome from Recent Studies of Manipulation

Study	Result
Evans et al., 1978[8]	SMT* > codeine phosphate
Rasmussen, 1979[9]	SMT > shortwave diathermy
Hoehler et al., 1981[10]	SMT > placebo
Godfrey et al., 1984[11]	SMT = massage & electrostimulation
Gibson et al., 1985[12]	SMT = shortwave & electrostimulation
Waagen et al., 1986[13]	SMT > placebo
Meade et al., 1986[14]	SMT > hospital treatment
Ongley et al., 1987[15]	SMT > placebo†
Hadler et al., 1987[16]	SMT > mobilization

* SMT—spinal manipulation therapy.
† Manipulation coupled with injection.

Patient descriptions fit typical categories of acute, subacute, and chronic disorders. The observed lengths of treatment for all three reports were well within the descriptions of natural history of these kinds of complaints.[21,22] Similar favorable findings were reported in a study of over 7,000 workmans' compensation cases.[23,24]

PRINCIPLES OF MANIPULATION MANAGEMENT

Manual treatment methods generally are employed in one or two ways. They are used to alleviate symptoms associated with aberrant joint flexibilities or they are directed toward subclinical abnormalities of joint function, with an eye to improving the quality of performance. The biomechanics and pathophysiology of the lesions are not well delineated, and the understanding of them is guided primarily by clinical observations. Various models have been proposed.[3,25–30] They all may be summarized as being mechanisms that cause the motion segment to be restricted at some point within the envelope of its normal range of motion. The blockage may be near its neutral position or only occur as the joint approaches its end-of-range. Persistence of the restriction is thought to bring about increased stresses in the joint and surrounding soft tissues, with potential for inflammation, pain, and degeneration.

Three kinds of barriers are proposed as responsible for limiting joint motion in some way. In the first, muscle can shorten through fibrosis, spasm, or voluntary contraction-restricting movement and increasing compressive joint stresses. Second, joint range may be limited by ligamentous shortening, formation of synovial tags within the facet articulations, or alteration of the passive tissue properties of the disc. Finally, osteophytic changes and ankylosis that cannot be affected by manipulation may be the cause of restriction. In cases where optimization of performance is desired, the assumption is made that restricted motion causes abnormal mechanics and reflex muscular incoordination that are normalized through manipulation.

In practice, limited joint motion can be found either as a primary disorder responsible for the patient's symptoms or as a coexisting complication of other disorders. For example, patients with spondylolisthesis and back pain frequently have abnormal flexibilities of the lumbosacral mechanics. Other discernible disorders with which symptom-contributing limitation of joint motion often arises include discopathy,[31,32] posterior facet syndrome, sacroiliac/piriformis syndrome, central spinal stenosis, intermittent lateral recess entrapments,[33] sprain/strain

TABLE 2. Categories of Manual Treatment Procedures

1. **Soft tissue techniques:** Methods include the various types of massage and are designed to improve venous and lymphatic drainage and relax muscle tension.
2. **Stretching:** These techniques attempt to selectively apply tensile forces along the length of specific ligaments or muscles. Loads used are quasistatic and are thought to bring about increased flexibility of the appropriate joint through passive means. Either relaxation of muscle spasm or creep deformity of the elastic elements in connective tissues of the joint are commonly assumed mechanisms of action.
3. **Mobilization:** Passive movement of specific joints or whole regions of the spine are sought. Smooth, slow-speed oscillating pressures are applied directly to the joint or region without use of high accelerations.
4. **Muscle "energy":** In quasistatic posture positioned at the end-comfort range of motion, the patient attempts a maximum voluntary exertion against resistance. Upon relaxation of the muscle, the joint is passively moved to comfortable limit and the exertion is repeated.
5. **High-velocity thrusting:** These methods are among the most common and are often exclusively referred to as manipulations to differentiate from less dynamic procedures. Performance incorporates the movement of the selected joint to its end range of voluntary motion, followed by the application of an impulse loading.

injuries, and myofascial pain syndromes.[34] Clinical experience with joint-motion abnormalities suggests that they may become episodic in nature once an injury has been sustained, much like the other disorders with which they may associate. Each episodic flare-up is approached therapeutically much the same as the initial-onset acute state.

The primary purpose for performing a manipulation treatment is to alter range of motion and reduce pain in symptomatic joints and surrounding soft tissues. The desired outcome is a reduction of symptoms and a normalization of motion segment kinematics. Five main categories of manual procedures are recognized. They are defined briefly in Table 2.

The treatment plan is divided into three phases (Table 3), each having distinct objectives that utilize both passive and active therapeutic measures. During acute distress, efforts to reduce soft tissue and joint stresses are applied so that inflammation and swelling may subside. A short term of reduced activity is often supportive. Passive forms of treatment such as manual and palliative procedures, including such modalities as cryotherapy, hydrotherapy, electrotherapy, transcutaneous nerve stimulation, trigger-point therapy, and acupuncture, are often combined with manipulation to speed the recovery.

TABLE 3. Treatment Staging

1. Acute intervention
   a. To promote anatomical rest
   b. To diminish muscular spasm
   c. To reduce inflammation
   d. To alleviate pain
2. Remobilization
   a. To increase pain-free motion
   b. To minimize deconditioning
3. Rehabilitation
   a. To restore local strength and endurance
   b. To increase physical work capacity

Once the sharper pain and discomfort of the acute phase have abated, the injured area is remobilized with low-speed, light-load exercises to preserve maximum joint flexibility. It is important that mechanical stresses be kept low throughout the effort to avoid inciting new inflammatory response. As range of pain-free motion is improved, a graded increase in exertional output can be implemented. When a full range of motion is achieved, a rehabilitation program designed to rebuild both strength and endurance of the part can be devised. It is beneficial to move to the rehabilitation stage quickly and to minimize the dependence upon passive forms of treatment. Often, complete resolution of pain is not readily achieved until the patient focuses on increasing his or her level of performance. Even then, some residual pain may persist, despite a return to full activity.

TREATMENT OF SPECIFIC INJURIES

Examples of common athletic injuries and the therapeutic approach using manipulative procedures presented here focus on the acute and remobilizing phases. The description begins with sprain/strain and incorporates current thinking on pathomechanics that applies to other injuries listed.

Strains/Sprains

The most common causes[35] for which a weekend athlete or professional player is clinically evaluated is the so-called low back strain and muscle spasm. Strains to the lower extremity also have a high incidence and are among the most disabling in sports.[36] Injuries of these kind arise particularly often from football, basketball, lacrosse, squash, and gymnastics. Muscle strain or tearing occurs at a critical tension that is proportional to stretch in the muscle and the rate at which it is applied.[37] Muscles that have a higher tensile capacity may absorb more energy than weaker ones before failure. Strains involve damage to the muscle, tendon, the musculotendinous junction, or the attachment of the tendon to the bone. Sprains involve damage to the ligamentous structure. The damage to a ligament may occur in its body or at its attachments. Both strain and sprain may be divided into 1st degree, 2nd degree and 3rd degree, or alternatively can be classified as mild, moderate, and severe.[38] Most back-related strain/sprain injuries fall into the 1st or 2nd degrees of severity.

Strain/sprain mechanisms can be simply grouped into three categories,[39] defined as follows: (1) acute injury—a sudden overloading of musculotendinous units, as might occur in sprinting or kicking; (2) chronic or overuse injury—a repeated overload and/or frictional resistance, which occurs in endurance training or other highly repetitive action, and (3) acute imposed on chronic injury—a sudden rupture in a persistent lesion; for example, the rupture in a chronic Achilles' tendonitis.

In strain, a progressive decline in capacity to develop tension is evident as the severity of injury increases. With ligamentous damage, protective spasm may arise. Reactive hypertonicity from overuse or trauma such as is seen with quadratus lumborum syndrome[40] has also been reported. In any case, the patient assumes characteristic adaptive postures and gaits that can add stress both at the level of injury and above it.[41] When primary muscles are involved, secondary muscles must substitute in order to control motion and govern flexibility,[42] and to alter the joint biomechanics. Painful abnormalities in joint motion may coexist with soft tissue injury, either as a primary effect of the inciting trauma or secondarily due to the altered kinematics of posture that result. Joint levels at the ankle, knee, sacroiliac, and lumbar spine are often involved.

Treatment. A main feature of the clinical evaluation is the search for hidden contraindication to manual treatment methods. These include muscular and bony avulsions[43–45] as well as fractures.[35]

Within the first 72 hours following an acute 1st or 2nd-degree sprain/strain, ice should be used.[39] Application is generally made for 30 minutes,[38] followed later by application for 20 minutes each hour as necessary. Care is needed when using cryotherapy for athletes who also have diabetes, circulatory disorders, cold allergies, or sensory neuropathies. To minimize the detrimental effect of inactivity on osseous and soft tissues,[39,46,47] it is desirable to mobilize the injured area as early as possible. Tiptan et al.[48] demonstrated that the strength of both intact and repaired ligaments was proportional to their mobility. Vailas et al.[49] have shown that controlled exercise, even with minimal mechanical loading, enhances ligament strength. Collagen fiber growth and realignment are stimulated by early tensile loading,[50] and the formation of adhesions between repairing tissues and adjacent structures, which otherwise might limit muscle and joint flexibility, is minimized by early movement.

In practice, these principles are assumed to apply equally to spinal and extremity joint structures. Mobility can be induced passively through manual procedures very early in the course of treatment. Depending upon the degree of inflammation and swelling that are present, any of the ancillary procedures, including massage, mobilization, or manipulation procedures, may be implemented. Stretching may be used for hyperactive muscles. Soft tissues are generally treated before joint mobilizations[51] are performed; otherwise, tight, soft tissue would resist the maneuver.

Physical modalities may be utilized, for example, acupuncture or acupressure, trigger-point therapy, muscle stimulation and interferential current, and transcutaneous nerve stimulation.[40] After the acute phase has resolved, active flexibility exercises in the pain-free range of motion are added. Reese and Vurruss[52] suggest that both the low back and the hamstrings must be stretched to allow full flexibility for either. They recommend the modified Williams flexion exercise routines. Finally, the rehabilitation of the patient's performance is sought by focusing upon strength and endurance.

Third degree strain/sprain when complete tearing occurs often requires surgical intervention. Efficient repair depends upon good apposition of the torn ligament attachments.

Lumbar Facet Syndrome

The facet syndrome is a painful irritation of the posterior elements of the motion segment, with the first report of this entity ascribed to Goldthwait[53] and later emphasized by Putti,[54] Ghormley,[55] and Badgley.[56] Potential risk to neural elements as they exit through the intervertebral foramen from capsular swelling was described by Danforth and Wilson in 1925.[57]

Kleynhans[58] classifies facet syndrome into three types. They are: (1) traumatic, (2) pathologic, and (3) postural. The traumatic form is associated with an acute onset and inflammation of the synovial linings of the joint with effusion, synovitis, and limitation of movement.[59] The pathologic classification is due to an apparent narrowing of the intervertebral disc space, which permits an approximation of the facet surfaces and precedes typical degenerative joint changes.

Perhaps this theory was best described by Kirkaldy-Willis[60] as a continuous process divided into stages of dysfunction, instability, and restabilization. The postural variety is said to be found in individuals with increased lumbar lordosis, poor abdominal musculature, and a protruding abdomen. Athletes who participate in sports involving repeated and forceful hyperextension of the lumbar spine appear to suffer a higher incidence of lumbar facet syndrome. Examples include involvement in football, gymnastics, diving, power lifting, and golf. Tennis players,[61] especially during a serve, and dancers participating in partner lift maneuvers seem particularly at risk.

Later changes from persistent or recurrent lesions include continued degeneration, with the formation of osteophytes and enlargement of both the inferior and superior facets. Canal stenosis either of the vertebral canal or of the lateral recesses may ultimately follow.[40]

Signs and Symptoms. The classic facet syndrome (1) is characterized by local paralumbar tenderness; (2) pain on hyperextension; (3) absence of neurological deficit; and (4) hip, buttock, or back pain on straight leg raising. Other diagnostic factors have been suggested by Banks[62] and include scleratogenous leg pain, supraspinous ligament tenderness, and absence of coronal plane analgesia. These patients often have pain when assuming an upright position following forward flexion of the lumbar spine. Kirkaldy-Willis[60] divides the symptoms into acute, subacute, or chronic, and indicates they are frequently localized to one side. Pain may be referred to multiple areas, including the groin, the greater trochanter, and to the posterior thighs as far as the knee. Generally, the pain is relieved by rest and made worse by movement.

Treatment. Acute facet disorders respond quickly to short terms of physiologic rest that can often be achieved by limiting activity. Bed rest up to 2 days may be necessary for some. Modalities such as ultrasound and interferential electrical currents passed through the inflamed area appear to give relief.

Using manual procedures for both acute and chronic cases, positioning of the patient is done passively in an effort to open the offending joint space. If there is no significant discomfort from positioning, specific mobilization and manipulation can then be applied. Mechanisms of improvement following manipulative methods are unknown. Especially where degenerative changes have occurred, periodic mobilization of the spinal joints for episodic flair-ups may be required.

Sacroiliac Disorder

The sacroiliac joint is one of the largest articulations in the body. Together, the bones of the pelvis form an inverted mortise that becomes inherently more stable as vertical load increases.[63] In contrast to size, its relative motions are remarkably small. They consist primarily of torsional movements about an axis passing through the joint surfaces. More complex accessory motions are believed to occur.[63,64] Three groups of trunk muscles and six groups of powerful hip and thigh muscles act on the pelvis. Motion at the sacroiliac is passive and based upon the resultant loads from muscle action and body mass. Ground reaction forces transmitted upward through the legs act on the pelvis at a different site than the downward acting forces from upper body weight.[65] The combined effect of a large pelvic structure with long levers for muscle attachments and the high body segment accelerations that athletes experience gives rise to large moments that act on the joint and restraining ligaments.

Acute lesions of the sacroiliac joint generally require a sudden forceful injury as might readily occur in a number of sports such as motor racing, football, soccer, rugby, hockey, basketball, and baseball. A misstep by a runner whose heel strike is made with the knee locked will transmit high loads to the pelvis, or one with significant difference in leg length[65] can precipitate a sacroiliac lesion. Cumulative effects of prolonged static or repeated low-grade stresses are not known. Symptoms commonly include pain in any of the regions encompassing the low back, buttocks, posterior thigh, or popliteal fossa.[66,67] Localized tenderness over the sacroiliac with asymmetry of intrapelvic movements is found on examination.[64,66,67] Tender and asymmetric landmarks at the symphysis pubis may be evident. Differential diagnosis includes a search for evidence of chordoma,[68] ankylosing spondylitis, or sacroilitis[69] by use of MRI, CT, or bone scan, as appropriate.

Treatment. As before, the management of sacroiliac lesions by manipulation includes a short initial period of physiologic rest. Pulsed ultrasound,[70] electrical stimulation, and acupuncture[65] have been recommended as adjunctive therapy to help reduce inflammation and control pain. Cryotherapy, followed later by penetrating heat, is often found useful. The type of manipulative maneuver that is selected depends upon the location and direction of motion limitation.

Remobilization is often aided by the fitting of a sacroiliac or trochanteric belt. No specific exercises are available for these joint dysfunctions, since none of the muscle groups crosses the joint. Hurdler stretches, extending the lumbar spine, pelvis, and hip joints, are sometimes used. Otherwise, exercising the appropriate trunk or leg groups that favorably load the pelvis to encourage restoration of normal motion, either on one or both sides, is based upon the limitations diagnosed.

Lumbar Disc Disorder

One of the most frequently implicated diagnoses for low back and leg pain is that of a disc lesion. Herniation is a regular occurrence in the athlete[71] and can occur during or after sports participation. Repeated injury and disc degeneration are common preceding events.[72] A snapping sensation in the back may follow a sudden movement or impact.[72,73] Low back pain is succeeded within 24–48 hours by radicular pain extending down the leg.

Diagnosis and imaging of disc disorders are topics well described elsewhere and are beyond the scope of this section.

Treatment. Because of the relatively limited amount of information previously available on the use of manipulation procedures in cases like this, listings of indications and contraindications reviewed from various sources are often contradictory. This probably arises because of limited experience in use of these procedures. With recent developments in the techniques available,[32,66,74–76] even some patients with radiating leg pain can be successfully treated. Acute onset or progressive neurological deficit and cauda equina syndrome are contraindications to manipulation.[67,73,77]

Supportive care, including modalities of electrotherapy, acupuncture, or TENS, is applied early for pain control. A rigid corset may also be used to restrict movement and aid in minimizing unguarded bending loads on the already-injured disc. For patients with evidence of nerve irritation or compression, an initial manipulative approach might include passive stretching and flexibility techniques such as those proposed by Cox.[74] For low back or leg pain without neurologic deficit, the full range of manipulation procedures, including high-velocity, short-lever thrust procedures, is available[32,66,74-77] if they are properly applied.

Leg-Length Inequality

Manipulation treatment of joint disorders is thought to concern itself with mechanical factors that contribute to the patient's symptoms. For that reason, the short-leg syndrome plays an important role in causing or aggravating existing spine-related disorders. A higher incidence of leg-length inequality has been noted in adult patients with lower back pain.[78] A relationship between reduced performance and pain of the spine and lower extremities with leg-length asymmetries has been described in athletes.[79,80] There is considerable controversy as to the relative difference necessary to be clinically meaningful. In the general population, a sample of authors felt that a minimum of 1 cm difference is needed before intervention is required.[81-84] Others, including those who have studied the effects in athletes specifically, tend to consider differences of 4 mm and up to be important.[79,80,85-90]

Differences in leg length are believed to shift the center of body away from the midline proportionate to the leg-length difference.[85,91] An unequal distribution of load is created between the two lower extremities. This is further accentuated when the athlete moves quickly and the stress transmitted through the skeleton is amplified by acceleration of the body mass. Thus, a small leg-length abnormality may be more biomechanically significant for athletes than for the general population. Symptoms emanating from the ankle, knees, hip, and low back all have been connected with leg-length differences. A therapeutic trial of correction may be warranted when symptoms are thus associated.[92]

Determinations of leg length is most often carried our manually. However, this procedure is highly prone to error.[93-95] Tape measure methods and manual comparison of leg lengths in both the recumbent and standing positions should be confirmed by radiography.[96,97] For adults, a standing modified Chamberlain's view x-ray with the tube level with the femur heads is sufficient to determine anatomical deficiency. For growing children, a scanogram measurement may be taken by successively exposing the hips, knees, and ankles on one film. Since each joint growth center is examined, any pathologic factors causing the length anomaly can be identified. Otherwise, repeating the measure once more after a year's growth will permit a prediction of final difference at the time of skeletal maturity.[98] Length disparity predicted to be greater than 2.5 cm is best treated surgically.[99,100]

Treatment. Treatment involves sufficient correction of length difference to relieve the symptom producing stresses. Manipulation of the symptomatic joints to restore normal flexibility is also carried out.[78-80,96] Pronation of the ankle can be controlled with orthotics to supply neutral arch control. Heel-lift therapy should be introduced in 3–5-mm increments, allowing a 2-week period of accommodation to each.[101] Lifts applied to the heel that are greater than 10 mm tend to distort foot biomechanics. Higher elevations should be made by adding dimension to the full length of the shoe sole. Most importantly, treatment should not be applied to a small length difference unless the patient's complaints are associated with the difference. Trial therapy permits this association to be uncovered or eliminated from consideration.

III. Acupuncture for Sports Injuries

S. James Montgomery, MB, BCh

Back pain is one of the oldest complaints known to man, so it is appropriate to consider one of the oldest treatments known to man, i.e., acupuncture. Acupuncture is 4,000 to 5,000 years old and is still being practiced widely in many parts of the world. Acupuncture can be of help in many sports injuries, including those of the back. In my experience it can ease some of the spasm and pain of the back and make the patient more mobile and more able to return to active participation.

THE HISTORY OF ACUPUNCTURE

It is inappropriate to consider any treatment with acupuncture without considering some of its history. Having originated many thousands of years ago, the original explanations were not scientific but were related to Chinese philosophy. The ancient Chinese philosophy of life postulated that there was a central life force called T'Chi. T'Chi was believed to travel through the body in a series of meridians. There were 12 meridians located on the body, and on these were a series of acupuncture points, originally 365. These acupuncture points were places where the flow of T'Chi through the meridians could be interrupted or changed. The second Chinese philosophy that came to bear was that of the Yin and Yang. This is the theory of life being a balance of opposites: male/female; high/low; inside/outside; everything was divided into the Yin-Yang philosophy. When Yin and Yang were in balance, the person was healthy. Disease therefore came about when Yin and Yang were out of balance, when one had too much Yin or too little Yang.

Acupuncture is the insertion of needles into the correct acupuncture points to balance the Yin and Yang and restore a healthy situation. In ancient China, medical examinations were very cursory, and the diagnosis was made by taking of a history and by feeling of the pulse. The Chinese physician made a diagnosis from the pulse, which was taken at the wrist with three fingers. The pulse diagnosis related where the disturbance was and which acupuncture points to use. Master acupuncturists were very good at diagnosing the pulse, and also they were experts in knowing where to position the needles. The greater the skill of the acupuncturist, the fewer needles used.[1]

There are many different needling techniques, with different insertion and stimulation methods. There is one form of acupuncture practiced in Japan in which a single needle is inserted in and taken out of acupuncture points in a very short period of time. In traditional Chinese acupuncture, the needles are left in sites for various periods of time. This method was (and still is) also combined at times with a treatment called moxabustion. In this treatment, the leaves of the moxa plant were ground up like tobacco and made into little balls, which were placed on the end of the needles and ignited. The moxa burns like incense on the end of the needle, allowing it to become slightly warm and adding the inhalation of moxa smoke to the treatment. In more modern times, the use of electricity has been added to acupuncture, and the needles are stimulated by an electrical current, either a DC current in Japan or an AC current with various different pulses in other techniques.

There is no anatomical evidence of meridians flowing through the body or any histological description of an acupuncture point. Modern theories on the mechanism of acupuncture range from Melzac and Wall's[2] gate theory to the release of endorphins from the body, thereby giving pain relief. However, in spite of the longevity of acupuncture and its varied uses, there is no accepted theory as to the exact method of its function. In any treatment based on the symptom of pain, it is difficult to get meaningful statistics on results.

Many years ago, I set out to satisfy my own curiosity by trying to prove that acupuncture had only a placebo effect. This was done in a pain clinic, with patients suffering from all types of chronic pain unrelieved by Western techniques. I recommended that I use some needles to see if I could locate the site of the pain. This was in the early 1970s, when acupuncture was not nearly so popular and many of the patients were not even sure that it was acupuncture. Nine of my first 14 patients noticed improvement. I have been practicing for many years since, and I have observed many patients who have had back pain for several years, with their back muscles tight and painful. Acupuncture often made these muscles more relaxed and pain was eased. I then began to use this treatment on patients with acute back pain and spasm. This was done for sports injuries from activities such as golf, running, tennis, and in particular the injuries of professional athletes associated with the Dallas Cowboys. Over the years I have observed that in many instances the spasm and pain can be lessened with acupuncture therapy.

PATIENT SELECTION

Patients selected for acupuncture treatment of the low back must of course have an adequate examination to establish that there is no acute surgical or neurological problem that should be corrected. The problem should be solely one of low back pain and spasm or weakness, with at most minor nerve root irritation. A typical patient is a lineman who continually irritates his back by heavy contact collisions day in and day out. He usually has no recovery time and the problem can persist for weeks. The patient could also be a golfer who injures his back while swinging, or various athletes who twist their back from time to time. The back pain takes enough edge off their game to make their performance mediocre, and for the amateur athlete it takes he enjoyment out of the activity. This, therefore, is a symptom well worth improving in order to make these patients more productive athletes. Physical examination shows that these patients have limited movement and a tender area in their low back, usually with some tightness and muscle spasm.

TREATMENT

Acupuncture treatment for this type of patient is very simple, with four or six needles placed on what would be the traditional bladder meridian. Two needles are placed on either side of the back in locations that represent the area of pain. If the pain is L4–5, then these two needles are put in the bladder meridian that is approximately 2 inches lateral from the midline straddling the L4–5 area. This is accompanied by two needles on the contralateral side in the same points. In some patients it is worthwhile adding two more needles on the bladder point in the middle of the posterior popliteal space, if there is a leg pain component.

Needles

Many years ago, it was quite difficult to get sterile disposable acupuncture needles, and I began to use 30 g hypodermic needles, which were readily available, sterilized, and disposable. I have continued to use these, even though disposable acupuncture needles are now available. An acupuncture purist would of course not accept these needles. However, my results are similar with both types of needles, and patient comfort is better with the disposable needles. They are also guaranteed sterile and are disposable, and this avoids any possible suggestion of hepatitis or AIDS from their use. The needles are placed after cleansing with an alcohol skin swab. I find it very convenient to treat the patients lying prone on their stomach in a relaxed position. The needles are placed in the acupuncture points; patients lie still for 10 minutes; the needles are turned slightly with the finger and thumb two or three times during the 10-minute period. Improvement may be delayed hours to days, and initially it may be temporary. Treatments are cumulative—three or more may be required—and can be on a daily basis or an every-other-day basis.

RESULTS

Treatment at an early stage of the injury, with two or three sessions before the next vigorous physical activity, yields 60 to 70% improvement among patients. The treatment is very simple and does not appear that it should work, yet many of the patients have obtained relief.[3] I have been doing this for about 14 years, and many of the professional football players seek it out, although most of them usually shy away from any needle. Many of them are very keen to have treatments repeated after experiencing the beneficial results. Many times a patient's back is tight and in spasm before a treatment, and after the treatment the back muscles look and feel more relaxed. This more relaxed feeling continues over the next few hours or days. Sometimes it is the second or third treatment before more significant relaxation is noted; however, it occurs in 60% or more of patients.

No one has yet found a reason why acupuncture works. If you put a needle into a muscle in spasm, there is a certain part of that muscle, if touched with the needle, that will fibrillate and relax. This can be demonstrated easily, particularly in groin or hamstring pulls in which the muscle will be much softer afterward. This does not usually happen in back patients, but it may play a part. About 25% of the patients feel a general relaxation during and after the acupuncture treatment. As with any treatment to improve pain, placebo does its part; however, in my experience, the placebo effect is normally approximately 30% of the total effect. In back pain, I have found that 60 to 70% of patients experience good relief, a much higher percentage than can be accounted for by placebo. Any treatment that improves 60 to 70% of patients and makes them more comfortable is definitely worth consideration. There are very few side effects to the acupuncture treatment. Very occasionally there is a little bleeding from one of the needle spots, which is very easily stopped with direct pressure. In a very small number of patients there is an occasional subcutaneous hematoma, which is usually not painful. With the use of sterile needles and proper insertion, there is minimal risk of infection. I instruct the patients to do whatever they would have done without the acupuncture treatment. Acupuncture will not affect any other treatments or their routine.

CONCLUSION

In conclusion, over a period of 14 years of experience with acupuncture in sports injuries, I have found that this simple treatment with very few side effects has improved the back pain in many athletes. I have excellent results with the Dallas Cowboys. I think that this is another form of therapy that should be considered in these injuries.

IV. Injections

RICHARD D. GUYER, MD

There are three basic injections that can be used for the injured athlete. They are (1) the local trigger-point injection, (2) the epidural steroid injection, and (3) the facet injection.

Trigger-point Injection

Local trigger-point myofascial injections entail the installation of a solution of local anesthetic with or without one of the various cortisone preparations in hope of alleviating the local injury, whether it be from a musculoligamentous attachment or from the "trigger point" to which the pain is referred. Melzack in 1981 enhanced our understanding of the relief of pain by injecting such trigger points. It was felt that this could be explained in terms of the gate control theory. By injecting the trigger point, one may affect the "central biasing mechanism" in the brainstem area and thus close the gated inputs from particular parts of the body.[7]

Garvey et al. have recently published a prospective double-blind evaluation of trigger-point injections and, in a group of low back pain patients, found that those receiving just acupuncture or vaporcoolant spray with acupressure had greater relief ($P < 0.09$) than those receiving lidocaine or lidocaine and steroid. It was concluded, therefore, that the injected substance apparently was not the critical factor, since direct mechanical stimulus of the trigger point seems to give symptomatic relief equal to that of the various types of medication.[3] Ready et al. reported that jet injection was preferable to conventional trigger-point injection due to the diminished pain of administration.[11]

These types of injections can be effective on a short-term basis and are only helpful for the athlete who has otherwise made an excellent recovery except for a lingering but nagging and reproducible pain. These techniques should not be used during the course of participation in order to get the athlete back to the field, as further damage can ensue without the sensory input of the tissues to warn the athlete of further injury.

Epidural Steroid Injection

This injection is reserved for the patient who has signs of nerve compression or radicular complaints along with lower back pain. In the athlete most likely this would be either from a ruptured disc or from isthmic spondylolisthesis in which there is secondary nerve root irritation. In the well-known study by Cuckler et al., it was shown on a double-blind basis that epidural steroids were not curative of patients having a ruptured disc.[2] There were obvious experimental deficits within the study itself. However, it should be understood that epidural steroids are used as a palliative modality, not as a curative one. The patient oftentimes is more comfortable after the injection. Frequently a series of three epidural steroid injections is used, spacing them 2 weeks apart.

In 1980, Jackson et al.[5] reported on a group of 32 athletes who had signs of a ruptured disc with both back pain and sciatica and found there was a dramatic abatement of symptoms after epidural steroid injections, with a significantly faster return to competition in 44%. It was felt that the results were encouraging, but much less than what was expected or reported in the literature. Even a 40%

success rate in chronic, symptomatic radicular problems may be reasonable when one considers the alternatives.[5] Solely from a scientific viewpoint, this is only slightly better than the placebo effect, however.

Despite this, an epidural steroid injection remains the last conservative measure in a patient who fails to respond to the other modalities. My own preference is to carry this procedure out through the sacral hiatus with an image intensifier, as there is less chance of a cerebral spinal fluid (CSF) leak followed by subsequent spinal headache and the ensuing morbidity. Through a 20-gauge spinal needle Depo-medrol 120 mg with 5 cc of sterile saline without preservatives is injected after an initial 5–10 cc of ½% Xylocaine without preservatives. Usually there will be reproduction of the radicular complaints during the injection. It is important to use x-ray control, because in a double-blind study by White, it was shown that placement of the epidural needle is incorrect 25% of the time.[15]

Facet Injections

Although the facet syndrome was first described in 1933 by Ghormley,[4] it was Badgley[1] who later emphasized the importance of the facet points in the production of low back and leg pain. Shealy and Rees in the 1970s promoted renewed interest in the role of the facet joints in the production of back pain.[12,13] It was Mooney in 1975 who popularized the concept of facet syndrome and showed that the injection of an irritant fluid into the facet joint can cause a referred pain pattern indistinguishable from that of patients having a ruptured disc. He found that straight leg raising and even reflexes could be affected.[8]

The theory behind the facet joints producing pain is explained by the triple innervation of the facet joints, as elucidated by Paris et al. in 1980.[9] They described an additional ascending branch of the posterior primary ramus. Before this report it was believed that each joint was only double innervated, receiving its nerve supply at its respective level from the medial branch of the posterior ramus as well as from the descending branch from the level above.[10,14]

Jackson et al. in 1988 reported a large prospective study showing that facet injections were not found to be effective.[6] However, from an empiric standpoint, if the pain can be lessened for resumption of palliative exercise as well as strengthening exercises, facet injections may aid in the athlete's recovery. The patients selected for this procedure should be those who complain primarily of low back pain, do not have any neurologic symptoms, have negative straight leg raising, and may have tenderness directly over the facet joint.

Generally the injection is carried out at the symptomatic level. If it is only right-sided, then the right-side facet joints are injected. Oftentimes the level above and below the affected joint is injected as well, due to multiple innervation. Each facet joint is injected with a solution of long-acting anesthetic, such as Marcaine, along with a steroid preparation. The injection is carried out under fluoroscopic control by passing a 20-gauge needle directly down to the facet joint. The initial response is usually one of amelioration of the pain from the anesthetic, followed by a slight exacerbation within the first 24 hours, and then finally a diminution of pain due to the steroid effect thereafter.

V. Psychological Intervention

DAVID T. HANKS, PhD

Early work in the field of athletic injuries focused attention to such critical variables as the context within which the injury occurred, kinds of protective equipment utilized, degree of physical contact involved in the sport, fatigue, and general levels of physical conditioning. Psychological factors have also been studied, with particular emphasis given to the personality of the athlete, the way the athlete interacts with others, and the athlete's perception of stress.[1-3,6] However, research to date has not identified one particular type of individual who seems more prone to injury than another.[2] Much has also been written on the effects of stress and how it influences the occurrence and likely response to injury.[2,3] Although the relationship between stress and injury is not well understood, there is a general emphasis in the field on helping those with pain problems to manage stress adaptively.[5]

Most athletes with acute spinal injuries typically respond well to standard treatment and will not likely need psychological assistance. Relative to the nature and degree of the injury, the athlete may be told to stop activity for a brief period in order to improve. As the original pain subsides, athletes are generally guided toward a gradual resumption of activity. In contrast, some spinal problems tend to persist or recur, leading the athlete to make even more difficult decisions regarding sports and physical activity. For most active people, this degree of change in physical function and activity is quite distressing. Many of these patients find they have to reduce the frequency of sports, modify performance of the activity, and possibly give up some athletic activities altogether and replace them with sports that are less stressful on spinal structures.

Concomitantly, it is generally accepted by those who treat spinal problems that some degree of exercise and physical conditioning is beneficial.[5] The phrase "no pain, no gain" is often used to emphasize the value of exercise for both improving physical tolerance and, at a minimum, to prevent patients from growing even weaker and further disabled. One of the beginning tasks is to help the patient to continue to be physically active, but in an intelligent way.

Most low back pain patients have either conscious or unconscious fears of reinjury and of becoming worse as a result of activity. These fears often lead to the development of guarding and bracing behaviors, as well as an excessive inner focus on bodily sensations. Consequently, it soon becomes important for athletes to learn to differentiate among their various aches and pains, so that they can know whether to continue or stop an activity. With guided practice and dialogue with a coach, therapist, or trainer, many of these initial fears subside. Likewise, as knowledge increases, the inner attentional focus tends to shift toward one of emphasis on relevant cues critical to performance. When these events do not occur, other strategies must be considered.

Nideffer observed that for optimal physical performance two things must occur: first, muscle tension needs to be controlled so that the athlete is ready for action, but also relaxed; secondly, the athlete must show appropriate external, performance-related attention.[3,4] He describes this process as becoming intense, but not tense.[4] Responding appropriately to tension may be particularly important in athletes with back pain, since the back is an area that is frequently affected by the pain-tension cycle.

A number of techniques are available that can help the patient learn the difference between being tense and intense. Among these tools are biofeedback, progressive relaxation, hypnosis, guided imagery, systematic desensitization, and attention control training. **Biofeedback** essentially involves monitoring a biological process such as heart rate or muscle tension with instrumentation. Information from the body is fed back to the patient through the instrumentation, typically via an auditory tone. Differences in the auditory tone correspond to measured increases and decreases in the bodily process being measured. Through the feedback process, a patient can then learn to gain better voluntary control of the bodily function being monitored.

Progressive relaxation is a technique that uses the principal of muscle fatigue and requires tensing and relaxing different muscle groups (such as muscles in the forehead and eyes, cheeks and jaw, neck, shoulders, right and left arms, chest, abdomen, buttocks, thighs, calves, and feet) to obtain a greater degree of physical relaxation. **Hypnosis**, usually self-hypnosis, involves the pairing of certain cues, such as a word or phrase, to a deeply relaxed and focused trance state. Practice allows the patient to quickly achieve a deep level of relaxation and to concentrate more effectively on the task at hand.

Guided imagery consists of mental rehearsal techniques, whereby an athlete can specifically review and concentrate on the desired behavior prior to performance. It is often useful with guided imagery to have the athlete image both the actual bodily movements as well as the feel of these movements when executed properly.

Systematic desensitization, while originally developed to treat irrational fears and anxieties, can be applied to realistic fears and anxieties as well. This technique has the patient develop a series of mental scenes that depict ever-increasing skill in the face of increased performance demand. Patients are taught to relax and maintain their relaxation while imagining the anxiety-arousing scene. Once graduated mental practice has been accomplished through the series of scenes, actual practice ensues.

Finally, **attention control training** is a technique that teaches the athlete to use deep breathing to reduce tension and to refocus attention to critical performance-related cues. At the very minimum, specific direction from a coach, trainer, or therapist to focus on specific technical or tactical cues related to the process of competing can also help reduce distracting inner thoughts regarding outcome.

For the less fortunate, the severity of spinal injury and associated pain virtually eliminates athletic activities altogether. Since participation in sports involves a variety of specific and nonspecific factors, finding substitutes for these needs is often a frustrating process of trial and error. Likewise, both psychological and physical progress are often slow and painful. Such individuals will need assistance through the process of adaptation, which includes grieving the loss of physical function and activity with an ever-increasing focus on developing other ways to maintain physical conditioning, productivity, achievement, competition, stress reduction, and affiliation with others. Teaching psychological and physical techniques to manage pain is usually required.

Initially, patients are likely to show shock, disbelief, and denial regarding the extent of their spinal injury. Professional or high-caliber athletes, in particular, may show even more in the way of denial and lack of regard for their bodies. They may have difficulty trusting the physicians and appear to be in a rush to return to sports. Finally, some athletes completely bypass the system and try to treat their own problem out of fear that the physician will direct them to stop the sport. In either case, considerable expertise is needed to help these patients make adaptive changes, live with residual pain, and accept the risks and fears of becoming worse without giving up on life.

The psychologist who specializes in the treatment of pain, adaptation to physical problems, and spinal injury can play an invaluable role with the physician. The skilled practitioner should be able to help the patient to set and achieve workable, realistic goals; to help expand or narrow the focus of treatment, depending on the issue at hand; to assist patients in moving from self-pity, helplessness, hopelessness, and blame to acceptance and adaptation; to help patients in taking different perspectives regarding their defined problems, thereby generating possible new solutions; to help them learn preventive strategies; and to be creative in terms of helping patients define themselves and their value to others in ways that are not likely to change with changes in physical function. It is also important that each patient be treated respectfully and helped in such a way that he or she can maintain a sense of pride, dignity, and productivity.

As patients begin to adapt and thereby show less focus on what they can no longer do, practical replacements and other changes in lifestyle can be introduced. For example, a person can learn to shift from being competitive in sports to competing with himself. Many of our patients at Texas Back Institute set daily and weekly goals of physical performance and learn to take pride in their accomplishments. As mentioned earlier, patients can also learn to replace high-risk activities with others such as swimming, walking, or bicycling, which reduce strain to the back. Finally, skill and expertise in performing or competing in sports can be transferred to teaching, coaching, or helping others develop those same skills. While care must be taken with this last suggestion to not forcing one's own needs and goals onto others, much satisfaction can be obtained in making a difference in another's life.

In summary, we believe there is a place and special role for everyone. There is life with back pain and people can adapt and change. Techniques are available to assist people in making these kinds of changes, and those treating patients with back pain, or spinal injuries, need to continually and tactfully influence patients toward the future, rather than the past.

REFERENCES

Modalities

1. Benson DR, Wolf AW, Shoji H: Can the Milwaukee brace patient participate in competitive athletics? Am J Sports Med 5:7–12, 1977.
2. Bernhardt DB: Sports Physical Therapy. New York, Churchill Livingstone, 1986.
3. Deyo RA, Diehl AK, Rosenthal M: How many days of bed rest for acute low back pain? A randomized clinical trial. N Engl J Med 315:1064–1070, 1986.
4. Grew ND, Deane G: The physical effect of lumbar spinal supports. Prosthet Orthot Int 6:79–87, 1982.
5. Hillman SK, Delforge G: The use of physical agents in rehabilitation of athletic injuries. Clin Sports Med 4:431–438, 1985.
6. Holm S, Nachemson A: Variations in the nutrition of the canine intervertebral disc induced by motion. Spine 8:866–874, 1983.
7. Jensen JE, Etheridge GL, Hazelrigg G: Effectiveness of transcutaneous electrical neural stimulation in the treatment of sports injuries. Sports Med 3:79–88, 1986.
8. Keene JS: Low back pain in the athlete from spondylogenic injury during recreation or competition.

9. Keene JS, Drummond DS: Mechanical back pain in the athlete. Compr Ther 11(1):7–14, 1985.
10. Kellett J: Acute soft tissue injuries: A review of the literature. Med Sci Sports Exerc 18:489–500, 1986.
11. Lehmann J, et al: Effects of therapeutic temperatures on tendon extensibility. Arch Phys Med 51:486, 1970.
12. Lehmann JS, Watten CG, Scham SM: Therapeutic heat and cold. Clin Orthop 99:207–249, 1974.
13. Meeusen R, Lievens P: The use of cryotherapy in sports injuries. Sports Med 3:398–414, 1986.
14. Micheli LJ, Hall JE, Miller ME: Use of modified Boston brace for back injuries in athletes. Am J Sports Med 8:351–356, 1980.
15. Nachemson A, Morris JM: *In vivo* measurements of intradiscal pressure: Discectomy, a new method for the determination of pressure on the lower lumbar discs. J Bone Joint Surg 46A:1077–1092, 1964.
16. O'Leary P, Boiardo R: The diagnosis and treatment of injuries of the spine in athletes. In Nichols JA, Hershman EB (eds): The Lower Extremity and Spine in Sports Medicine, Vol. 2. St. Louis, C.V. Mosby Company, 1986.
17. Oakley EM: Dangers and contraindications of therapeutic ultrasound. Physiotherapy 64:173, 1978.
18. Reese RC Jr, Burruss TP: Principles of therapeutic modalities: Implications for sports injuries. In Nichols JA, Hershman EB (eds): Lower Extremity and Spine in Sports Medicine, Vol. 1. St. Louis, C.V. Mosby Company, 1986, pp 196–244.
19. Saal JA, Saal JS: Nonoperative treatment of herniated lumbar intervertebral disc with radiculopathy: An outcome study. Spine 14:431–437, 1989.
20. Stanish W: Low back pain in middle-aged athletes. In Clancy EG (ed): Symposium: Low Back Pain in Athletes. Am J Sports Med 7:367–369, 1979.
21. Stewart HF, Abzug JL, Harris GR: Consideration in ultrasound therapy and equipment performance. Phys Ther 60:424, 1980.
22. Teitz CC, Cook DM: Rehabilitation of neck and low back injuries. Clin Sports Med 4:455–476, 1985.
23. Urban JPG, Holm S, Maroudas A, Nachemson A: Nutrition of the intervertebral disc: An *in vivo* study of solute transport. Clin Orthop 129:101–114, 1977.
24. Urban JPG, Holm S, Maroudas A, Nachemson A: Nutrition of intervertebral disc: Effect of fluid flow on solute transport. Clin Orthop 170:296–302, 1982.
25. Wilson FD, Lindseth RE: The adolescent swimmer's back. Am J Sports Med 10:174–176, 1982.

Manipulation

1. Williams J, Sperryn P (eds): Sports Medicine, 2nd ed. Baltimore, Williams & Wilkins, 1976.
2. Backx F, Erich W, Kemper A, Verbeek A: Sports injuries in school-aged children. An epidemiological study. Am J Sports Med 17:234–240, 1989.
3. Haldeman S: Spinal manipulative therapy in sports medicine. Clin Sports Med 5:277–293, 1986.
4. Schafer R: Chiropractic Management of Sports and Recreational Injuries. Baltimore, Williams & Wilkins, 1982.
5. LeBlanc F (ed): Scientific approach to the assessment and management of activity-related spinal disorders. Spine 12:16–21, 1987.
6. Mulley A, Eagle K: What is inappropriate care? JAMA 260:540–541, 1988.
7. Wennberg J, Barnes B, Zubkoff M: Professional uncertainty and the problems of supplier-induced demand. Soc Sci Med 16:811–821, 1982.
8. Evans B, Burke M, Lloyd K, et al: Lumbar spinal manipulation on trial. Part 1. Clinical assessment. Rheum & Rehab 17:46–53, 1978.
9. Rasmussen T: Manipulation in treatment of low back pain (a randomized clinical trial). Man Med 1:8–10, 1978.
10. Hoehler F, Tobis J, Burger A: Spinal manipulation of low back pain. JAMA 224:1835–1838, 1981.
11. Godfrey C, Morgan P, Schatzker J: A randomized trial of manipulation for low-back pain in a medical setting. Spine 9:301–304, 1984.
12. Gibson T, Grahame R, Harkness J, et al: Controlled comparison of short wave diathermy treatment with osteopathic treatment in non-specific low back pain. Lancet ii:1258–1260, 1985.
13. Waagen G, Haldeman S, Cook G, et al: Short term of chiropractic adjustments for the relief of chronic low back pain. Man Med 2:63–67, 1986.
14. Meade T: Comparison of chiropractic and hospital outpatient management of low back pain: A feasibility study. J Epidemiol Community Health 40:12–17, 1986.

15. Ongley M, Kleing R, Dormain T, et al: A new approach to the treatment of chronic low back pain. Lancet 143–146, 1987.
16. Hadler N, Curtis P, Gillings B, Stinnett S: A benefit of spinal manipulation as adjunctive therapy for acute low-back pain: A stratified controlled trial. Spine 12:703–706, 1987.
17. Phillips R: Physician selection in low back pain patients. Doctoral dissertation, Univ. of Utah, Dept. of Sociology, 1987.
18. Phillips R, Butler R: Survey of chiropractic in Dade County, Florida. J Manipulative Physiol Ther 5:83–89, 1982.
19. Phillips R: A survey of Utah chiropractic patients. ACA Journal of Chiropractic 15:113–128, 1981.
20. Guifu C, Zonmin L, Zhenzhong Y, Jinaghuz W: Lateral rotary manipulative maneuver in the treatment of subluxation and synovial entrapment of lumbar facet joint. J Tradit Chin Med 4:211–212, 1984.
21. Frymoyer J: Back pain and sciatica. JAMA 318:291–300, 1988.
22. Mayer T, Gatchel R: Functional Restoration for Spinal Disorders—Sports Medicine Approach. Philadelphia, Lea & Febiger, 1988.
23. Wolk S: An analysis of Florida workers compensation medical claims for back related injuries. (in preparation).
24. Wolk S: Chiropractic versus medical care: A cost analysis of disability and treatment for back-related workers compensation cases. (in preparation).
25. Jull G, Bogduck N, Marsland A: The accuracy of manual diagnosis for cervical zygapophyseal joint pain syndromes. Med J Aus 148:233–237, 1988.
26. Jirout J: The effect of mobilization of the segmental blockade on the sagittal component of the reaction on lateral flexion of the cervical spine. Neuroradiology 3:210–215, 1972.
27. Lewit K: Manipulative Therapy in Rehabilitation of the Motor System. London, Butterworths, 1985.
28. Grieve G: Common Vertebral Joint Problems. New York, Churchill Livingstone, 1986.
29. Paterson J, Burn L: An Introduction to Medical Manipulation. Lancaster, MTP Press, 1985.
30. Kirkaldy-Willis W, Hill R: A more precise diagnosis for low back pain. 4:102–108, 1979.
31. Raftis K, Warfield C: Spinal manipulation for back pain. Hospital Practice 89–108, 1989.
32. Quon J, Cassidy J, O'Connor S, Kirkaldy-Willis W: J Manipulative Physiol Ther 12:220–227, 1989.
33. Kirkaldy-Willis W, Hill J: A more precise diagnosis for low back pain. Spine 4:102, 1979.
34. Bernard T, Kirkaldy-Willis W: Recognizing specific characteristics of nonspecific low back pain. Clin Orthop Rel Res 217:266–280, 1987.
35. Yost JG Jr, Ellfeldt JH: Basketball injuries. In Nicholas JA, Hershman EB (eds): The Lower Extremity and Spine in Sports Medicine, Vol. 2. St. Louis, C.V. Mosby, 1986, p 1442.
36. Garrett WE: Basic science of musculotendinous injuries. In Nicholas JA, Hershman EB (eds): The Lower Extremity and Spine in Sports Medicine. St. Louis, C.V. Mosby, 1986, pp 43–51.
37. Skalak R, Chien S: Handbook of Bioengineering. New York, McGraw Hill, 1987, pp 6.1–7.26.
38. O'Donoghue DH: Treatment of Injuries to Athletes, 4th ed. Philadelphia, W.B. Saunders, 1984, pp 51–66.
39. Kellett J: Review: Acute soft tissue injuries. In A Review of the Literature, Medicine and Science in Sports and Exercise, Vol. 18, #5. 1986, pp 489–500.
40. Kirkaldy-Willis WH: Managing Low Back Pain. Edinburgh, Churchill Livingstone, 1983, p 177.
41. Schaffer F: Clinical Biomechanics, Musculoskeletal Actions and Reactions. Baltimore, Williams & Wilkins, 1983, p 75.
42. Parnianpour M, Nordin M, Kahanovitz N, Frankel V: The triaxial coupling of torque generation of trunk muscles during isometric exertions and the effect of fatiguing isoinertial movements on the motor output and movement patterns. Spine 13:, 1988.
43. Webber A: Acute soft tissue injuries in the young athlete. Clin Sports Med 7:617–623, 1988.
44. Garrett W, Califf J, Bassett F: Histochemical correlates of hamstring injuries. Am J Sports Med 12:98–103, 1984.
45. Nicholas J, Hershman E: The Lower Extremity and Spine in Sports Medicine. St. Louis, C.V. Mosby, 1986.
46. Astrin PO, Rodahl K: Textbook of Work Physiology. New York, McGraw-Hill, 1973, pp 411–420.
47. Zarins B: Soft tissue injury and repair—biomechanical aspects. Int J Sports Med 3(Suppl 1):9–11, 1982.
48. Tiptan CM, James SL, Megner W, Tcheng T: Influence of exercise on strength of medial collateral knee ligaments of dogs. Am J Physiol 218:894–902, 1970.

49. Vailas AC, Tiptan CM, Matthew RD, Gart M: Influence of physical activity on the repair process of medial collateral ligaments in rats. Connect Tis Res 9:25–31, 1981.
50. Oakes BW: Acute soft tissue injuries: Nature and management. Aust Fam Physician 10(Suppl):3–16, 1982.
51. Kulund DN: The Injured Athlete, 2nd ed. Philadelphia, J.B. Lippincott, 1988, p 242.
52. Reese RC, Vurruss TP: Athletic training techniques and protective equipment. In Nicholas JA, Hershman JB (eds): The Lower Extremity and Spine in Sports Medicine, Vol. 1. St. Louis, C.V. Mosby, 1986, p 323.
53. Lippitt AB: The facet joint and its role in spine pain: Management with facet joint injection. Spine 9:746–750, 1984.
54. Putti V: Lady Jones' lecture on new concepts in the pathogenesis of sciatic pain. Lancet 2:53–60, 1927.
55. Ghormley RK: Low back pain with special reference to the articular facets with presentation of an operative procedure. JAMA 101:1773–1777, 1933.
56. Badgley CE: The articular facets in relation to low back pain and sciatic radiation. 23:481–496, 1941.
57. Danforth MS, Wilson PD: The anatomy of the lumbosacral region in relation to sciatic pain. J Bone Joint Surg 7:, 1925.
58. Kleynhans AM. Facet syndrome. J Aust Chiro Assoc 10(14): 1976.
59. Farfan HF: Symptomatology in terms of the pathomechanics of low back pain and sciatica. In Haldeman S (ed): Modern Developments in the Principles and Practice of Chiropractic. New York, Appleton-Century-Croft, 1980.
60. Kirkaldy-Willis WH: Managing Low Back Pain. New York, Churchill Livingstone, 1983, p 25.
61. Marks MR, Hass SS, Wiesel SW: Low back pain in the competitive tennis player. Clin Sports Med 7:277–287, 1988.
62. Banks SD: Lumbar facet syndrome. Spinographic assessment of treatment by spinal manipulative therapy. J Manipulative Physiol Ther 6:175–180, 1983.
63. White A, Panjabi M: Clinical Biomechanics of the Spine. Philadelphia, J.B. Lippincott, 1978, p 264.
64. Bourdillion JF, Day EA: Spinal Manipulation, 4th ed. London, William Heinneman, 1987.
65. Sim FH, Scott SG: Injuries of the pelvis and hip in athletes' anatomy and function. In Nicholas JA, Hershman JB (eds): The Lower Extremity and Spine in Sports Medicine, Vol. 2. St. Louis, C.V. Mosby, 1986.
66. Greenman P: Principles of Manual Medicine. Baltimore, Williams & Wilkins, 1989, p 231.
67. Schneider W, Dvorak J, Dvorak V, Tritschler T: Manual Medicine Therapy. New York, Theime Medical, 1988, pp 41–46.
68. Yochum TR, Rowe LJ: Essentials of Skeletal Radiology. Baltimore, Williams & Wilkins, 1987.
69. Stanish W: Low back pain in athletes and over use syndrome. Clin Sports Med 6:341, 1987.
70. Kulund DN: The Injured Athlete, 2nd ed. Philadelphia, J.B. Lippincott, 1988.
71. O'Leary P, Boiardo R: The diagnosis and treatment of injuries of the spine in athletes. In Nicholas JA, Hershman EB (eds): The Lower Extremity and Spine in Sports Medicine. St. Louis, C.V. Mosby, 1986, pp 1213–1216.
72. Kulund DN: The Injured Athlete. Philadelphia, J.B. Lippincott, 1988, p 417.
73. Roy S, Irvin R: Sports Medicine—Prevention, Evaluation, Management and Rehabilitation. Englewood Cliffs, NJ, Prentice-Hall, 1983, pp 275–278.
74. Cox JM: The facet syndrome. In Low Back Pain. Mechanism, Diagnosis and Treatment. Baltimore, Williams & Wilkins, 1985, p 238.
75. Kirkaldy-Willis WH: Managing Low Back Pain. New York, Churchill Livingstone, 1983, pp 25, 96.
76. Chrisman OD, Miyynacht A, Snook GA: A study of the results following rotary manipulation in the lumbar intervertebral disc syndrome. J Bone Joint Surg 46A:517, 1964.
77. Quo PP, Loh ZC: Treatment of lumbar intervertebral disc protrusions by manipulation. Clin Orthop 215:45–55, 1987.
78. Giles LG: Anatomical Basis of Low Back Pain. Baltimore, Williams & Wilkins, 1989.
79. Roy S, Irvin R: Sports Medicine—Prevention, Evaluation, Management and Rehabilitation. Englewood Cliffs, NJ, Prentice-Hall, 1983.
80. Subotnick SI: Limb length discrepancies of the lower extremity (the short leg syndrome). J Orthop Sports Phys Ther 3:11–15, 1981.
81. Maigne R: Orthopedic Medicine: A New Approach to Vertebral Manipulation. Springfield, IL, Charles C Thomas, 1972.

82. Fisk JW, Baignet ML: Clinical and radiologic assessment of leg length. NZ Med J 81:477–480, 1975.
83. Siffert RS: Current concepts review. Lower limb-length discrepancy. J Bone Joint Surg 69:1100–1105, 1987.
84. Anderson WV: Modern Trends in Orthopedics. New York, Appleton-Century-Crofts, 1972, pp 1–22.
85. Mahar RK, Kirby FL, MacLeod DA: Simulated leg length discrepancy: Its effects on knee center-out pressure position and postural sway. Arch Phys Med Rehabil 66:22–24, 1985.
86. Beal MC: The short leg problem. JAOA 76:745–751, 1977.
87. Heilig D: Principle of lift therapy. JAOA 76:745–751, 1977.
88. Peter J: Short leg and sciatica. (letter) JAMA 242:1257–1258, 1979.
89. Rush WA, Steiner A: A study of lower extremity length inequality. Am J Roent 55:616–623, 1946.
90. Schwab WA: Principles of manipulative treatment. JAOA 31:384–388, 1932.
91. Kendall H, Kendall F, Boynton D: Posture and pain. Huntington, NY, Kreiser Publishing, 1977.
92. Reid DC, Smith B: Leg length inequality: A review of etiology and management. Physiother (Can) 36:177–182, 1984.
93. Clark GR: Unequal leg length: An accurate method of detection and some clinical results. Rheumatol Phys Med 11:385, 1972.
94. Fisk JW, Baignet ML: Clinical and radiological assessment of leg length. NZ Med J 81:477, 1978.
95. Giles LG: Low back pain associated with leg length inequality. Spine 6:510–521, 1981.
96. Danbert RJ: Clinical assessment and treatment of leg length inequalities. J Manipulative Physiol Ther 11:290–295, 1988.
97. DeBoer KF, Harmon RO, Savoie S, Tuttle CO: Inter- and intra-examiner reliability of leg length differential measurement: A preliminary study. J Manipulative Physiol Ther 6:61–66, 1983.
98. Moseley C: A straight line graph for leg length discrepancies. Clin Orthop Rel Res 136:33–40, 1978.
99. Winquist R, Hansen S, Pearson R: Closed intramedullary shortening of the femur. Clin Orthop Rel Res 136:41–48, 1978.
100. Stephens D, Herrick W, MacEwen G: Epiphysiodesis for limb length inequality: Results and indications. Clin Orthop Rel Res 136:561–564, 1978.
101. Banks SD: Leg length inequality. Lt Rev 1:1–7, 1985.

Acupuncture

1. Mann F: Acupuncture: The Ancient Chinese Art of Healing and How It Works Scientifically. New York, Random House, 1972.
2. Melzack R, Wall PD: Pain mechanisms: A new theory. Science 150:971–979, 1965.
3. Montgomery SJ: Acupuncture in an American pain clinic. Paper read at Sixth World Congress of Anesthesiology, Mexico City, 1976.

Injections

1. Badgley CE: The articular facet in relation to low back pain and sciatic radiation. J Bone Joint Surg 23:481, 1941.
2. Cuckler JM, Bernini PA, Wiesel SW, et al: The use of epidural steroids in the treatment of lumbar radicular pain. J Bone Joint Surg 67A:63–66, 1985.
3. Garvey TA, Marks MR, Wiesel SW: A prospective, randomized, double-blind evaluation of trigger-point injection therapy for low back pain. Spine 14:962–964, 1980.
4. Ghormley RK: Low back pain with special reference to the articular facets with presentation of an operative procedure. JAMA 148:1773, 1933.
5. Jackson DW, Rettig A, Wiltse LL: Epidural cortisone injections in the young athletic adult. Am J Sports Med 8:239–243, 1980.
6. Jackson RP, Jacobs RR, Montesano PX: Facet joint injection in low back pain: A prospective statistical study. Spine 13:966–971, 1988.
7. Melzack R: Myofascial trigger point: Relation to acupuncture and mechanisms of pain. Arch Phys Med Rehabil 62:114–117, 1981.
8. Mooney V, Robertson J: The facet syndrome. Clin Orthop 115:149–156, 1976.
9. Paris SV, Nyberg R, Mooney VT: Three-level innervations of the lumbar facet joints. Paper presented at the Seventh Annual Meeting of the International Society for the Study of the Lumbar Spine, New Orleans, 1980.

10. Rashbaum RF: Radiofrequency facet denervation: A treatment alternative in refractory low back pain with or without leg pain. Orthop Clin North Am 14:569–575, 1983.
11. Ready LB, Kozody R, Barsa JE, Murphy TM: Trigger point injections vs. jet injection in the treatment of myofascial pain. Pain 15:201–206, 1983.
12. Rees WS: Multiple bilateral subcutaneous rhizolysis of segmental nerves in the treatment of intervertebral disc syndrome. Ann Gen Prac 26:126, 1974.
13. Shealy CN: Percutaneous radiofrequency denervation of spinal facets: Treatment for chronic back pain and sciatica. J Neurosurg 43:448–451, 1975.
14. Shelokov AP, Rashbaum RF: Injection therapy for conservative management of low back pain. Spine: State Art Rev 3:83–89, 1989.
15. White AH: Injection techniques for the diagnosis and treatment of low back pain. Orthop Clin North Am 14:553–567, 1983.

Psychological Intervention

1. Hair JE: Intangibles in evaluating athletic injuries. JACHA 25:228–230, 1977.
2. Kerr G, Fowler B: The relationship between psychological factors and sports injuries. Sports Med 6:127–134, 1988.
3. Nideffer RM: The injured athlete. Psychological factors in treatment. Orthop Clin North Am 14:373–385, 1983.
4. Nideffer RM: Concentration and relaxation in sports. Sports Med Digest 7:1–3, 1985.
5. Stith WJ, Ohnmeiss DD, Carranza C, Hanks D: Rehabilitation of patients with chronic low back pain. Spine: State Art Rev 3:125–138, 1989.
6. Taerk GS: The injury-prone athlete: A psychological approach. J Sports Med 17:187–194, 1977.

Chapter 24

PERCUTANEOUS DISCECTOMY

Stephen H. Hochschuler, MD

The concept of a percutaneous approach for the surgical treatment of a herniated disc in the athlete is quite appealing. Despite the fact that percutaneous discectomy is a procedure that at this point has limited applicability, the athlete might well prove to be the ideal candidate. In most instances one cannot question the motivation of the athlete. His goal is to return to an active lifestyle. Perhaps the most difficult aspect of the management of the athlete is trying to contain his energies and give his clinical situation time to resolve. As with any patient with a herniated disc, the conservative approach should be the line of first defense. However, if this proves ineffective, then percutaneous discectomy should be considered. The young athlete is perhaps the ideal candidate for this procedure. He is less likely to have significant degenerative changes associated with stenosis and his disc is better hydrated and perhaps more responsive to this form of operative intervention.

A successful percutaneous discectomy is probably the result of:

1. Decreasing the intradiscal pressure secondary to decompressing the disc.
2. Removal of some large fragments causing mechanical nerve root compression.
3. Decreasing chemical irritation secondary to lavage.

HISTORY OF THE PROCEDURE

Ottolenghi first described the posterior lateral approach in an article in JAMA 1948.[18] Thereafter, Craig described the approach for vertebral body biopsies.[2] In 1950 Hult described a series of 30 patients who had relief of both low back pain and sciatica after fenestration of the annulus and nucleus via an open retroperitoneal approach.[7] In 1975, Hijikata described the use of a 5 mm cannula inserted by the posterior lateral approach percutaneously, entering the disc space and thereafter utilizing modified pituitary rongeurs and other instruments to decompress the disc space.[6] He described a 72% satisfied patient population. A similar technique has been used by Parviz Kambin, who has had an 87% success rate in 100 prospective cases.[11]

Other approaches have also been described. Jacobsen and Friedman employing a 10 mm cannula, described a true lateral approach.[4] This was fraught with complications, as described by Friedman in a report in *Neurosurgery* in 1983.[4] More recently, Gary Onik, using the surgical nucleotome, described a technique utilizing a 2.8 mm cannula to introduce a 2 mm suction, cutting, and irrigating device.[14] In a multi-center study, which included the Texas Back Institute, the success rate was initially reported as 75%.[15]

Unfortunately, clinical results with the surgical nucleotome for percutaneous lumbar discectomy have varied from center to center. Some reports, such as that by Kahanovitz at a recent North American Spine meeting (Quebec City, Canada, 1989) reported a success rate of approximately 50%.[8] Nevertheless, in the properly selected patient the appropriate procedure might still prove efficacious.

INDICATIONS FOR PERCUTANEOUS DISCECTOMY

The advantages of percutaneous discectomy over other surgical procedures are multiple. Despite the fact that chymopapain had proved to be a successful treatment modality, several reported cases of anaphylaxis and neurologic complications caused both the patient and the surgeon some hesitancy in its acceptance. Subsequently, and despite the fact that it is a reasonable treatment alternative, chymopapain has not been widely utilized.

In contrast to a simple laminectomy/discectomy, percutaneous discectomy has the theoretical advantage of decreased perineural fibrosis, as well as a decreased incidence of epidural bleeding. In addition, the approach does not compromise ligamentous stability nor prohibit future surgical intervention, if necessary, through virgin tissue. It is performed as an outpatient procedure, is less expensive, and does not require the use of general anesthesia. It is thought that the incidence of significant reherniation is diminished secondary to the establishment of a fenestration in the posterolateral aspect of the annulus that affords egress of any future disc material preferentially through this site rather than into the spinal canal. In fact, Hijikata demonstrated in two postoperative discograms that indeed the fenestration remained patent at 4- and 9-month intervals.[6]

Who Is a Candidate for Percutaneous Discectomy?

The ideal patient presents with a history of lumbar radicular syndrome (i.e., back pain and leg pain), with the leg pain being worse than the back pain. Ideally, the patient should be one who has not had previous surgery at this disc level, although William Davis reported an 80% success rate in this subgroup of patients.[3] Prior to any type of operative intervention, including percutaneous discectomy, a thorough trial of conservative modalities must be undertaken. At the Texas Back Institute this includes analgesics, nonsteroidal anti-inflammatories, and muscle relaxants. A thorough trial at physical therapy, which might include Williams flexion exercises, McKenzie extension exercises, various modes of traction therapies, etc., should be undertaken. Bed rest, when appropriate, is utilized, but not for prolonged periods. A course of epidural steroid injections is likewise often undertaken in an attempt to avoid operative intervention.

On physical examination, the patient should demonstrate clear-cut evidence of lumbar radicular syndrome. One would like to find evidence of sensory, motor, or reflex changes, positive root tension signs, and a lack of histrionics. The clinical findings should be corroborated by objective, diagnostic studies. In our institution, either the CT scan or MRI scan is most commonly utilized. Electromyographic (EMG) testing has likewise been of assistance. It is quite important to ascertain not only the disc level involved, but indeed to demonstrate that the herniated disc remains in continuity and that one is not dealing with a free fragment lying within the spinal canal. The importance of this is self-evident. The posterolateral approach cannot afford access to such a fragment. In those cases where it remains doubtful as to the exact disorder, myelography with a post-myelographic CT scan can prove helpful. In addition, discography with post-discographic CT scanning likewise is utilized when indicated.

Contraindications

Percutaneous discectomy is to be avoided in patients presenting with cauda equina syndrome. In addition, it plays no present role in the treatment of spinal stenosis, tumors, or sequestered discs. Relative contraindications include the previously operated spine, a significantly high-riding iliac crest, and a patient with significant psychological problems. Percutaneous discectomy is performed under local anesthesia and requires considerable patient cooperation, which is difficult for most patients and might prove impossible for the individual with significant psychological problems. In addition, most investigators feel that the technique should only be utilized for a herniated disc. Nevertheless, in January 1989 Hijikata reported satisfactory results in a subgroup of patients with back pain consistent with degenerative disc disease.[5]

ANATOMY

Perhaps the best description of the surgical anatomy can be found in an article by Parviz Kambin in *Surgical Rounds for Orthopaedics,* December 1988.[12] It is to be noted that the lumbar spinal nerve exits the neuroforamen, hugging the inferior aspect of the pedicle, and thereafter migrates anteriorly and distally across the intervertebral disc space (Fig. 1). Thereafter, the nerve descends anterior to the transverse process below (Fig. 2). Fully understanding the anatomy is crucial to the successful performance of a percutaneous discectomy. The clear zone, therefore, is a triangular target that is inferior and posterior to the exiting nerve root. The approach should be medial to the nerve root itself. The clear or target zone should be that portion of disc just lateral to the superior facet of the inferior vertebral body, just cephalad to the endplate of the inferior vertebral body, and posterior and medial to the exiting nerve root. The iliac arteries and veins, as well as the sympathetic nerve root fibers, are located anterior to the vertebral body and therefore are not violated with the correct operative approach (Fig. 3).

In using the posterolateral approach, it is generally agreed that a point somewhere between 8 and 12 cm lateral to the midline should be the point of entry. One should approach the disc from the involved side. The direction of the

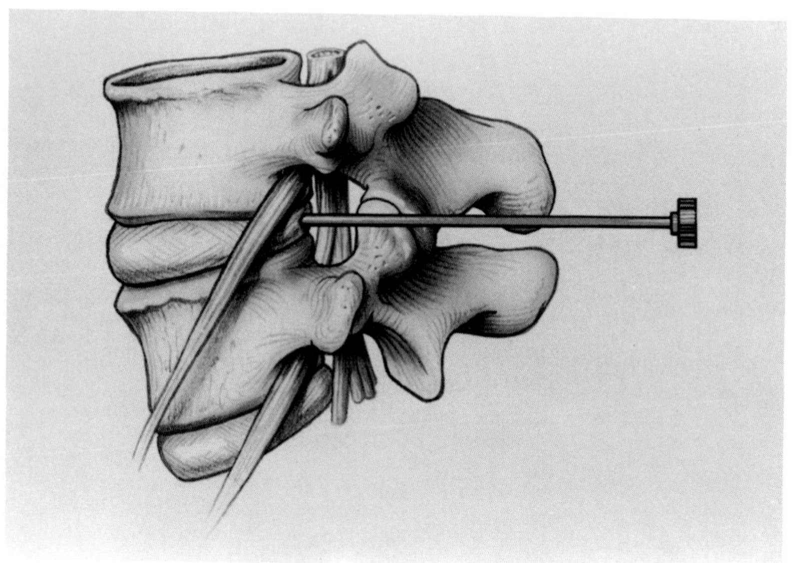

FIGURE 1. The path of the lumbar spinal nerve root as it exits the neuroforamen.

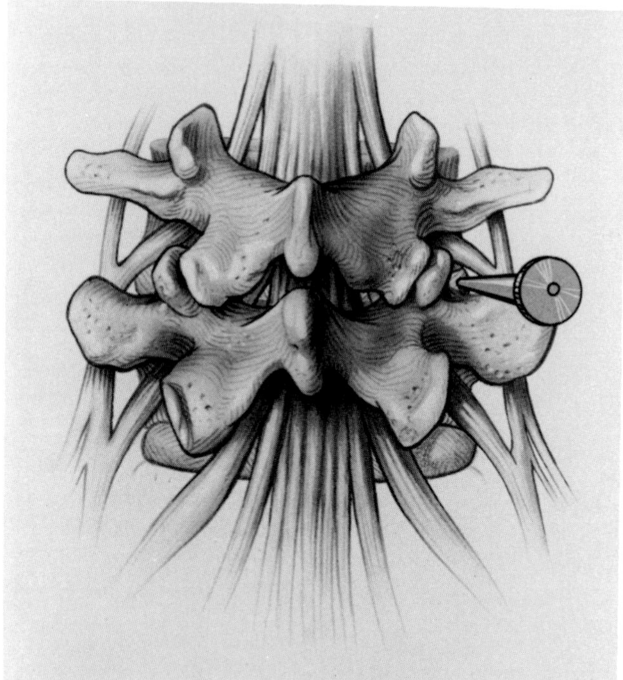

FIGURE 2. The relationship of the exiting spinal nerve to the transverse process.

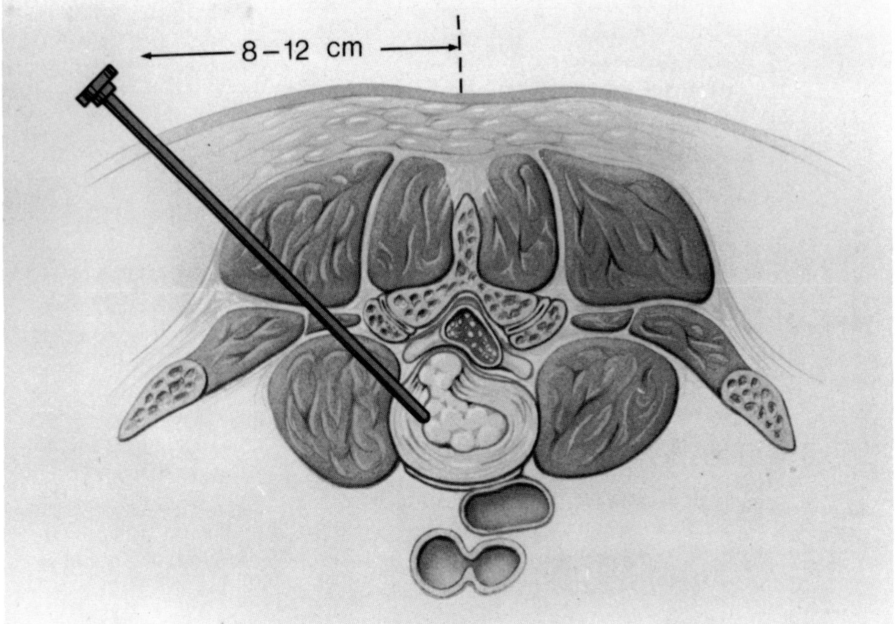

FIGURE 3. Axial view of probe pathway in performing percutaneous discectomy.

probe is at approximately 45°, parallel to the disc space. This trajectory will penetrate subcutaneous tissue, fascia, quadratus lumborum muscles, and thereafter pass between the transverse processes and the contiguous vertebrae, penetrating the psoas major muscle prior to entering the disc space itself. One needs to vary the approach slightly for the L5–S1 interspace, in that it is not possible to approach it in a parallel fashion in most instances.

ANESTHESIA

It is generally accepted that percutaneous discectomy should be performed under local anesthesia. As the technique evolves, however, and various satisfactory means are established to identify the spinal nerve roots, general anesthesia might be appropriate sometime in the future. This will be discussed later in the chapter.

Most surgeons performing percutaneous discectomy use monitored anesthesia care (MAC). At the Texas Back Institute we utilize a combination of fentanyl and midazolam (Versed). It is important that the patient is comfortable but responsive, and able to respond if indeed the instruments are violating the exiting spinal nerve. Lidocaine is injected in the skin and the subcutaneous tissue in addition to anesthetizing the fascia. One must be cautious, however, not to penetrate too deeply with the lidocaine to avoid anesthetizing the exiting spinal nerve. Once the disc space itself has been successfully entered, stronger sedation might be warranted to make the patient more comfortable.

TECHNIQUE

The patient is positioned in either a lateral or prone position with the abdomen decompressed. The procedure is performed under sterile conditions. At our institution, prophylactic antibiotics are given. Depending on the technique, the procedure is performed either on an inpatient or outpatient basis after proper preoperative and postoperative instructions.

As mentioned previously, various techniques have been described for percutaneous discectomy, including Jacobsen's lateral approach using a larger cannula, which was fraught with significant complications.[4] This approach seems to have been generally abandoned. The posterolateral approach, as initially described by Hijikata, is utilized for both the automated percutaneous discectomy as well as the more traditional technique described by Hijikata and advocated by Kambin. The difference in the two procedures seems to be the size of the operating sleeve as well as the size of the instruments. In addition, the positioning of the instruments advocated by these two groups is also somewhat different.[11,13] Surgical Dynamics has advocated the use of a small probe measuring approximately 2 mm and positioning the instrument in the center of the disc, as demonstrated on AP and lateral x-ray control. Kambin has advocated utilization of a larger sleeve measuring approximately 5 mm and positioning the discectomy equipment in the posterior medial aspect of the disc itself, not the central portion. He believes that the larger fenestration, using the 5 mm instruments, affords a more adequate decompression of the disc itself, as well as allowing a larger portal of exit for future potential herniations. In addition, Kambin feels that the placement of the dissecting instruments in the posteromedial aspect of the disc allows one to decompress the area where the herniation has occurred more effectively. Proper instrument placement is probably a very important component of this procedure, as it directly influences success or failure. Hijikata reports one case of a poor result because too much disc was taken anteriorly, as seen on postoperative discography, but when a second procedure was performed placing the instruments in a more posterior position, a good result was attained.[5]

It has been our experience that some variation of the Hijikata and Kambin approach utilizing automated instruments as well as hand held instruments positioned in the more posterior central region is more effective. It is to be noted that in performing the procedure, biplaner image intensification is mandatory. One must be absolutely certain of the positioning of one's dissecting instruments prior to performing the discectomy itself. Usually 1 to 3 g of disc material are extracted.

POSTOPERATIVE CARE

A successful procedure usually will be noted by the patient immediately postoperatively, although in some instances patients have noted gradual improvement over the ensuing several days. Patients might experience some back discomfort associated with settling and inflammation, though this is usually minor. They are generally discharged with a minor pain medication as well as an anti-inflammatory medication and thereafter progressed to gentle aerobic exercise and a stretching program. Over the ensuing several weeks, a strengthening program is instituted. The patient is schooled in proper body mechanics and cautioned as to any excessive strenuous activities for the preliminary 6-week period. In general, the patient is returned to a sedentary-type occupation within a week to 10 days postoperatively or to more strenuous labor within a 4- to 6-week period.

In the event of an unsuccessful result, conservative modalities are once again employed, including anti-inflammatories, physical therapy, and epidural steroids.

If they do not prove efficacious, open operative intervention may be indicated but is usually not undertaken prior to 6 weeks.

COMPLICATIONS

Complications in general have been few and far between. However, those that do occur can be significant. There have been reports of postoperative infection.[1,5] One investigator advocates the use of a lavage cocktail of Depo-Medrol, lidocaine, and gentamicin (40 mg gentamicin, 40 mg Depo-Medrol, 2 cc Marcaine 0.5%),[17] in addition to which several investigators, including the Texas Back Institute, give prophylactic antibiotics.[1] Other reported complications include hematoma formation for which some have used Gelfoam and others a single tube Hemovac.[11,17] In addition, nerve root injury has been described as well as vascular injury.[5,16] Consequently, though complications are infrequent, they can indeed occur and the procedure should be treated with respect.

RESULTS

As mentioned previously, the results vary from 50 to 87%. There is concern with regard to potential overutilization of the technique. The procedure should be used within strict parameters, as outlined earlier, but it can prove to be quite efficacious when discriminately selected.

THE FUTURE

I believe there is a future for percutaneous discectomy, and we will see the evolution of various techniques involving previously proven arthroscopic technology, as well as many new and innovative variations. Schreiber et al., as well as others, have described the use of discoscopy utilizing elongated arthroscopic instruments.[16] The development and evolution of spinal operating arthroscopes will occur. The concept of laser percutaneous discectomy is also being addressed, in addition to which some investigators have been developing percutaneous fusions as well as percutaneous lumbar intervertebral disc replacements. The exact role of lumbar myeloscopy for the treatment of an extruded fragment, perhaps employing a laser through the fiberoptiscope, will itself evolve. The future is bright, but one must be cautious in the development of any new technique to avoid overutilization.

REFERENCES

1. Blankstein A, Rubinstein E, Ezra E, et al: Disc space infection and vertebral osteomyelitis as a complication of percutaneous lateral discectomy. Clin Orthop 225:234–237, 1987.
2. Craig FS: Vertebral body biopsy. J Bone Joint Surg 38A:93, 1956.
3. Davis WG: Clinical experience with automated percutaneous lumbar discectomy. In Onik G, Helms LA (eds): Automated Percutaneous Lumbar Discectomy. San Francisco, Radiology Research and Education Foundation, 1988, pp 111–117.
4. Friedman WA: Percutaneous discectomy: An alternative to chemonucleolysis. Neurosurgery 13:542–547, 1983.
5. Hijikata S: Percutaneous nucleotomy. Clin Orthop 238:9, 1989.
6. Hijikata SA: A method of percutaneous nuclear extraction. J Toden Hospital 5:39, 1975.
7. Hult I: Retroperitoneal disc fenestration in low back pain and sciatica. Acta Orthop Scand 20:342–348, 1950.
8. Kahanovitz N, Viola K, Watkins R, et al: A multicenter analysis of automated percutaneous discectomy. Presented at the North American Spine Society. Quebec City, Canada, June 1989.
9. Kambin P, Brager MD: Percutaneous posterolateral discectomy: Anatomy and mechanism. Clin Orthop 223:145, 1987.

10. Kambin P, Gellman H: Percutaneous lateral discectomy of the lumbar spine: A preliminary report. Clin Orthop 174:127, 1983.
11. Kambin P, Schaffer JL: Percutaneous lumbar discectomy: Review of 100 patients. Clin Orthop 238:24, 1989.
12. Kambin P: Surg Rounds for Orthop, Dec, 1988.
13. Mooney V: Percutaneous discectomy. In Guyer RD (ed): Lumbar Disc Disease. Spine: State of the Art Reviews 3(1):103–112, 1989.
14. Onik G, Helms C, Ginsberg L, et al: Percutaneous lumbar discectomy using a new aspiration probe. AJNR 6:290, 1985.
15. Onik G, Maroon J, Helms C, et al: Automated percutaneous diskectomy: Initial patient experience. Radiology 162(1):129–132, 1987.
16. Schreiber A, Suezawa Y, Leu H: Does percutaneous nucleotomy with discoscopy replace conventional discectomy? Clin Orthop 238:35, 1989.
17. Shepperd JAN, James SE, Leach AS: Percutaneous disc surgery. Clin Orthop 238:43, 1989.
18. Valls J, Ottolenghi EC, Schajowicz F: Aspiration biopsy in diagnosis of lesions of vertebral bodies. JAMA 136:376, 1948.

Chapter 25

LAMINECTOMY AND FUSION IN THE ATHLETE

Arthur H. White, MD

A number of special circumstances unique to the lifestyle and expectations of professional athletes need to be considered when lumbar surgery is anticipated.

Time is usually of the essence. A recovery period following surgery lasting even one month longer than necessary could cause an athlete to miss an entire season or circuit, and possibly end his or her career. Moreover, the physical demands athletes experience are clearly greater than those of the average patient. These physical demands, along with trauma to the spine and to the operative site, increase the potential of recurrent herniated disc, spinal stenosis, and instability.

On the brighter side, the physical condition of an athlete is usually better than that of the average patient. Furthermore, athletes generally understand the importance of physical fitness, strength, and flexibility for the particular sport in which they are involved, and often have extensive assistance and training available to them.

Thus, athletes often have physical attributes, expectations about their current or future job or play requirements, and time factors and outside influences, all of which may affect the decisions a surgeon makes regarding the timing and extent of surgery, and the technique to be used. However, as with other patients, pre- and postoperative training is unquestionably the strongest tool for successful surgery in the athlete.

It must be remembered that the injuries suffered by professional athletes are, in essence, work-related injuries, and many of the rules for treating patients with occupational disorders apply. For example, secondary gain is known to be a factor that impedes a patient's return to work. Factors motivating a patient to return to work include job satisfaction, fair treatment, good communication on the job, and good relations with supervisors. Professional athletes, as with other patients, are more likely to return to work if they are treated honestly and fairly. However, the stakes are higher when working with professional athletes than when working with the average industrial patient. Although the motivation of professional athletes may be very high because of their desire to resume play, and their potential income is much higher than that of the average industrial patient, if they are barely making the team and have a good disability policy, they may give in to their pain and not return to work.

There are at least four factors that might give a surgeon cause to alter an athlete's normal plan of treatment:

Conditioning. Athletes may be extremely strong and flexible. They may have a high pain tolerance and be greatly motivated.

Demand. Athletes may expect and demand a return to peak function, e.g., when playing contact sports. A professional football player may want to return to this high level of athletic function for the remainder of his normal career. At times, athletes may be aggressive, impatient, and eager for rapid, physical solutions to anything that interferes with their athletic activities.

Outside Influences. Athletes frequently have other individuals, such as trainers, coaches, family, and teammates, who may be motivating them beyond their own abilities or desires. Such pressures can set up conflicts that leave the athlete frustrated, confused, and psychologically overburdened.

Time Factors. Athletes may frequently be caught in a time frame that may cause them to lose their position on a team, miss an entire season of play, or lose their chance at a professional career.

SURGICAL DECISION-MAKING FOR THE ATHLETE

There are basically two surgical procedures that can be performed for lumbar spine disease in the athlete, namely, decompression or fusion. And for each of these, there are many different techniques. Decompression, regardless of the technique, is successful as long as it relieves the neural compressive disorder. Likewise, fusion, no matter what technique is employed, is only successful if it becomes stable.

When considering surgery for an athlete, two questions need to be answered for a given athlete:

- Is *any* surgery on the spine indicated?
- What is the disorder upon which one is operating?

If surgery is indicated, the appropriate surgical technique will be determined by the athlete's spinal pathology, the sport played, and the level of athletic performance demanded.

Sports-specific Decision Making

The specific demands of a particular sport and the position an athlete plays on the team are important factors affecting a surgeon's decision about the type of surgery to be performed on an athlete. The first question a surgeon asks is whether the sport played is a contact sport. If the athlete plays a contact sport, the surgeon needs to know the degree of control a player has of his body mechanics.

When a football player is hit unaware, or a water skier topples off of a ski at 40 miles per hour, or a gymnast misses the mark taking a hard fall, there is no time for their conscious protective mechanisms to come into play. The damaged vertebral segment takes the brunt of the accident. A stenotic foramen crashes closed, a herniated disc protrudes further, or an unstable vertebral segment reaches a new extreme of instability. The neural elements are no longer protected by conscious stabilizing mechanisms the athlete may have developed. Inflammation and pain ensue, and the athlete may be out of play for an undetermined period.

Fortunately, most sports can be performed "in control," i.e., players can practice their sport with particular body mechanics that protect the underlying physical pathoanatomy that they suffer. These body mechanics that stabilize the spine come naturally to athletes and may even improve their performance. An athlete using these stabilizing body mechanics, who does not play contact sports, may undergo a lesser surgery with success. Fusions, for example, are not usually necessary in athletes who do not play contact sports and are able to play "in control." Particularly interesting is that minor spinal pathology may present with major limiting consequences in athletes playing contact sports in an "out-of-control" manner. Whereas major spinal pathology can be tolerated quite well in trained athletes who learn and maintain stabilization throughout their athletic endeavors.

THE DIAGNOSTIC WORKUP

It is imperative that the diagnosis of an athlete be unquestionably demonstrated before surgery is undertaken. Identifying a herniated disc in an athlete without verification of concomitant stenosis, internal disc disruption, instability, and other levels of disease might mean the end of his or her career. Consequently, it is worthwhile to have more diagnostic tests performed and to get a second opinion prior to surgery.

Multiplanar CT scans of good quality are necessary to identify spinal stenosis. It is not appropriate to perform a discectomy without adequate prophylactic decompression, because future stenosis is one of the principal reasons for surgical failure. All too frequently, an athlete has surgery simply on the basis of a myelogram or MRI scan, which are not adequate to reveal the extent of spinal stenosis or the true source of the pain.

Discograms are essential if fusion is being contemplated. They should be performed in all cases of anticipated disc excision when there is no radiculopathy.

Electrodiagnostics are important when determining whether there is chronic or acute neurological involvement, although neurological deficit is not in itself an indication for surgery. Many athletes develop neurological deficit and then regain their ability to perform the most difficult athletic tasks without surgery.

Diagnostic blocks are extremely helpful in the treatment of athletes. Many athletes will only have pain at peak functional levels. Examination in a doctor's office may not reveal any symptoms. Testing them, even in a gym or exercise room, may not produce significant pain. It can sometimes take hours to produce the pain as it is usually experienced by them. For example, note the professional golfer currently under treatment who has pain only after approximately 15 holes of highly competitive, professional golf. On a daily basis, he is pain-free, and in the examining room he has only a slight weakness. His discograms are positive at the lower two lumbar levels. He has slight spondylolisthesis at L5–S1, and a narrowed L5–S1 intervertebral foramen.

What surgery is to be performed? Can the intervertebral foramen simply be enlarged? Does one or another of his painful discs need to be removed? Should he have a fusion at the level of spondylolisthesis or at both lower lumbar levels? Can this professional golfer return to full athletic function after a two-level lumbar fusion? The answers to these types of questions require complete diagnostics.

When the information that an EMG demonstrates L5 radiculopathy and that a selective nerve root block at L5 gives the golfer in our example relief is added to what is already known, the surgical options are narrowed. It is essential in such a case to have impeccable multiplanar CT scans to identify the exact degree of narrowness of the L5 foramen and the position of the nerve root within that foramen.

In the case of the golfer, an epidural block or even a selective nerve root block performed in the office will yield no information. The patient should receive a block when he is feeling pain, i.e., at a time when he is actually competing at his peak level. Thus, facilities where selective nerve root blocks can be performed should be available wherever the patient is playing in a professional tournament. Such logistics are virtually impossible. However, this is the only way to be absolutely certain that surgery will give the patient relief he needs to meet the demands of his sport.

INDICATIONS FOR LUMBAR SPINAL SURGERY IN AN ATHLETE

The global question that needs to be answered is whether an individual, who is otherwise healthy, productive and happy, should consider lumbar spine surgery solely because he or she wants to perform high level athletic activities. What is the likelihood that surgery will return such an individual to athletics?

Given a definite diagnosis of spinal pathology, e.g., spinal stenosis or herniated disc, an athlete may want surgery. Surgery can return individuals to athletic activities in at least 50% of the cases, and in well-selected and well-trained individuals, the success rate can be as high as 90%. Training level, athletic pursuit, the extent of the underlying disorder, and the athlete's motivation and psychological set are the factors that will determine whether surgery is appropriate. With appropriate surgery, training and an encouraging psychological setting, an athlete may return to his chosen sport most of the time.

INDICATIONS FOR FUSION

Once committed to performing a fusion, a surgeon cannot step back and do a foraminotomy or disc excision. Thus, the sport played and the performance levels athletes are demanding of themselves are important factors affecting a surgeon's decision about the type of surgery to be performed. Although fusions are generally indicated in the average population for situations where there is gross instability, i.e., deformity, damage, or pain by vertebral displacement of more than 3 mm, many athletes perform quite well under those conditions. When the demands of a contact sport become so great that instability prevents competent performance in play, any surgery short of fusion is unlikely to offer relief. A discectomy will most likely create additional instability. Decompression might relieve pain, but it also carries the probability of additional instability.

Unfortunately, most professional athletes have multilevel degenerative disc disease. Even young athletes in their early twenties seen in our practice have evidence on scan of at least two segments of degenerative disc disease. Therefore, fusing one segment carries the risk of additional stress on adjacent segments. Discograms on those adjacent segments are frequently abnormal. Degenerative discs may have been present and asymptomatic for years and are probably still asymptomatic during play. After a fusion, however, they may become symptomatic. Furthermore, in an average nonathletic patient, prophylactic restrictions would be employed. For these reasons, fusions in athletes return them to their sport in only about 50% of cases. Surgeons need to be highly selective and totally candid in the process of obtaining informed consent when fusion is anticipated.

Since time is extremely important for professional athletes, internal fixation may offer more rapid recovery. Anterior interbody fusions are notoriously slow to become solid and should be supported, in addition, with posterior fusion and internal fixation.

Good posterior intertransverse fusions of one level supported with a body jacket can consolidate and return athletes to play in 3 to 4 months. An athlete can continue heavy weight-training during the first 3 months and then progressively return to play in the forth and fifth months, reaching peak performance 6 months following surgery. Such was the case of one professional cornerback who had a spondylolysis at L5–S1. He developed pain sprinting backwards and turning around at full speed to deliver full contact to the receiver. He received relief from pain with local anesthetic blocks. An L5–S1 intertransverse fusion with copious amounts of bone graft was performed on him. He wore a body jacket with a leg extension for 3 months. Three months after surgery, he had not lost any upper extremity strength or conditioning. He had been jogging in his body jacket. His fusion had solidified, and he was able to return to full, unrestricted play 5 months after surgery.

EXTENSIVE SPINAL DISEASE

For those playing contact sports, the disease process in the spine may be extensive, even in relatively young athletes. Rarely are athletes in competition seen with low back pain and only one level of disease. It is common to see them with multilevel congenital lumbar spinal stenosis and superimposed multilevel bulging or small herniated discs. They may have occasional bouts of low back pain, but this may not include any neurological involvement. Myelograms and scans of athletes often present results that are quite serious even in average individuals. Yet, these athletes, many of them quite young, will continue to play football and basketball at peak levels, and will frequently have expectations of a professional career.

What is to be done with such individuals? Whatever surgical decompression is performed on a disc at one level will leave the next level in great jeopardy. Local decompression or single-level disc excision is not likely to make them much better and is even more likely to weaken the spine enough to make them worse. From a medical and legal standpoint, it is difficult to clear such individuals for contact sports. They should be restricted from contact sports or heavy labor. Instead, they are playing competitive athletics at risk without *major* symptoms.

However, many of these athletes frequently do not have another professional career or a good income. Their livelihood depends on their sport or on their return to nonathletic endeavor. Many of them continue their professional athletic career for 5 to 10 years. In our experience no catastrophic incident has ever occurred from the return of this type of player to competitive athletics, although there is a much greater risk of catastrophe in the case of injuries to the cervical spine than to the lumbar spine.

Probably their extensive conditioning allows these individuals to continue their sport. Similar injuries in the normal population prevent even light athletics and all labor. A physician finds it hard to accept the restrictions placed on the nonathletic patient disabled with extensive spinal disease when a 250-pound professional lineman continues to play on a daily basis having the disease to the same extent. Surgery is rarely indicated in individuals like the professional lineman. Multilevel decompressions and disc excisions are certainly not the answer, nor are multilevel fusions. If we are able to identify a single level of stenosis or a single herniated disc in the mass of other abnormalities, there is a fair hope of success with a limited surgical procedure. However, surgeons are still faced with the conflict of returning a patient with extensive disease back to the playing field.

SUMMARY

Although there are occasional dramatic recoveries of professional athletes with lumbar surgery, such as Joe Montana, our athletic patients should not be encouraged to expect such successes. As with all lumbar spine surgery, there are intangible characteristics of each individual that play a more important role than the surgical procedure. Such intangibles are pain tolerance, mental attitude, coordination and physical conditioning. In general, athletes should not be encouraged to have surgery in order to return to abusive and potentially dangerous activities. In certain circumstances, however, when an athlete's professional career is at stake, and not merely his competitive drive, spine surgery may be indicated for pain and for the inability to perform at peak athletic levels. In such cases, the diagnosis must be unquestionably accurate. The type of surgery selected should be the least invasive type that could reasonably relieve symptoms in the face of the highly trained individuals who are willing to make any sacrifice to return to their sport. Fusions are rarely necessary, because athletes have high pain tolerance and can be trained to stabilize minor degrees of instability and pain from degenerative segment disease.

REFERENCES

1. Brady TA, Cahill BR, Bodnar LM: Weight training-related injuries in the high school athlete. Am J Sports Med 10:1–5, 1982.
2. Day AL, Friedman WA, Indelicato PA: Observation on the treatment of lumbar disk disease in college football players. Am J Sports Med 15:72–75, 1987.
3. DeLong WB: Microdiscectomy. In White AH, Rothman RH, Ray CD (eds): Lumbar Spine Surgery: Techniques & Complications. St. Louis, C.V. Mosby, 1987.
4. McCarroll JR, Miller JM, Ritter MA: Lumbar spondylolysis and spondylolisthesis in college football players: A prospective study. Am J Sports Med 14:404–405, 1986.
5. Micheli LJ: Sports following spinal surgery in the young athlete. Clin Orthop Rel Res 198:152–157, 1985.
6. Morris J, Onik G: Percutaneous nuclectomy. In White AH, Rothman RH, Ray CD (eds): Lumbar Spine Surgery: Techniques & Complications. St. Louis, C.V. Mosby, 1987.
7. Ray CD: Laminectomy vs. Laminotomy. In White AH, Rothman RH, Ray CD (eds): Lumbar Spine Surgery: Techniques & Complications. St. Louis, C.V. Mosby, 1987.
8. Simmons JW: Chemonucleolysis. In White AH, Rothman RH, Ray CD (eds): Lumbar Spine Surgery: Techniques & Complications. St. Louis, C.V. Mosby, 1987.

Chapter 26

THE REHABILITATION OF ATHLETES FOLLOWING SPINAL INJURIES

Clinton Maxwell, MD, and Amy Spiegel, BA

The incidence of spinal injuries in athletes has been reported by various authors to be between 5 and 15%. Additionally, many spinal injuries do not come to the attention of medical personnel because they are self-limiting and result in little change in the athlete's performance. Of the spinal injuries that require treatment, only a small number require surgical intervention. The rehabilitation of athletes with spinal injuries, therefore, will involve mostly conservative methods. The thrust of this chapter will be toward conservative treatment.

The initial evaluation of spinal injuries should involve careful history-taking. Many nonmechanical sources of pain can only be suspected following an accurate history from the patient. Information from onlookers will also assist in arriving at a diagnosis. A good history serves as a guide during the physical examination. The diagnostic tests should be tailored to the individual injury and should follow the path suggested by the history and physical examination. Diagnostic tests such as x-ray studies, CT scanning, myelography, electrodiagnostics, and laboratory tests have been well discussed elsewhere and will not be dealt with in this chapter. Suffice it to say that the tests should all be selected on an individual basis.

Fractures of the bony elements of the spine should be well healed before the athlete begins exercising. While they are healing, however, the patient may begin exercises that do not excessively strain the defect. For example, a patient in a cast or body jacket may begin isometric exercises that are limited by pain. At the same time, general conditioning should continue.

Injuries to the cervical spine are relatively few in number.[8] The noncatastrophic ones usually involve only soft tissue. Soft tissue injuries can be separated into those with radicular components and those without. The radicular symptoms direct attention to the neural elements. They may involve a disc herniation or cervical nerve disorders from the nerve root distally. Immobilization, anti-inflammatories, and/or analgesics may be all that are needed to resolve the symptoms within a few weeks. Soft collars are used on patients with cervical injuries. It must be remembered that the soft collar does not prevent motion of the cervical spine; it only serves as a reminder to the patient to avoid excessive motion.[10] Most conventional braces do restrict less than 50% of flexion at the atlantoaxial joint. Halos restrict about 75% of motion. When cervical arthroses are required, they should be carefully selected on the basis of amount of desired motion. If the symptoms subside, the patient may progress with rehabilitation. If not, a more in-depth look should be taken at the etiology of the problem.

Thoracic spinal injuries in athletes are rare.[8] These are caused, for the most part, by high-velocity sports and may result in compression fractures of the vertebrae. Soft tissue injuries of the thoracic spine usually respond to conservative care more rapidly than other spinal injuries because of the relative immobility. Rest, anti-inflammatories, and analgesics will frequently decrease the symptoms in a matter of days rather than weeks.

The most common bony injuries to the lumbar spine are spondylolysis, spondylolisthesis, compression fracture, and fractures of the transverse processes. More unstable injuries such as burst and chance fractures may occur and frequently involve surgical intervention or extensive in-patient care. Soft tissue injuries to the lumbar spine are more disabling than those involving the cervical and thoracic spine. Injuries with neurologic involvement not requiring surgery are treated as they are elsewhere in the spine. Rest, non-weight-bearing positions, analgesics, and anti-inflammatories may be used to heal the soft tissue spinal injuries prior to exercise and range of motion therapy.

APPROACH TO TREATMENT OF SOFT TISSUE INJURIES

The main goals of rehabilitation are to restore range of motion, strength, and endurance. At the same time, restoration of fine motor skills and cardiovascular function must be addressed.

In the acute phase of therapy, symptomatic relief of pain is the first step. Absolute or relative immobilization must be carried out immediately, but it should be tailored to the individual and the sport's requirement. With significant soft tissue injury, bed rest may be indicated. This is probably the most frequently prescribed for periods of from 2 to 10 days. In Europe, 7 to 10 days of bed rest are frequently recommended. In this country, the lower end of the scale is coming more into use. Two to four days is typical for a common uncomplicated injury.[3] Absolute bed rest eliminates bathroom privileges. This should be avoided if possible and most certainly should be prescribed for as short a time as possible. The effects of immobilization apply to the spine as well as to the extremities. Rest will assist in pain relief and will afford an opportunity for the healing process to begin.

Prolonged bed rest results in generalized deconditioning. As in any immobilization, it also results in atrophy. Mueller reported that, in the absence of any contraction of the muscle, strength decreases at the rate of about 5% per day.[13]

On the other hand, he reports that the rate of increase in strength with maximum exercise is about 12% per week, increasing linearly up to 75% and progressing downward to 0 at maximum limiting strength. Fischbach and Robbins found that immobilization of a muscle fixed at resting length resulted in a 5–15% change in the EMG activity.[6] Adaptive shortening of the muscle and periarticular tissues also occurs when the tissues are immobilized in the shortened position.[4] Additionally, during immobilization slow-twitch fibers develop characteristics of fast-twitch fibers.[1]

It is clear that immobilization of muscles will result in atrophy. Atrophy, in turn, will prolong recovery, especially in athletes. Three important ways to prevent atrophy during immobilization have been identified. First, muscles should be maintained in a lengthened position. Second, isometric exercises may be used, along with the third method, electrical muscle stimulation.

It is the opinion of the authors that the shortest possible bed rest interval should be used, preferably 2 to 3 days. This should be accompanied by the above-mentioned methods of preventing atrophy. The motion of the spine may be increased by using pain tolerance as a guide.

PHYSICAL THERAPY

Ice

To decrease swelling, ice is used in conjunction with immobilization. Ice (cryotherapy) has been shown to help reduce swelling by causing superficial vasoconstriction.[10] It also increases muscle metabolism. Additionally, ice is used to reduce spasms secondary to underlying disorders, as in low back syndromes or nerve root irritation. Pain relief using cryotherapy is thought to be brought about by elevating the pain threshold as a direct effect of temperature reduction on nerve fibers and receptors. The effect on muscle spindles is the basis for treatment of muscle spasm.[11]

Ice may be used crushed, or as flakes or cubes. It should be put on the patient, not the patient on the ice. This will prevent thermal damage to the skin. It is commonly used for a period of 20 to 30 minutes. Ice massage may be used for 10 to 20 minutes. This may be easily accomplished by freezing a large cup and then pealing down the cup so that it may be used to rub the ice over the injured musculoskeletal structure. Cold baths or whirlpools between 50 and 60° F may be used for 20 minutes. Evaporative cooling with ethyl chloride or fluorimethane may be used on the skin surface over the injury. Travell has reported success by using evaporative cooling followed by massage of the area.[15] In addition to its use during the acute phase, ice may also be used in the post-acute phase of rehabilitation. Some patients are able to tolerate ice and some are not. Ice and heat may be used interchangeably or substituted for one another in many cases.

Heat

The two major techniques of heating are superficial and deep. These can be subdivided into modes of heat transfer and types of modality (Table 1).

In **conduction**, heat is transferred from one object to another by direct contact (e.g., heating pad, hot packs, etc). With **convection**, heat is transferred by fluid moving past the object (e.g., whirlpool or between a surface and air). **Radiation** involves the transfer of energy through space by means of electromagnetic waves (e.g., heat lamp). **Conversion** "converts" one form of energy into

TABLE 1. Heat Modalities

Type	Equipment	Method
Superficial heat	Hot packs Paraffin bath	Conduction
	Fluidotherapy Hydrotherapy Moist air	Convection
Deep heat	Radiant heat	Radiation
	Microwaves Shortwaves Ultrasound	Conversion

another (e.g., nonthermal into thermal). A specific example is sound waves entering tissue where they act as heat (i.e., any diathermy [microwave, shortwave or ultrasound]). Since conduction and radiation transfer heat only as a result of temperature difference, they are in the strictest sense the only fundamental mechanisms of heat exchange.

The desirable effects of therapeutic heat include increase of extensibility of collagen tissues, decrease in joint stiffness, relief of muscle spasm, pain relief, increase in blood flow, and assistance to resolution of inflammatory infiltrates. The selection of the type of modality should depend on the desired effect, patient tolerance, indications, and available sources.

Vigorous heating is required to achieve certain therapeutic responses, such as increase in extensibility of connective tissue, to obtain maximal blood flow, and to resolve inflammatory processes.[11] In the most acute phase of an injury, mild or no heat should be recommended. By way of example, if a muscle spasm is secondary to a herniated disc that is compressing a nerve root in the intervertebral foramen, vigorous heating may cause hyperemia and edema in a confined area, increasing the symptoms. On the other hand, superficial heat may be applied, reflexly producing a decrease in muscle spasm without affecting the underlying injury. If mild heating effects are desired, one may use the modality that can result in the highest temperature throughout the tissue at the site of the injury, but reduce the output so that lower temperatures are obtained. One may also choose a superficial heating modality to obtain a limited response at the site of the deep disorder. Heat may be used for a broad spectrum of desired effects, from relieving muscle spasm and inflammation to simply warming a muscle prior to exercise to prevent injury.

Following acute care with immobilization, medication, and appropriate modalities (i.e., heat, cold, etc.), and after early range-of-motion exercises have been initiated, attention is then directed toward the increase in strength and endurance. At this point, however, it is not uncommon to have focal areas of persistent pain that have not responded to therapy. Since ligament and tendon injuries usually require longer recovery periods than muscle, they should be investigated as a source of the pain, and more modalities and medication may be required. It has been well documented that these tissues tend to contract with injury. The therapist must then direct attention to increasing extensibility and length of the connective tissues. This may be achieved by using heat and stretching. Lehmann et al., using rat tails, documented that exclusive heat or stretching does not produce elongation of the collagen tissue.[11] However, a combination of a sustained load and heat does produce a significant increase in the residual length of tendons. It is beneficial, then, to use heat and gentle sustained stretching wherever possible when treating ligaments and tendons. It must be remembered that these tissues do not have the generous blood supply of muscles, and this fact alone results in longer treatment periods.

Focal trigger points are frequently isolated after the acute care is completed. These may respond well to injection with a steroid and lidocaine. Larger areas of spasm do not respond as well. Ice or ethyl chloride may be used followed by massage and/or stretching.

Another source of pain may be the facet joints. Inflammation and/or degeneration may occur, and even in younger athletes early degeneration can occur. Anti-inflammatory medications, ultrasound, and injections of the facet joints may relieve the pain.

Strength and Endurance

Strength and endurance are the next focus of rehabilitation. Muscular strength is defined as the ability to generate maximum muscle force one time. It is a single-dimension value and should not be confused with work and power, which introduce the additional parameters of distance and distance-time, respectively. Muscular endurance is defined as the ability to maintain a less than maximal force for an extended period of time. During any exercise program there will be an overlap in the development of strength and endurance. This must always be considered when rehabilitating muscles.

Isometric, isotonic, and isokinetic exercises can be used singly or in combination to increase strength and endurance. Commonly, isotonic exercises are used with some isometrics for increasing strength and endurance. They are more commonly used in rehabilitation of the extremities than the spine. As pointed out above, isometric exercises are very helpful during immobilization. Typically, the exercises are used in continuous training (CT) and intermittent training (IT) techniques. Intermittent training is reported to give equal or greater improvement in the patient's maximum aerobic capacity.[7] This depends to a great extent on the level of the patient's fitness. In addition, athletes are frequently more compliant with IT than with CT. Either CT or IT may be used effectively.

The goal of any exercises protocol should be a ratio of 1.3 to 1.0 for extensor strength to flexor strength. The selection of the type of equipment used to achieve this ratio should be left up to the rehabilitation team. There are many available types.

Hydrotherapy

At this point a special emphasis will be placed on hydrotherapy, a modality whose importance is frequently overlooked. The second author of this chapter has developed special expertise in hydrotherapy and is responsible for this review.

At the Texas Back Institute, we have determined that hydrotherapy is an effective complement to the many therapeutic modalities offered to back patients. There are certain aspects of hydrotherapy that uniquely enhance the overall objectives of any back exercise program. Basically, the objectives of muscular strength and endurance, aerobic capacity, and flexibility are specific to rehabilitation programs.

A characteristic of hydrotherapy versus similar land-based exercises is that specific properties of water remove barriers (such as pain, tension, and joint stress) when a patient enters the water. This allows the patient to achieve full range of motion and exercise potential.

Several studies have shown that water exercise is a less stressful mode of therapy, yet achieves the objectives of rehabilitation. Due to the resistance and buoyancy factors of water, it is possible to expend high energy with little movement and strain on the lower extremities.[2,5,9,16] Oxygen utilization (VO_2) and heart rates were also found to be higher during water exercise when compared to land-based exercises.[2,5,9,16] We can therefore surmise that patients are capable of achieving the same exercise benefits of land-based exercise with less work and strain on the joints, yet still acquiring the benefits of aerobic conditioning.

The properties of water that produce hydrotherapeutic benefits are as follows:

Buoyancy. Archimedes' Principle states that as a body is immersed in water, it experiences an upward thrust. This effect produces work in the opposite direction of land-based exercises, which work against gravity. In comparison, the weight-bearing stress on joints is reduced by the buoyant effect of water immersion.[14] In depths of 4 to 5 feet of water, patients are bearing only approximately 10% of their body weight. In terms of rehabilitation, the force of buoyancy is found to assist movements toward the surface, resist downward movements, and is nonfunctional in horizontal movements.[9]

Hydrostatic Pressure. Pascal's Law states that water pressure is equally exerted on the surface of an immersed body at rest at a given depth. This property aids in weightlessness, decreases swelling, and inhibits the blood from pooling in the lower extremities.[9]

Viscosity. Viscosity is friction that occurs between water molecules and causes resistance to the flow of water. This is one of the dominant forces affecting movement of the body during water exercise.[9] Even limited movement offers substantial physical resistance.[2]

At Texas Back Institute, we utilize these properties in an organized hydrotherapy program as a complement to other modalities. Since it is easier to commence rehabilitation with hydrotherapy prior to land exercises, we begin with ambulation and active range of motion. Basically, patients begin with all-directional walking and upper and lower extremity exercises. Upper-extremity exercises consist of horizontal adduction, abduction, extension, flexion, and circumflexion. Lower extremity exercises consist of hip flexion, adduction, abduction, and circumflexion. As tolerated, patients are encouraged to increase rate, time, and extremity movements. If symptoms intensify, techniques are assessed and subjective complaints are evaluated to determine severity of symptoms. This first stage of hydrotherapy allows the therapist to determine the patient's functional capabilities and assists the patient in interrupting the pain cycle. Once this is accomplished, the program focuses on muscular strength and endurance with the implementation of swimming.

Swim strokes are incorporated into the walking program on a walk/swim work ratio (i.e., 2:1 = 2 laps walking, 1 lap swimming). The walk/swim ratio changes to increased swim time as the patient gains muscular strength and endurance. Although there are exceptions based on diagnosis, the first stroke used is the elementary back stroke. This is the easiest stroke to learn, yet allows the spine to remain neutral while exercising the upper and lower extremities. The kick-board is utilized for spinal extension and lower extremity endurance. On a graduated level and according to desired joint movements, additional strokes are added—freestyle, back stroke, and breast stroke (Table 2).

TABLE 2. Joint Movements and Swimming Skills*

		Neck	
Flexion	*Extension*	*Lateral Flexion*	*Rotation*
Elem. back stroke Breast stroke	Free style Breast stroke Back float	Side stroke	Free style Side breathing
		Trunk	
Flexion	*Extension*		
	Free style Breast stroke Back float		
		Shoulder	
Flexion	*Hyperextension*	*Abduction*	*Adduction*
Free style Breast stroke Back stroke	Free style	Side stroke Breast stroke Elem. back stroke Back stroke Finning Sculling	Side stroke Breast stroke Elem. back stroke Back stroke Finning Sculling
Internal Rotation	*External Rotation*		
Free style Back stroke Sculling	Breast stroke Back stroke Sculling		
		Elbow	
Flexion	*Extension*	*Pronation*	*Supination*
Side stroke Free style Breast stroke Elem. back stroke Back stroke Finning Sculling	Side stroke Free style Breast stroke Elem. back stroke Back stroke Finning Sculling	Side stroke Breast stroke Elem. back stroke Back stroke Sculling	Side stroke Breast stroke Back stroke
		Wrist	
Flexion	*Extension*		
Side stroke Free style Breast stroke	Breast stroke Elem. back stroke Back stroke Finning Sculling		
		Hip	
Flexion	*Hyperextension*	*Abduction*	*Adduction*
Flutter kick Scissor kick Breast stroke kick Walking	Walking Flutter kick Scissor kick	Breast stroke kick	Breast stroke
Internal Rotation	*External Rotation*		
Breast stroke	Breast stroke		
		Knee	
Flexion	*Extension*		
Flutter kick Breast stroke kick Bobbing Walking Scissor kick	Flutter kick Bobbing Breast stroke kick Walking Scissor kick		
		Foot and Ankle	
Dorsi Flexion	*Plantar Flexion*	*Eversion*	*Inversion*
Scissor kick Breast stroke kick	Flutter kick Scissor kick Breast stroke kick	Breast stroke	Flutter kick Breast stroke kick

* From Rehabilitation Institute of Chicago, Feb. 1983, with permission.

We have found the use of resistive devices, such as UE hydrotone belts, to be an effective exercise method for muscular strength training. While isolating the upper extremities, the trunk and buttocks are forced to stabilize the spine, thus simulating various land-based exercises.

Psychology

During the course of rehabilitation of an athlete, the psychological components of care are frequently underrated or overlooked. Since athletes, especially those with high levels of competence, are high achievers and have good physical and mental discipline, it is assumed that the psychological problems will be overcome without effort. It must be remembered, however, that the athlete faces the same type of psychological barriers as nonathletes. Anyone sustaining an illness or injury resulting in a change of lifestyle will go through three general phases: denial, depression, and recovery. The recovery will depend largely on how well they overcome the denial and depression. The denial is frequently subtle but may well retard recovery. Denial may simply be nonacceptance. For example, a patient with a cast or brace may feel a great deal of aggravation at not being able to do things he or she used to do and may not yet have accepted limitation. Depression can range from mild to severe but almost always occurs. This is especially true when rehabilitation goes on for an extended period of time. Depression has a significant negative effect on the athlete's motivation. Most athletes expect to be restored to their highest level of performance and they want it quickly.

When patients overcome denial and depression, they generally have little difficulty coping with the rehabilitation process. The key to helping athletes get through these phases is to begin discussing how they feel about the injury from the onset. Having patients discuss their feelings will afford the therapist the opportunity to help solve problems as they arise. The athlete wants to compete and achieve, and is frequently intolerant of therapy over any length of time. The patient must be informed frequently that the rehabilitation process will require time and patience, and at the same time must be given positive input. Most athletes will need psychological support from injury to recovery. The medical team is best equipped to achieve success in this area.

Aerobic Capacity

During the entire post-acute stages of rehabilitation, cardiovascular and respiratory fitness must be addressed. Aerobic exercises in the form of treadmill, cycling, and swimming are most useful in achieving greater aerobic capacity.

SUMMARY

The approach to rehabilitation of athletes with spinal injuries must include emphasis on conservative treatment, with educational and psychological support. After a diagnosis is made, the patient is treated with modalities and medication. This is followed by range of motion and increase in strength and endurance. The rehabilitation should be a gradually progressive process with the goal of a high performance level and return to competition.

A vital part of rehabilitating any athlete is an emphasis on education and prevention of future injury. This should be stressed throughout the rehabilitative process.

REFERENCES

1. Booth FW: Effect of limb immobilization on skeletal muscle. J Appl Physiol 52(5):1113–1118, 1982.
2. Costill DL: Energy requirements during exercise in water. J Sports Med 11:87–92, 1971.
3. Deyo RA, Diehl AK, Rosenthal M: How many days of bed rest for acute low back pain? A randomized clinical trial. N Engl J Med 315:1064–1070, 1986.
4. Downey JA, Darling RC: Physiological Basis of Rehabilitation Medicine, 3rd ed. Philadelphia, W.B. Saunders, 1971.
5. Evans BW, Cureton KJ, Purvis JW: Metabolic and circulatory response to walking and jogging in water. Res Q 49:442–449, 1978.
6. Fischbach GD, Robbins N: Changes in contractile properties of the solius muscle. J Physiol 201:305–320, 1969.
7. Glisan B, Stith WJ, Kiser S: Physiology of active exercise in rehabilitation of back injuries. Spine: State Art Rev 3(1):146–149, 1989.
8. Huurman WW: The spine in sports. In Mellion MB (ed): Office Management of Sports Injuries and Athletic Problems. Philadelphia, Hanley & Belfus, 1988, pp 199–212.
9. Johnson BL, Strome SB, Adamczyk JW, Tennoe KO: Comparison of oxygen uptake and heart rate during exercises on land and in water. Phys Ther 57:273–278, 1977.
10. Johnson RM, Hart DL, Simmons EF, et al: Cervical orthoses: A study comparing their effectiveness in restricting cervical motion in normal subjects. J Bone Joint Surg 59A:332–339, 1977.
11. Lehmann JF: Therapeutic Heat and Cold. Baltimore, Williams & Wilkins, 1982.
12. Lehmann J, et al: Effects of therapeutic temperatures on tendon extensibility. Arch Phys Med Rehabil 51:486, 1970.
13. Mueller EA: Influence of training and inactivity. Arch Phys Med Rehabil 51:449–462, 1970.
14. Sheldahl L: Special ergometric techniques and weight reduction. Med Sci Sports Exerc 18:25–30, 1985.
15. Travell J: Ethylchloride spray for painful muscle spasm. Arch Phys Med Rehabil 33:291, 1952.
16. Whitley JD, Schoene LL: Comparison of heart rate responses: Water walking versus treadmill walking. Phys Ther 67:1501–1504, 1987.

PART IV

CASE REPORTS

Case Report 1

HERNIATION OF LUMBAR DISC IN A FOOTBALL ATHLETE WITH SPINAL STENOSIS

David F. Fardon, MD

Disc herniation, uncommon among young people, can be especially troublesome when it occurs into a small vertebral canal. When an athlete suffers such a combination of problems, management decisions are particularly difficult.

CASE REPORT

The patient, a 20-year-old university football athlete, felt a sudden "pop" in his lower back while attempting to power clean 280 pounds during a routine weight-training session. He said that pains radiated into both arms and both legs and that his lower back pain was so intense that he could not move for 30 minutes.

A star high school football and basketball player, he had been recruited to a major university football program where he anticipated starting as an offensive tackle. He had had no prior trouble with back pain.

Orthopedic examination revealed that he was a very muscular, 6-foot 2-inch, 290-pound man, who moved as though he were in distress. He maintained a flattened lumbar lordosis and a list to the left. He could not tolerate motion of his back or tension sign testing. His neurologic functions were intact. He was treated with corticosteroids, rest, and passive therapy.

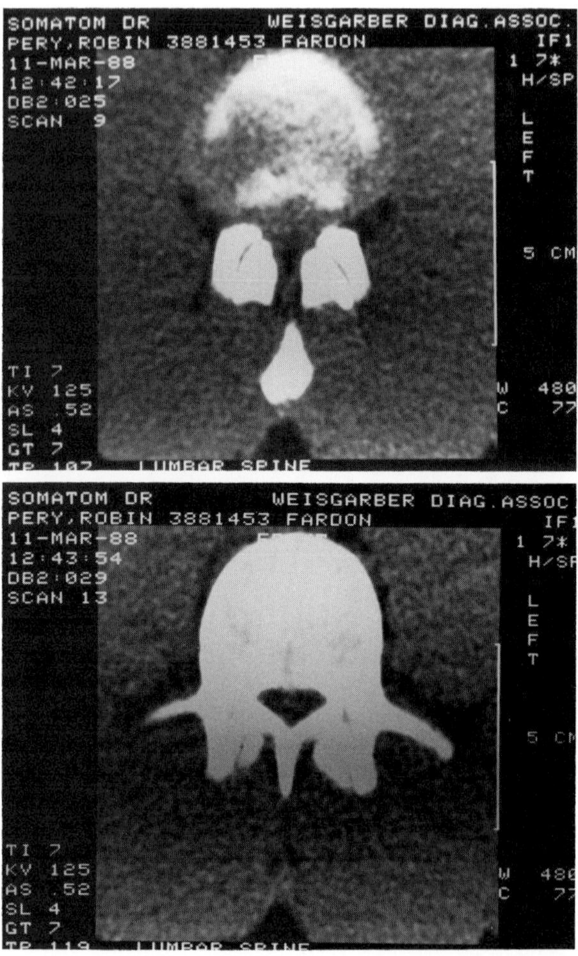

FIGURE 1. CT axial images 2 weeks after onset of symptoms: *A,* through the L3–4 disc, which is protruding posteriorly. *B,* through the mid-pedicle level of L4, demonstrates the very small spinal canal and short, thick pedicles.

Three weeks later, he complained that he was unable to walk comfortably, felt cramping pain in his right hamstrings, and had pain that radiated from his low back to, but not below, the right knee, and to, but not below, the left buttock. He could not permit passive supine straight leg raising beyond 30 degrees in either leg. His neurologic functions remained normal. His CT scan (Fig. 1A, B) demonstrated posterior protrusion of the L3–4 disc and severe developmental stenosis of the vertebral canal from L2 through L5. Myelography (Fig. 2A, B) showed a complete block at L3–4.

At surgery, done under general anesthesia in the crouch position, the ligamentum flavum was removed, the superior edges of the laminae excised, and the anterior surface of each lamina was trimmed with an ultrasonic curette, along with resection of the medial edge of each facet. This procedure was

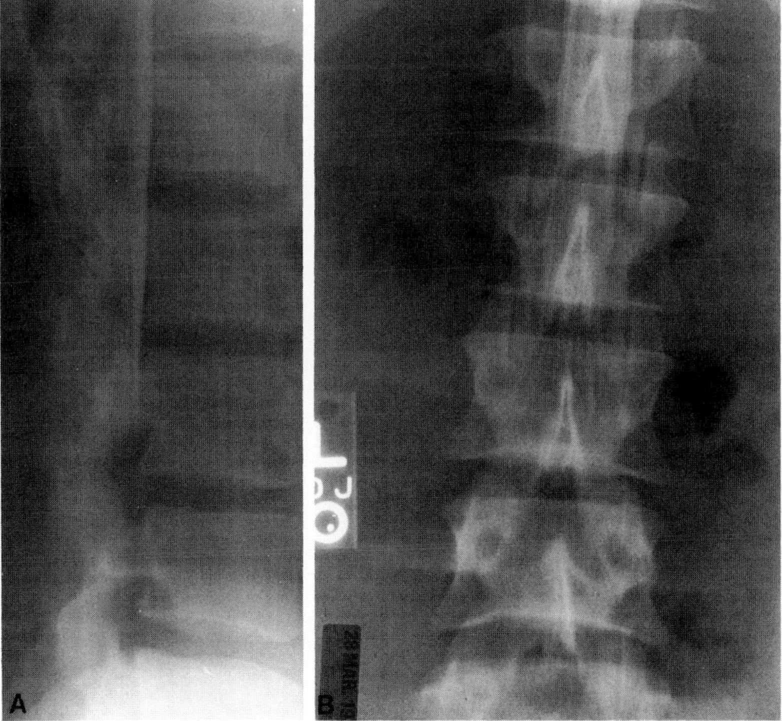

FIGURE 2. Myelogram 3 weeks after symptoms began: *A,* the lateral, demonstrates the short pedicles and narrow sagittal diameter of the canal. *B,* the anteroposterior, shows complete block at L3–4.

performed bilaterally from L2 through L5 in an effort to enlarge the spinal canal (Fig. 3A, B). The interspinous and supraspinous ligaments were preserved as well as facet capsules, except for those fibers that had to be sacrificed during the medial facetectomies.

The L3–4 disc was protruding into the canal, but the nucleus was still contained within anulus fibers that did not appear to be severely attenuated. The anulus was incised and the nucleus removed with rongeurs. The nucleus looked healthy except for its position. It was adherent, intimately mixed with anulus fibers, and resectable only in small pieces. The other discs looked normal.

The patient experienced immediate relief of leg pain but continued to have back pain. His neurologic functions remained normal except for dysesthesias in the distribution of the left lateral femoral cutaneous nerve, which were relieved by local infiltration of Xylocaine near the anterior superior iliac spine.

Two weeks later, the patient's back pain had diminished. After 1 month, the meralgia paresthetica had ceased to bother him, though he still had some hypesthesia. By the third month, he reported that he could do light weight training and some jogging, that his legs felt a little uncoordinated when he jogged, and that he had occasional catches of pain in his back during exercise. At 6 months, he was able to bend to touch his toes with no discomfort, and other motions of his back were fluid and painless.

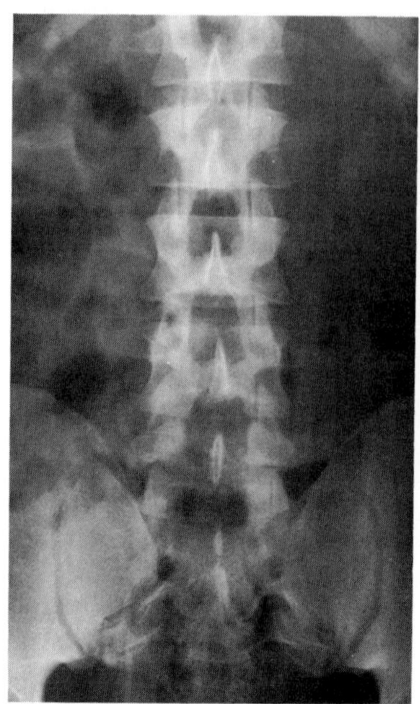

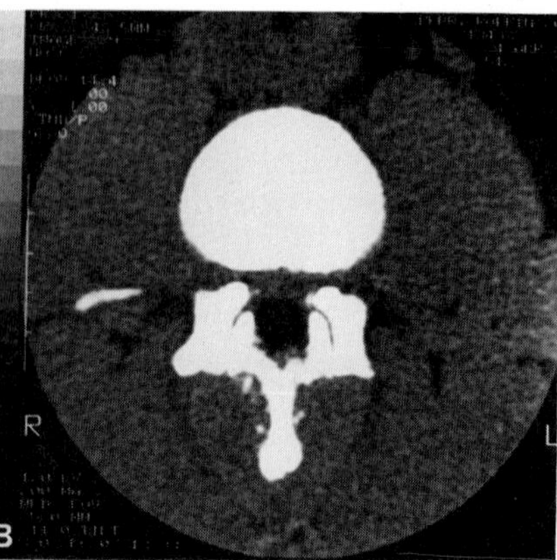

FIGURE 3. Studies done after surgery. *A,* an AP radiograph, shows the surgical increase in interlamina and interfacet distances. *B,* a CT axial image, demonstrates some thinning of the L4 lamina due to curettage of its anterior surface.

One year after surgery, the patient was weight training regularly, running, and playing intramural basketball. After vigorous workouts, he experienced some pain and stiffness in his back. Occasionally, after heavy exercise involving a lot of jumping, he noticed transient dysesthesias in his feet. After a conference with his surgeon and his trainer, he decided to give up the idea of playing collegiate or professional football.

Two years after his surgery, he was in school, participating in intramural athletics and experiencing minimal symptoms, for which he required no care. Examination revealed excellent muscle development, normal back motion, negative tension signs, and no neurologic deficit. Radiographs showed the anticipated postoperative changes, with slight translational motion at L3–4 on flexion and extension lateral xrays, and no degenerative changes.

DISCUSSION

Back injuries are common among college football athletes; perhaps 30% lose playing time due to lumbar pain. It has been suggested that linemen may often sustain back injuries while weight-training.[9]

Our case illustrates the dilemma of the young patient with lumbar disc herniation into a stenotic canal, further complicated by the fact that this young man was a football athlete with a promising college career and the potential to play professionally. Although his pathological problem was not rare, it was unusual enough that well-studied solutions do not exist. Therefore, management decisions had to be based upon anecdotal reports, understanding of the anatomy and physiology, and evaluation of the peculiar needs of the patient.

Only about 1% of disc herniations occur in the second decade of life. According to Epstein et al., herniated disc tissue in young people is usually firm, fibrous, and tightly adherent,[3] quite unlike the extrusions of degenerated nucleus seen in adults. Many young patients with disc herniation have a history of trauma and clinical findings limited to positive tension signs with normal neurologic functions.[4]

Developmental spinal stenosis, a term introduced by Verbiest, refers to a narrow sagittal diameter of the vertebral canal, with short, thick laminae and short pedicles, apparently the result of a genetically determined disturbance in the growth of the neural arch.[11] Eisenstein found 6% of skeletons to have a sagittal diameter of less than 15 mm, measured radiographically.[2] Bolender et al. suggest that a cross-sectional area of the dural sac of less than 100 mm^2 is a more reliable clinical parameter of a too small canal than is measurement of the sagittal diameter.[1]

Since the apparent incidence of developmental stenosis is much greater than indicated by the small number of young patients in reported series of stenosis surgery, it must be true, as Kornberg suggested, that most young individuals with developmental stenosis are not symptomatic unless there is a co-existent condition such as a herniated disc.[6] Even so, their small canals must place their roots at increased jeopardy from what might be a minor injury in a patient with a normal canal. As suggested by Epstein, simple protrusion without rupture of the peripheral fibers of the anulus may precipitate symptoms.[3] The situation, as applied to athletes, would be somewhat analogous to that in the cervical spine, where transient cord dysfunction following relatively minor acute athletic injury has been linked to canal stenosis.[10]

When symptoms from lumbar central stenosis warrant surgery, the standard treatment consists of posterior decompression by bilateral laminectomy, spinous process excision, and partial facetectomy. Common sense would lead one to worry that such surgery would reduce the strength and stability of the spine. Some clinical reports document the validity of such worries.[5,7] One study suggested that young age may predispose to such a complication,[12] perhaps because the young will subject their spines to more prolonged and vigorous stress, or because they are less well protected by the tethering effects of hypertrophic and degenerative changes. Some would be concerned, in a case such as ours, about the added destabilizing effects of a torn and surgically incised anulus.

As with other sports-related injuries, we had to consider our patient, first, as an otherwise healthy young man, and second, as an athlete. It was clear that he required disc excision and canal decompression so that he could return to school and to ordinary activities. Judgment about his athletic future influenced our thinking about the extent of his decompression and about his rehabilitation.

As an interior lineman, his back would be subjected to frequent and extraordinary stresses during play and more so during weight-training—stresses that would thicken the bones of his lumbar spine. In view of his very small vertebral canal, simple disc excision did not seem adequate, though perhaps it would have sufficed for short-term symptom relief. To enlarge his canal without subjecting him to the prolonged uncertainties of osteotomy or fusion procedures required that bone be removed. By removing only that bone in proximity to the canal and preserving all other bone and ligamentous structures, we hoped to strike a compromise that would meet our patient's needs. We succeeded, short of his returning to collegiate football.

Major college or professional football requires a single-minded determination that few uninjured people possess. The occurrence of a frightening injury, major surgical procedure, and prolonged convalescence test such determination severely. The maturing experience of such an injury and all that follows broadens the life-scope of many young athletes beyond the single-minded pursuit of a football career. Though we agree with the general recommendation that, after back surgery, a player who has regained full painfree strength and flexibility may be permitted to return to playing football,[8] we recognize that the player who does so takes an added risk and that return should be permitted only if he well understands that risk and seems to be making a realistic decision after he has measured the risk against the potential benefits.

Our patient was quite young and early in his career as a football player. When he weighed the potential gain from playing, therefore, he had to face several uncertainties other than adjustment to his injury. His youth and enrollment in school left many options open to him, a fact of which he became more aware during his convalescence. His particular ability, that of an interior lineman, placed him at even greater risk of further back difficulty than would be true for most other athletes, including football players at other positions. Although he had obtained an excellent functional result, we knew the anatomy of his lumbar spine was far from normal.

In spite of the fact that we had, from the first, allowed the possibility that he might someday return to football, when the time came it seemed right to all concerned for him to give up the idea of doing so. Pursuit of that goal as a possibility had stimulated his rehabilitation and given him time to adjust. Realization from the first that it was only a chance prevented a feeling of failure at the end.

Return to university or professional football is not a realistic requirement of a "good result" from treatment of a complicated back injury. Surgeons, therapists, and trainers should not, while they strive to keep such an option open to the patient, lead the patient to feel that he must achieve the unreasonable to satisfy their expectations of him. After all parties evaluate the many physical, mental, and motivational factors, a decision should be made in the best interest of the patient. If the patient has a good result by ordinary standards, a decision to discontinue the sport should not leave surgeon, trainer, or patient with a sense of failure.

Acknowledgement. The author wishes to acknowledge William T. Youmans, M.D., team orthopedist, and Tim Kerin and Mike Rollo, team trainers, of the University of Tennessee, Knoxville, for their assistance in the care of this patient.

REFERENCES

1. Bolender NF, Schonstrom NS, Spengler D: Role of computed tomography and myelography in the diagnosis of central spinal stenosis. J Bone Joint Surg 67A:240–246, 1985.
2. Eisenstein S: Measurements of the lumbar spinal canal in two racial groups. Clin Orthop 115:42–46, 1976.
3. Epstein JA, Epstein NE, Marc J, et al: Lumbar intervertebral disk herniation in teenage children: Recognition and management of associated anomalies. Spine 9:427–432, 1984.
4. Epstein NE, Epstein JA, Carras R: Spinal stenosis and disc herniation in a 14-year-old male. Spine 13:938–941, 1988.
5. Johnson KE, Wilner S, Johnsson K: Postoperative instability after decompression for lumbar spinal stenosis. Spine 9:541–545, 1985.
6. Kornberg M, Rechtine GR, Dupuy TE: The treatment of a herniated lumbar disc in a young adult with developmental spinal stenosis. Spine 9:541–545, 1985.

7. Lee CK: Lumbar spinal instability (olisthesis) after extensive posterior spinal decompression. Spine 8:429–433, 1983.
8. Micheli LJ: Sports following spinal injury in the young athlete. Clin Orthop 198:152–157, 1985.
9. Saal JA: Rehabilitation of football players with lumbar spine injury. Phys Sports Med 16:61–67, 1988.
10. Torg JS, Pavlov H, et al: Neuropraxia of the cervical cord with transient quadriplegia. J Bone Joint Surg 68A:1354–1370, 1986.
11. Verbiest H: Further experiences on the pathological influence of a developmental narrowing of the bony lumbar vertebral canal. J Bone Joint Surg 37B:576–583, 1955.
12. White AA, Wiltse LL: Spondylolisthesis after extensive lumbar laminectomy. Presented at the 43rd Annual Meeting of the American Academy of Orthopedic Surgeons in New Orleans, Louisiana, 1976.

Editor's Note

Dr. Fardon's analysis of the dilemma surrounding the athlete's return to sports is well stated. The individual's medical well-being is what is of primary importance. Risks regarding returning to sports need to be fully explained and reviewed with all concerned.

Case Report 2

SUCCESSFUL SURGICAL OUTCOME IN AN ATHLETE

Arthur H. White, MD

S.B. is a 26-year-old professional football offensive lineman. He is 6-feet, 4 inches tall and weighs 250 lbs. He had no difficulty playing football in college and was drafted professionally. After 1 year of playing, he developed back pain that prevented him from achieving his normal stance and weakened his ability to play so much that he sought medical attention. X-ray studies demonstrated a Grade II isthmic spondylolisthesis of L4 on L5. A CT scan demonstrated, in addition, moderate spinal stenosis at the L4–5 level.

Extensive conservative training with stabilization and heavy weight training did not improve the patient's ability to play. In fact, he became worse and could not even play lighter athletics normally or comfortably. Epidural blocks gave him temporary relief but did not allow him to play.

Because the patient's professional career lay in the balance, he sought several consultations with spine surgeons who deal with athletes. A discogram was done at L3–4, which was normal, and at L5–S1, which created slight pain and the area was slightly degenerated. Opinions rendered by the consultants were as follows:

1. Do not consider surgery and attempt to enable the patient to return to professional football. There is no neurological deficit and the stenosis is not severe enough to require surgery. The instability could be fused, but the likelihood of the patient returning to professional football is poor.

2. Fuse only the L4–5 and L5–S1 segments with internal fixation. This carries the possibility of failure of fusion as well as the possibility of further significant symptoms at the L5–S1 segment.

3. Fuse both the L4–5 and L5–S1 segments with internal fixation. This approach has the highest likelihood of short-term success, because it eliminates all of the known pain generators. It does, however, create the potential for new problems, such as breakdown at the level above the fusion with the future stresses of professional football. It also carries with it a higher infection rate because of the internal fixation and other complications of multilevel internal fixation.

As with many professional athletes, this one sought multiple opinions and then made his own decision. He knew that he had been playing high level athletics for years with degenerative discs and even spondylolisthesis. He knew that most of his teammates were playing with abnormalities equivalent to the one at his L5–S1 segment as demonstrated by discogram. He was convinced that his spondylolisthesis created an unstable and insecure feeling that prevented him from full performance, and he wanted only that level fused. He also wanted, as most professional athletes do, the most rapid return to athletic activity. He assumed, which may be valid, that internal fixation allows a higher likelihood of fusion with a faster return to athletic activities. He requested and received a one-level fusion of L4–5 with pedicle screw internal fixation.

He left the hospital after 7 days and was participating in active gym weight lifting and stabilization rehabilitation at 3 weeks postoperatively. By 1 month, he was walking 5 miles and doing a full workout in his body jacket. By the end of 3 months, he was jogging and doing broken field jogging in his body jacket. He started football training at this point as he weaned from his body jacket. He scrimmaged at the high school level of football for 1 month,, then at a college level for 1 month. Then, at 5 months postoperatively, he began to play with his own professional team. At 6 months postoperatively, he was released to full, unrestricted professional football competition.

There were some spine surgeons who recommended removal of the internal fixation devices for fear of breakage or to reduce the rigidity of his fusion. Flexion and extension views, of course, demonstrated no movement. He has played for 1 year with the devices in place and without significant pain or apparent complications from the L5–S1 level. Only time will tell whether the metal or the L5–S1 segment will stand up under the heavy rigors of professional football. The patient remains in top physical condition and peak stabilization capabilities.

This case illustrates the great diversity of opinions that can occur in this field. Interestingly enough, no consultant recommended an anterior interbody fusion or an anterior-plus-posterior interbody fusion, which is done in many centers for patients needing maximum assurance of success.

Editor's Note

1. This case demonstrates the difficulty in reaching the treatment decision. This athlete had many treatment avenues available. The important thing to note is that there is no one right answer. The patient must be a part of the decision-making process. He must make an informed and understood decision.

2. Professional athletes oftentimes make medical choices that the highschool or college athlete might be better advised against. The risks must be fully explained.

3. Rehabilitation in this case was begun early. The patient was allowed to return to contact at 3 months and professional athletic endeavors at 5 months following surgery. One cannot help but compare the interesting parallel to the work-injured patient, when often the patient is pampered for 12 to 18 months or longer.

Case Report 3

HERNIATED NUCLEUS PULPOSUS OF THE LUMBAR SPINE IN AN ELITE ATHLETE

John H. Peloza, MD, David K. Selby, MD
and J. Richard Steadman, MD

Disabling low back pain in athletes is becoming more common, as reported in the media. Herniated nucleus pulposus (HNP) of the lumbar spine sidelined at least three professional athletes in 1989 alone. Until recently, this condition was widely regarded as career-ending. To our knowledge, there is no series in the literature addressing the problem of HNP in an elite athlete. We describe a case of HNP in an elite skier, who eventually had a successful outcome. A treatment regimen of laminectomy and discectomy, along with an aggressive physical training based on principles of sports medicine, was utilized.

CASE REPORT

A 25-year-old U.S. Ski Team racer complained of intractable low back and right leg pain. The patient was racing when he hit a bump on a giant slalom course in December 1987. The patient did not fall, but he felt a soreness in his back as well as stiffness. The soreness increased to pain by the next day, but he continued racing. Over the next several days, he complained of increasing back pain and stiffness as well as right leg pain down the buttocks, lateral thigh, and shin. He was evaluated at that time, diagnosed with "back sprain," and was prescribed physical therapy and a nonsteroidal anti-inflammatory drug.

The patient refrained from competitive ski racing for about 2 weeks. When he returned to racing, he exacerbated his back injury. He complained of increasing back and right leg pain, but without paresthesias or weakness. Plain radiographs at this point were normal. Because the Olympic Games were only 1 month away, a nonoperative treatment course was recommended. The patient was started on physical therapy, flexibility exercise, and a "Contour Form" brace.

The patient continued racing with persistent back and right leg pain and reinjured himself 1 week prior to the Olympic Games. He rested during the week preceding the Olympics, continued NSAID therapy, and received traction and ultrasound treatments. He competed in the Olympic giant slalom but did poorly secondary to back and leg pain.

At this point, a CT scan revealed an L4–5 HNP. He was started on another PT program, NSAID therapy, and chiropractic adjustments. The patient improved; however, 4 months later, in his next ski camp, the back injury recurred. In June 1988, he underwent a percutaneous discectomy. Postoperatively, the patient resumed physical therapy, NSAID, and chiropractic adjustments. He improved slightly but continued to have significant back and right leg pain. He also complained of right leg weakness. His condition did not change for approximately 6 months. Repeat CT scan revealed a large L4–5 lateral HNP with compression of the L5 nerve root (Fig. 1).

At this point the patient was referred to our clinic. In addition to the above history, his physical exam revealed a well-muscled, 25-year-old, white male. He had decreased range of motion of the spine in flexion and lateral side-bending, especially to the right, but without obvious spasm or tenderness. He did list to the left side. Neurologically, his sensation was intact, reflexes were normal, and motors were 5/5 and symmetric except for 4/5 weakness in the extensor hallucis longus. The patient also had a positive straight leg raise at 60 degrees on the right side. Again, the repeat CT scan revealed an HNP at L4–5 on the right, with obliteration of perineural fat of the L5 root. The patient had a laminectomy and discectomy with medial facetectomies at L4–5 in March 1989. It was noted at the time of the procedure that there was severe tension on the right L5 nerve root with a large lateral HNP. The patient tolerated the procedure well without complications. Postoperatively, he was immediately started on a training program described in Tables 1 and 2.

Six months postoperatively, the patient had no back or leg pain. He was playing competitive basketball and tennis. He was doing long-distance swimming, bicycling, and waterskiing. He reported no difficulty with grass agility drills or running. He stated that he was in "the best shape of my life." He returned to the U.S. Ski Team dry land camp without difficulty and competed later in the winter.

DISCUSSION

Herniated nucleus pulposus of the lumbar spine accounts for only a small percentage of all causes of low back and leg pain. However, it is becoming more common in athletes. Until recently, this was considered a career-ending injury. However, after the recovery of Joe Montana in 1986, this poor prognosis needs reevaluation. The successful outcome depends on proper diagnosis, appropriate nonoperative or surgical therapy, and aggressive rehabilitation based on spine biomechanics, flexibility, strength training, and aerobic conditioning.

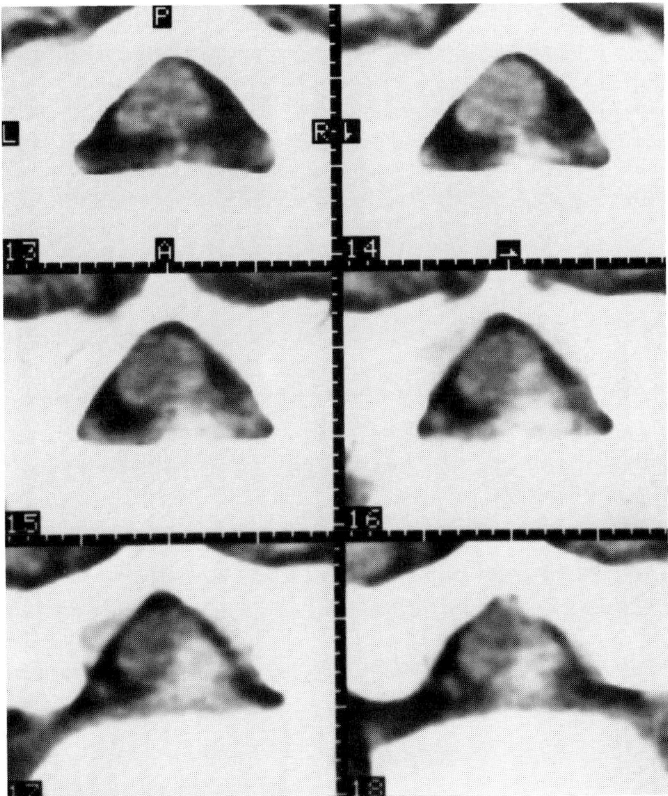

FIGURE 1. *A,* Axial section of L4–5 shows large HNP (right) compressing the L5 nerve root. *(Figure continued.)*

In addition, a maintenance rehabilitation program must be incorporated in the management plan.

A proper diagnosis requires accurate history, physical examination, and imaging studies. The details of history and physical exam for HNP are well documented elsewhere and will not be discussed. A comparison between MRI and CT shows that they are equal in diagnostic accuracy for HNP (82.3% vs. 83.0%) and superior to metrizamide myelography (71.4%).[36] The combination of MRI and CT is equal to CT and metrizamide myelography (92.5% vs. 89.4%).[36] MRI and CT are both noninvasive. Preference for a diagnostic test or a combination of tests rests with the treating physician. This information must be kept in perspective and combined with history and physical exam to obtain accurate diagnosis.

A serious consequence of back injury is deconditioning. The physiologic response to soft tissue immobilization can be catastrophic, Joint contractures, muscle atrophy, tendon/ligament weakening, and cartilage degeneration are well documented.[1–4,9,10,15,22,23,34,37,40,41,43,44,47–49] This must not be allowed to occur in any patient with low back and/or leg pain, but it is especially devastating to an athlete. Deconditioning can be prevented by appropriately aggressive rehabilitation based on the physiology of healing tissue.[24,43,44] These modalities

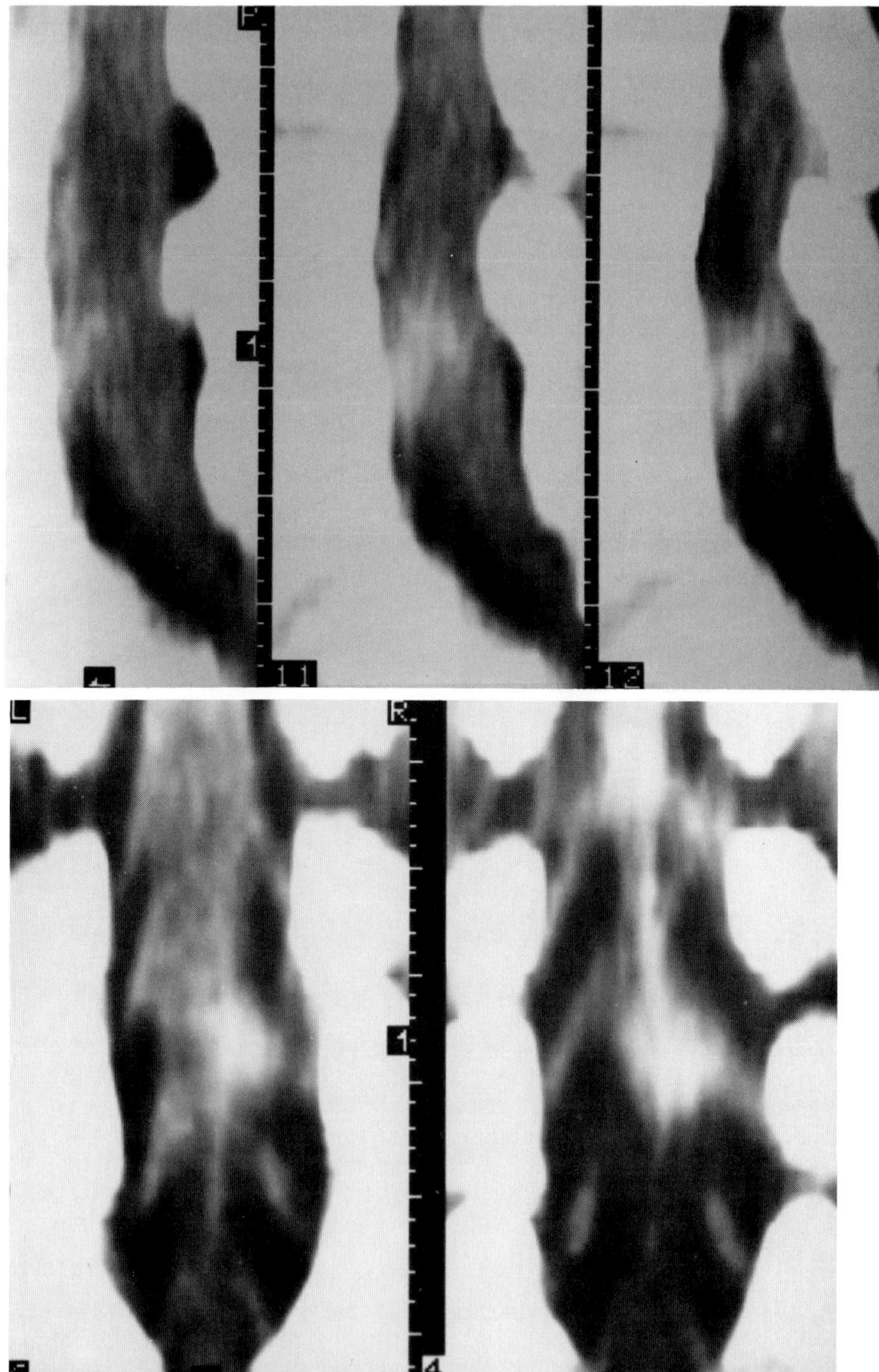

FIGURE 1. *(Continued). B,* (top) Sagittal reformat shows large noncontained HNP at L4–L5. *C,* (bottom) Coronal section shows large HNP L4–5 (right).

TABLE 1. Spine Rehabilitation

- I. Flexibility—daily
  - A. Hamstring stretch (one set, 12 reps. slowly)
  - B. Quadriceps stretch (one set, 12 reps. slowly)
  - C. Hip flexors (one set, 12 reps. slowly)
  - D. Gastrocsoleus (one set, 12 reps. slowly)
  - E. McKenzie extension (three sets, 12 reps. slowly)
- II. Strengthening
  - A. Trunk extensors
    - 1. Prone over pillows
      - a. Leg raises
      - b. Trunk raises
      - c. Trunk and leg raises
      - d. Sport Cord extension exercises
  - B. Abdominals
    - 1. Floor curls
    - 2. Floor curls diagonally
    - 3. Floor curls 90/90
    - 4. Roman chair
    - 5. Sport Cord
      - a. Rectus
      - b. Obliques
  - C. Lower extremity—Sport Cord
    - 1. Single knee dips (3 minutes each leg)
    - 2. Seated hamstrings (three sets, 20 reps.)
    - 3. Inside/outside leg toners (three sets, 20 reps.)
    - 4. Hip pulls (three sets, 20 reps.)
    - 5. Gluteal strengtheners (three sets, 20 reps.)
- III. Aerobic Conditioning (30 minutes, 5 times per week); choice of:
  - A. Stationary bicycling
  - B. Stairmaster
  - C. Nordic track
  - D. Swimming
  - E. No running until 3 months postop

include pain control, flexibility,[47] muscle strength training,[16,33,35,48,50] and aerobic conditioning.[11,12]

Pain management is achieved by controlling the products of inflammation. Inflammation can be decreased by NSAIDs, which are useful in acute, low back, and leg pain.[5,6,18,19] Another efficacious therapeutic modality is epidural steroid injections.[21,28,51] This provides increased local concentration of steroid anti-inflammatory medication around inflamed neural tissues. Although there is some controversy about epidural steroids,[17,21,28,51] we feel that they are extremely useful in clinical practice.

A thorough knowledge of biomechanics is essential in order to design an effective rehabilitation program. However, details of biomechanics are beyond the scope of this presentation. It is essential that patients be instructed in body mechanics; we use a "back school" for this purpose. In addition, stretching and flexibility exercises are done daily to prevent soft tissue contracture;[40,44,47] increase bone, ligament, and tendon strength (i.e., Wolff's Law);[44,47,49,50] promote cartilage nutrition;[41,44,47] and increase a sense of well-being.

Strength training is the cornerstone to any rehabilitation program. Significant muscle atrophy occurs after injury (primarily type I, slow twitch, aerobic endurance fibers), compounded by immobilization.[23,43,44] These changes take

TABLE 2. Rehabilitation Progression

I. Week One
   A. Flexibility daily
   B. Alternate days, trunk extensors and abdominals
   C. Trunk extensors, exercises 3 days/per week (one set, 20 reps.);
      Sport Cord extensors (one set, 25 reps.)
   D. Abdominals—3 days per week (one set, 25 reps.),
      Roman chair (two sets, 20 reps.),
      Sport Cord (one set, 25 reps.)
   E. Lower extremities—4 days per week, Sport Cord
   F. Aerobic conditioning—30 minutes/5 times per week, any day

II. Week Two
   A. Flexibility daily
   B. Trunk extensors (two sets, 20 reps.), Sport Cord (two sets, 25 reps.)
   C. Abdominals—all exercises (two sets, 20 reps.),
      Sport Cord (two sets, 20 reps.),
      Roman chair (two sets, 20 reps.)
   D. Lower extremities (two sets, 20 reps.)
   E. Aerobic Conditioning (two sets, 20 reps.)

III. Week Three–Six
   A. Flexibility daily
   B. Trunk extensors—all exercises (three sets, 20 reps.),
      Sport Cord (three sets, 50 reps.)
   C. Abdominals—all exercises (three sets, 20 reps.),
      Roman chair (three sets, 20 reps.),
      Sport Cord (three sets, 50 reps.)
   D. Lower extremities—(three sets, 50 reps.)
   E. Aerobic conditioning—(three sets, 50 reps.)

IV. Week Seven–Nine
   A. Same as weeks three–six
   B. Add forward and backward running against Sport Cord 5 minutes each way, 4 days per week

V. Week Ten–Twelve
   A. Same as weeks seven–nine
   B. Add Sport Cord side to side lateral agilities (two sets, 50 reps. each way, 4 days per week)

place within 2 weeks and require up to a year of aggressive training to overcome.[35,37,43,44] Muscle atrophy is especially worrisome, since the decreased endurance of trunk extensor muscle is a predictor of low back pain and is associated with both initial onset and recurrent episodes of pain.[7,8,20,30,31] Gracovetsky has also demonstrated the importance of abdominal, gluteus, and quadricep muscles in powering spinal/trunk movements and in spinal stabilization.[26]

Our strength training program primarily strengthens the abdominals, gluteus, and quadricep muscles, and to a lesser extent spinal musculature. We use isotonic exercises with emphasis on proper form and prolonged repetitions. We also stress eccentric as well as concentric contraction and proprioception to obtain maximum strength gains. our clinic deemphasizes machines and relies on a simple rehabilitation device called the Sport Cord. This device is similar to surgical tubing but is much more versatile. Resistance can be varied; eccentric and concentric contraction as well as proprioception can be incorporated. The device is inexpensive, easy to use, easy to transport, and a proven rehabilitation tool in a sports medicine rehabilitation model.[43] Because it is so easy to use and versatile, patient compliance is much greater. Patients are not programmed to rely on machines and technology, but instead take responsibility for their rehabilitation.

Aerobic exercise is essential to return a back patient to health. Aerobic fitness decreases the incidence of low back pain, speeds recovery, and reduced recurrence.[11,12] Additionally, aerobic exercise can increase pain tolerance by activating the central endorphin systems.[13,14,39,45] This alters pain perception[42] and, in combination with strength training, increases functional capacity.[14,52]

If conservative care fails, then surgical therapy may be indicated. Persistent pain secondary to well established HNP, in spite of maximal pain control efforts, physical rehabilitation, behavioral therapy, and time, is an acceptable indication for surgical intervention. When to operate must be individualized, depending on specific circumstances. The only absolute surgical indications are cauda equina syndrome and progressive motor loss.[32] Pain is a relative indication. Surgery to relieve pain does not change the natural history of HNP.[46] However, early surgery may be more appropriate in an elite athlete. This is because the athlete cannot control his activity level and remain competitive. In addition, there is increased incidence of recurrence of pain in the nonoperated group.[27] Early surgery is the preferred option in order to return an athlete with an HNP to competition quickly, with the least chance of recurrence and without deconditioning.

In order to fully rehabilitate a patient with HNP and keep him well, he or she must be continued on a maintenance rehabilitation program. Body mechanics, flexibility, strength, and aerobics must be reinforced to prevent recurrence or additional injury. A good maintenance program should include constant awareness of body mechanics (possibly a back school refresher), daily stretching, and strength training with aerobics 3–4 times per week.

SUMMARY

In this case report, an elite skier had acute low back pain with radicular leg pain suggesting HNP. Diagnosis was delayed approximately 3 months, and rehabilitation was more consistent with that for a deconditioned, chronic low back pain patient than for an elite athlete. The patient was returned to competition without a diagnosis or effective treatment. He had several recurrent injuries prior to diagnostic workup. Percutaneous discectomy was performed on a noncontained HNP with predictable result.[38] This case emphasizes the importance of appropriate surgery. The patient was returned to an inadequate rehabilitation program for approximately 6–7 months without any improvement.

Repeat CT scan revealed a large L4–5 HNP that was consistent with the history and physical exam. Appropriate surgery was performed. Surgery was followed by immediate, aggressive physical training based on the physiology of inflammation control, healing, spinal biomechanics, strength training, aerobic fitness, and maintenance. This athlete has returned to competitive status. We feel that an aggressive approach to athletes with HNP is appropriate and has a much greater likelihood for success than conventional treatment.

REFERENCES

1. Akeson WH, Amiel D, La Violette D: The connective tissue response to immobility: A study of the condroitin 4 and 6 sulfate and dermatan sulfate changes in periarticular connective tissue of control and immobilized knees of dogs. Clin Orthop 51:183–197, 1967.
2. Akeson WH, Woo SL-Y, Amiel D: Biomechanical and biochemical changes in periarticular connective tissue during contracture development in the immobilized rabbit knee. Connect Tissue Res 2:315–323, 1974.
3. Akeson WH, Woo SL-Y, Amiel D, et al: The connective tissue response to immobility: Biochemical changes in periarticular connective tissue of the immobilized rabbit knee. Clin Orthop 93:356–362, 1973.
4. Akeson WH, Woo SL-Y, Amiel D, et al: Rapid recovery from contracture in rabbit hindlimbs: A correlative biomechanical and biochemical study. Clin Orthop 122:359–365, 1977.
5. Anlie E, Weber H, Holme I: Treatment of acute low back pain with proxicam: Results of a double-blind placebo controlled trial. Spine 12:473–476, 1987.
6. Arvidsson RI, Eriksson E: Double-blind trial of NSAID versus placebo during rehabilitation. Orthopedics 10:1007–1014, 1987.
7. Bierng-Sorensen F: A one-year prospective study of low back trouble in the general population; prognostic value of low back history of physical measurement. Dan Med Bull 31:362–375, 1974.
8. Bierng-Sorensen F: Physical measurements as risk indicators for low back trouble over a one year period. Spine 9:106–119, 1984.
9. Booth FW: Effective limb immobilization on skeletal muscle. J Appl Physiol Respir Environ Exerc Physiol 52:1113–1118, 1982.
10. Booth FW, Gollnick PD: Effective disuse on the structure and function of skeletal muscle. Med Sci Sports Exerc 15:415–420, 1983.
11. Cady LD, Bischoff DP, O'Connell ER, et al: Strength and fitness in subsequent back injuries in firefighters. J Occup Med 21:69 272, 1979.
12. Cady LD, Thomas PC, Karwasky RJ: Program for increasing health and physical fitness in firefighters. J Occup Med 27:110–115, 1985.
13. Chuang-Shyu B, Andersson S, Thoren P: Endorphin-mediated increase in pain threshold induced by longlasting exercise in rats. Life Sci 30:833–840, 1982.
14. Colte E, Wardlaw S, Frantz A: The effect of running on plasma B-endorphin. Life Sci 28:1637–1640, 1981.
15. Cooper R: Alterations during immobilization and regeneration of skeletal muscle in rats. J Bone Joint Surg 54A:919–953, 1972.
16. Costill DL, Coyle EF, Fink WF, et al: Adaptations in skeletal muscle following strength training. J Appl Physiol Respir Environ Exerc Physiol 46:96–99, 1979.
17. Cuckler JN, Bernini P, Wiesel S, et al: Use of epidural steroids in the treatment of lumbar radicular pain. J Bone Joint Surg 67:63–66, 1985.
18. Dahners LE, Gilbert JA, Lester DE, et al: The effect of non-steroidal anti-inflammatory drug on the healing of ligaments. Am J Sports Med 16:641–646, 1988.
19. Dapas F, Hartman S, Martinez L: Baclofen for the treatment of acute low back syndrome. Spine 10:345–349, 1985.
20. DeVries HA: EMG fatigue curves in postural muscles. Possible etiology for idiopathic low back pain. Am J Phys Med 47:175–181, 1968.
21. Dilke T, Burry H, Grahame R: Extradural corticosteroid injections in the management of lumbar nerve root compression. Br Med J 2:635–637, 1973.
22. Enneking WF, Horowitz M: The intra-articular effects of immobilization on the human knee. J Bone Joint Surg 54A:973–985, 1972.
23. Eriksson E, Haggmark T: Comparison of isometric muscle training and electrical stimulations supplementing isometric muscle training and the recovery after major knee ligament surgery. Am J Sports Med 7:169–171, 1979.
24. Falch JA: The effect of physical activity on a skeleton. Scand J Social Med 29(supp):55–58, 1982.
25. Gould N, Donnermeyer D, Pope N, et al: Transcutaneous muscle stimulation as a method to retard disuse atrophy. Clin Orthop 164:215–220, 1982.
26. Gracovetsky S, Farfan HF: The optimum spine. Spine 11:543–573, 1986.
27. Hakelius A: Progress in sciatica. Acta Orthop Scand 129:6–76, 1970.
28. Heyse-Moore G: A rational approach to the use of epidural medication in the treatment of sciatric pain. Acta Orthop Scand 49:366–270, 1978.
29. Higgins RW, Steadman JR: Anterior cruciate ligament repair in world class skiers. Am J Sports Med 15:439–447, 1987.

30. Hoyt WH, Hunt HH, DePouw MA, et al: Electromyographic assessment of chronic low back syndrome. J Am Osteopath Assoc 80:57–59, 1981.
31. Jayasinghe WJ, Harding CH, Anderson JAD et al: EMG investigation of postural fatigue in low back pain—a preliminary study. Electromyogr Clin Neurophysiol 18:191–198, 1980.
32. Kostuik JP, Harrington I, Alexander D, et al: Cauda equina syndrome in lumbar disc herniation. J Bone Joint Surg 68:386–391, 1986.
33. Kramer WJ, Deschenes MR, Fleck SJ. Physiological adaptations to resistance exercise: Implications for athletic conditioning. Int J Sports Med 6:246–256, 1988.
34. Larios GS, Tipton CM, Cooper RR: Influence of physical activity on ligament insertions in the knees of dogs. J Bone Joint Surg 53A:275–286, 1971.
35. McDonagh MJ, Davies CT: Adaptive responses of mammalian skeletal muscle to exercise with highloads. Eur J Appl Physiol 52:139–155, 1984.
36. Modic MT, Masaryk T, Boumphrey F, et al: Lumbar herniated disc disease and canal stenosis: Prospective evaluation by surface coil MR, CT, and myelography. AJNR 7:709–717, 1986.
37. Noyes F, Torvik PF, Hyde WB, et al: Biomechanics of ligament failure—WWI. Analysis of immobilization, exercise, and reconditioning effects in primates. J Bone Joint Surg 56A:1406–1418, 1974.
38. Onik G, Helms C (eds): Automated Percutaneous Lumbar Discectomy. San Francisco, Radiology, Research and Education Foundation, 1988.
39. Puig M, Laorden M, Moiralles F: Endorphin levels in cerebral spinal fluid of patients with postoperative and chronic pain. J Anesthesiol 57:1, 1982.
40. Salter RB, Hamilton HW, Wedge JH, et al: Clinical application of basic research on continuous passive motion for disorders and injuries of the synovial joint: A preliminary report of a feasibility study. J Orthop Res 1:325–342, 1984.
41. Salter RB, Simmonds DF, Malcolm EW, et al: Biologic effects of continuous passive motion on the healing of fullthickness defects in articular cartilage: A experimental investigation of the rabbit. J Bone Joint Surg 62A:1232–1251, 1980.
42. Scott V, Gijsbers K: Pain perception in competitive swimmers. Br Med J 283:91, 1981.
43. Silfverskoild JP, Steadman JR, Higgins RW, et al: Rehabilitation of the anterior cruciate ligament in the athlete. Int J Sports Med 6:308–319, 1988.
44. Steadman JR, Bodner RJ, Rodkey WG: Protective role of training and conditioning in sports induced inflammation; early return to function after major knee injury or surgery (submitted for publication).
45. Terenius L: Endorphins in pain. Fornt Horm Res 8:162–167, 1981.
46. Weber H: Lumbar disc herniation: Controlled prospective study with 10 years of observation. Spine 8:31–141, 1983.
47. Woo SL-Y, Buckwalter JA, eds: Injury Repair of the Musculoskeletal Soft Tissues. Parkridge, IL, American Academy of Orthopaedic Surgeons, 114–117, 1988.
48. Woo SL-Y, Gomez MA, Seguchi Y, et al: Measurement of mechanical properties of ligament substance of bone-ligament-bone preparation. J Orthop Res 1:22–29, 1983.
49. Woo SL-Y, Gomez MA, Sites TJ, et al: The biomechanical morphological changes in the medial collateral ligament of the rabbit after immobilization and remobilization. J Bone Joint Surg 69A:1200–1211, 1987.
50. Woo SL-Y, Ritter MA, Amiel D, et al: The biomechanical and biomechanical properties of Swann tendons—longterm effects of exercise on the digital extensors. Connect Tissue Res 7:177–183, 1980.
51. Yates DW: Comparison of the types of epidural injection commonly used in the treatment of low back pain and sciatica. Rheumatol Rehabil 17:181, 1978.
52. Young R: The effect of regular exercise on cognitive functioning in personality. Br J Sports Med 13:110–117, 1979.

Editor's Note

1. The authors appropriately stress the importance of strength, flexibility, and endurance. An aggressive approach based on an accurate diagnosis is essential to avoid deconditioning and optimize results.
2. Percutaneous discectomy, although often quite successful in the athlete, is contraindicated in the situation of a noncontained herniated disc.

Case Report 4

AN ADOLESCENT SKIER WITH INCREASING LOW BACK PAIN

John W. Frymoyer, MD

A 15-year-old male, Junior Olympic contender in downhill skiing presented 5 years ago with a 3-month history of increasing low back pain. Initial physical examination was normal except for mild tenderness over the S1 spinous process and limitation of straight leg raising to 80 degrees because of hamstring tightness. Initial radiographs showed a questionable unilateral spondylolysis at L5. A bone scan revealed bilateral increased uptake at the pars interarticularis. He was treated with an anterior-opening Boston brace, which was used consistently for 3 months. The back pain gradually diminished.

Four months after the onset of symptoms, oblique spinal radiographs showed definite bilateral spondylolytic defects. He had resumed his training regimen during the 4-month interval, except for avoidance of bench presses and forced twisting exercises, and also had won a number of major competitions. In the ensuing 8 months he continued to wear his brace when he was racing competitively or doing weight training.

One year after the onset of symptoms the patient's back pain acutely increased. Physical examination was unchanged except for increased hamstring tightness, but spinal radiographs now suggested a 3 to 4 mm anterior slip at the L5–S1 level. After a 1-week period of bedrest, he gradually resumed training and intermittently used his brace while racing.

Over the ensuing 3 years, the patient improved his national junior standing and reported only mild back pain, usually relieved by stretching. Radiographs at

1-year intervals showed no increase in the degree of slip. He entered college, raced competitively at the intercollegiate level, and trained each summer with the Olympic team. In his junior year he decided to enter the Pro-Am program. During the summer between his junior and senior year in college, he worked as a surveyor's assistant and also was intensively training. After a day of carrying heavy equipment, acute onset of right leg pain was noted, which increased in severity over the next 24-hours. His family physician treated him with bedrest, analgesics, and anti-inflammatory medications for a period of 1 week. Physical examination then revealed loss of lumbar lordosis, restricted spinal motion, straight leg raising productive of sciatica at 30 degrees, absence of the right ankle reflex, plantar flexor weakness, and diminished sensation in the S1 distribution. An MRI was ordered. He refused an epidural block and was treated by a rapidly tapered dose of oral steroids and encouraged to begin walking, bicycling, and swimming, in combination with intermittent bedrest.

After 2 weeks the patient's symptoms were less but his physical examination remained unchanged except for the straight leg raising test, which was now allowed to 50 degrees. The plain radiographs also were unchanged from those taken 1 year previously. Flexion-extension films showed no increase in the spondylolisthetic slip, and the MRI revealed an L5–S1 sequestered disc herniation.

Over the next 3 weeks the athlete continued the walking/bicycling program. A second period of 5 days of bedrest did not relieve his symptoms and his examination remained unchanged. He was offered the option of continued conservative treatment or surgical intervention and elected the latter. The surgical findings confirmed the MRI findings, with a large L5–S1 root. A Gill procedure, removal of the sequestered disc fragment, and intertransverse process fusion were performed from L4 to the sacrum. The L5 nerve roots were visualized and were not compressed. He was discharged from the hospital in 4 days with a Boston brace and resumed his walking and bicycling program at 10 days. It was anticipated he would begin vigorous weight training at 3 months but be kept from downhill competition until the fusion mass was mature, which was expected to be 6 months after his operation.

His current physical examination shows negative straight leg raising; weakness and sensory loss are no longer present; and apart from mild incisional pain, he has no complaints.

DISCUSSION

This case has a number of interesting and, in my experience, unusual features. There is little question that this athlete's isthmic spondylolysis was a fatigue failure as described by Wiltse,[5] based upon the symptom onset and bone scan. Appropriate early treatment of this condition in athletes, once acute symptoms have subsided, is the use of a rigid orthosis and resumption of athletic training. I have tended to discourage exercise programs that involve any repetitive flexion-extension or axial rotation because of the biomechanics of the forces producing the fatigue failure, and I have also minimized axial compressive forces based on the premise that they will translate into shear forces at the L5–S1 lordotic level. The fact that the initial radioisotope uptake was modest, combined with the radiographic findings at 3 months, indicated the potential for healing was probably minimal. Would bedrest or inactivity allow healing in this early phase? Were we too lenient in his initial management? Presented with the same history in a highly competitive athlete, I would not change the approach that was used in this patient's management, but others will probably disagree.

The second unusual feature of this patient was the acute recurrence of symptoms 1 year later, combined with radiographic evidence of slip. In a 16-year-old patient, increased slip can occur, usually combined with severe hamstring spasm (the spondylolisthetic crisis). However, this athlete had none of the radiographic features or abnormal measurements that place an individual at greater risk for this event. I am also reassured by Fredrickson's longitudinal observations of a large cohort of children and adolescents, none of whom had progressive slip over a 15-year period of observation.[1] It is worth pointing out that the L5–S1 slip, which has little propensity for increase in the late adolescent and virtually no risk for increase in the adult, is distinctly different from the less common L4–L5 isthmic lesion.

Grobler, Wiltse and I[3] have reported a series of 54 patients with the L4–L5 lesion, a significant number of whom had progressing slips, usually during their fourth decade of life. Again, we can question if avoidance of this patient's athletic program or a different exercise program, such as the McKenzie extension protocol, would have avoided this increased slip. There is no convincing evidence to guide the clinician with regard to this issue.

The third unusual feature of this patient was the disc herniation at the L5–S1 level. The risk of this development has been debated, but I have seen no patient previously with this lesion. By far the most common radiculopathy involves the L5 root, from compression either by fibrous or bony overgrowth at the level of the pars defect. In a number of skiing professionals, I have seen the combination of spondylolisthesis and L4–L5 disc herniation. These patients have profound radiculopathy, possibly because of the "double crunch" phenomenon.

Given the relative absence of low back pain over a 3-year interval, the radiographic stability of the spondylolisthesis, and the unequivocal clinical and imaging evidence of S1 radiculopathy due to disc herniation, it can be argued this patient could have been adequately treated by disc excision alone or disc excision with fusion from L5 to sacrum only, both of which would have allowed him to resume training earlier. Without certain proof, I am convinced that fusion should be part of the treatment of spondylolisthesis, except in the population over the age of 50, who present with the later symptoms of radiculopathy. Fusion from L5 to sacrum remains an operation for which my indications are uncertain. In our long-term follow-up studies of fusion,[2] L5 to sacrum fusions were associated with a 20% later occurrence of symptomatic L4–L5 disc disease that required reoperation. In comparison, only 3 to 4% of L4 to sacrum fusions required further surgery for new disease above the previous operation.

Lastly, it can be debated if the operative intervention would have been enhanced if we had used pedicle fixation. The proponents of this technique argue it gives a higher and more rapid rate of fusion and quicker relief of symptoms, which would permit, in this case, earlier return to a competitive status. Although the clinical data are not yet convincing, McAfee's elegant laboratory experiments show unequivocal evidence for the enhancement of fusion through the use of rigid fixation.[4]

In a young nonsmoker with inherent stability of the diseased level, I will continue to avoid fixation devices because: (1) they add to the operative risk, even with experienced surgeons, as measured by infection, screw misplacement, and nerve injury; (2) the S1 level is more difficult and the fixation less certain, although many of these problems can be overcome by proper screw placement; (3) a percentage of these patients will require later removal of the fixation device; and (4) basic laboratory studies indicate a risk of osteoporosis of the vertebral body due to stress shielding. Although we are discounting these long-term risks, why take a chance? Moreover, my experience with highly motivated athletes, including professional skiers and hockey players, convinces me that a rigorous training program and return to competition can be achieved in the 3- to 5-month interval following and L4 to sacrum fusion.

REFERENCES

1. Fredrickson BE, Baker D, McHolick WJ, Yuan HA, Lubicky JP: The natural history of spondylolysis and spondylolisthesis. J Bone Joint Surg 66-A:699–707, 1984.
2. Frymoyer JW, Hanley E, Howe J, Kuhlmann D, Matteri R: Disc excision and spine fusion in the management of lumbar disc disease: A minimum ten-year followup. Spine 3:1–6, 1978.
3. Grobler L, Haugh L, Wiltse L, Frymoyer J: L4–5 isthmic spondylolisthesis: Clinical and radiological review of 52 cases. Presented at the meeting of the International Society for the Study of the Lumbar Spine, Kyoto, Japan, 1989.
4. McAfee PC, Farey ID, Sutterlin CE, Gurr KR, Warden KE, Cunningham BW: Device-related osteoporosis with spinal instrumentation. Spine 14:919–926, 1989.
5. Wiltse LL, Widell EH Jr, Jackson DW, Fatigue fracture: The basic lesion in isthmic spondylolisthesis. J Bone Joint Surg 57-A:17–22, 1975.

Editor's Note

An interesting and well-documented clinical review. Dr. Frymoyer's decision to include the L4–5 segment in the fusion is discussed. Some would have evaluated this segment with discography to help decide treatment.

Although, as in this case, a herniated nucleus pulposus can occur at the level of the spondylolysis, it is more commonly associated with the level above.

Case Report 5

A 19-YEAR-OLD COLLEGE FRESHMAN TENNIS STAR WITH SECOND DEGREE ISTHMIC SPONDYLOLISTHESIS

Leon L. Wiltse, MD

A 19-year-old Caucasian man in his first year at a major university, on a tennis scholarship, was considered extremely talented, and he was aiming toward a professional career. He had a 4-year history of back trouble, but until the previous year the pain had not been severe enough to preclude him from sports. However, during the preceding year his pain had become worse. When first seen by us, he had been off tennis 8 months. He had been able to attend school but could not participate in any sports.

His chief complaint was pain in the low back, radiating into the left leg to the outer side of the left ankle (Fig. 1). No right leg pain was experienced. His pain was much worse with activity and was relieved by rest, especially when lying down.

Physical examination showed a thin male, 6-feet, 1-inch tall, weighing 172 pounds. His back appeared straight. There was no list and no visible change in body contour. He could bend to bring his fingertips within 4 inches of the floor. Straight leg raising was mildly limited, left greater than right. Sciatic tension tests were negative on the right and mildly positive on the left. Chest expansion was 3½ inches. Muscle strength was normal, and the patient was neurologically negative.

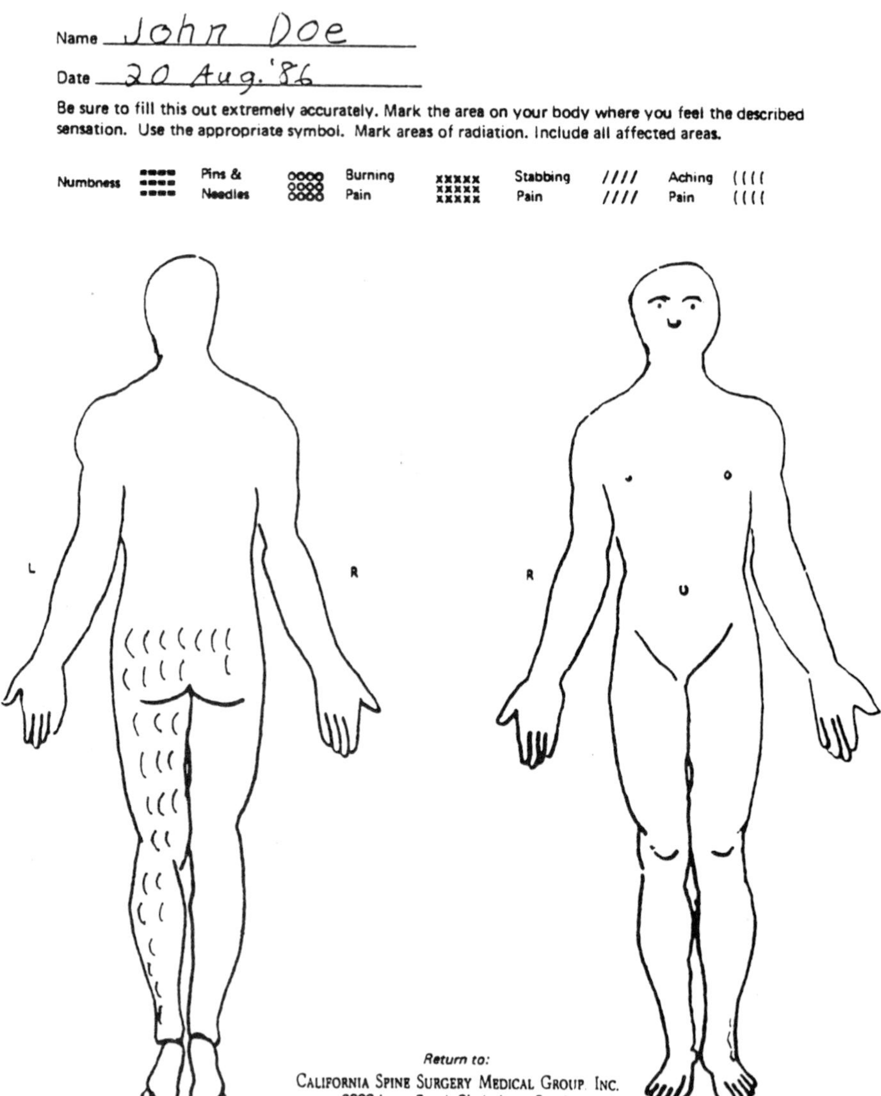

FIGURE 1. Pain drawing made by the patient on the first day seen.

X-ray studies (Fig. 2) showed a 32%[4] slip of L5 on S1, with marked disc space narrowing at L5. Above L5, the discs appeared normal on a plain x-ray film. The electromyogram was negative and the sedimentation rate was normal. Arthritis studies (RA latex and HLA B27) were negative. Bone scan showed moderate uptake in the posterior elements of L5. The sacroiliacs appeared

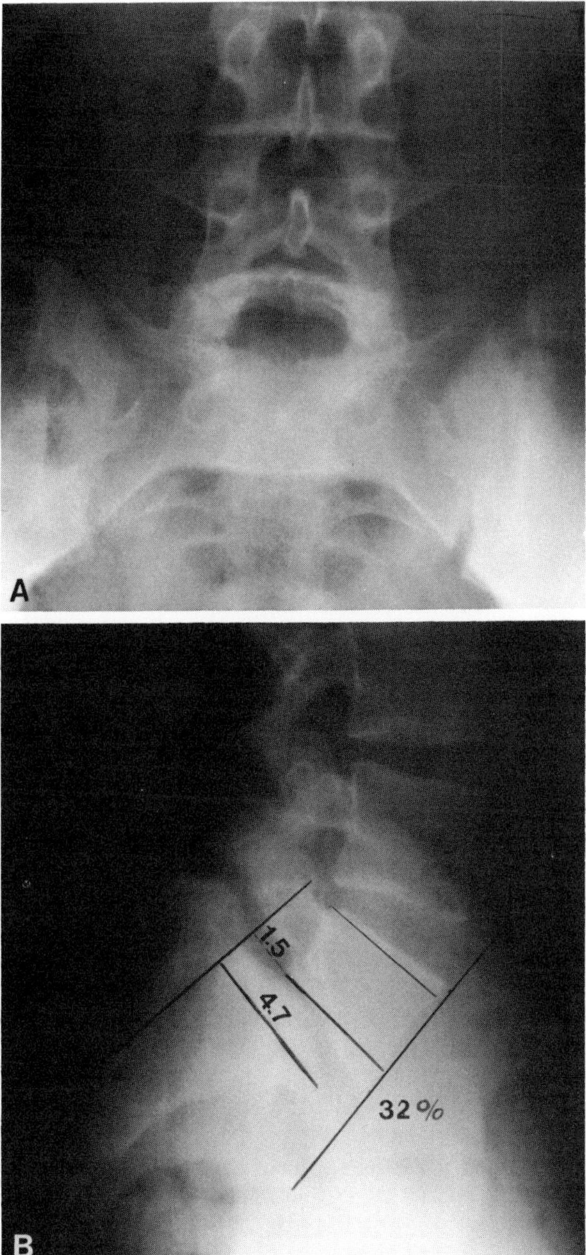

FIGURE 2. *A,* Standing AP film on the first day seen. *B,* Standing lateral film shows 32% slip. Note method of measurement of degree of slip.

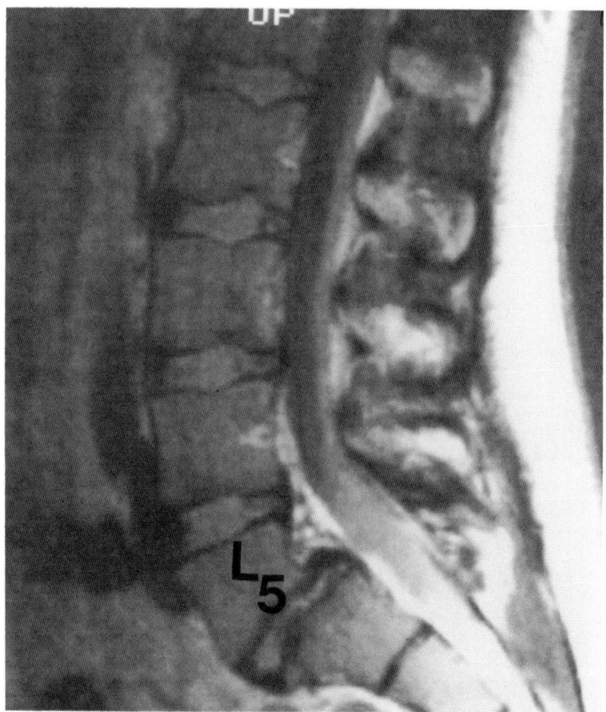

FIGURE 3. MRI before surgery. Note that the discs above L5 appear normal.

normal. Standing x-rays taken over the previous 3 years showed no increase in slip. MRI (Fig. 3) showed the L2, L3, and L4 discs to be normal in appearance, with the L5 being clearly degenerated.

Treatment had consisted of stabilization exercises, anti-inflammatories, back school, a small Velcro corset, and two epidural injections. An injection of the pars had given him 75% relief for 3 hours.

OPTIONS FOR TREATMENT

1. Continue conservative therapy and disallow athletics, hoping that patient would improve with time.
2. Surgery: If surgery were chosen, the following decisions had to be made, assuming that any surgery would include a spinal fusion.
   a. One- or two-level fusion.
   b. Decide whether or not to decompress the painful side (considering negative EMG and negative neurological exam).
   c. Whether to select the paraspinal or midline approach.
   d. Whether to use autologous or homologous bone.
   e. If autologous bone, which crest should be used?
   f. Should a discogram be done at L4 before operation?
   g. Should a bone stimulator be implanted at surgery or should a transcutaneous bone stimulator be used postoperatively?
   h. Should internal fixation be used?

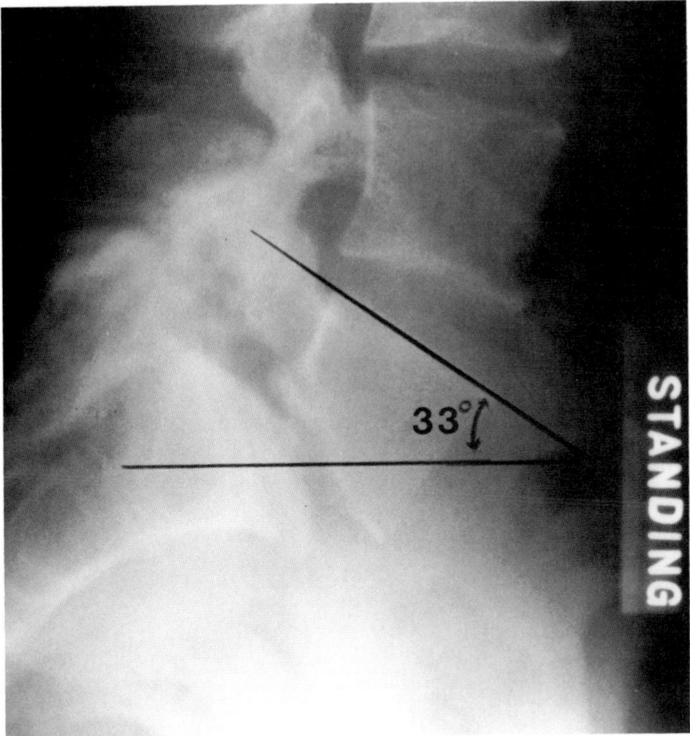

FIGURE 4. "New sacrohorizontal angle." When there is a solid fusion between L5 and S1, the angle of the top of the body of L5 with the horizontal becomes the functional sacrohorizontal angle.

DECISIONS REGARDING TREATMENT

1. It was decided to do an L5 to S1 fusion for the following reasons.
   a. The angle of the top of L5 with the horizontal was only 32%. We include L4 in the fusion only if this "new sacrohorizontal angle" is greater than 55° (Fig. 4).[4]
   b. We did not use a discogram on the patient because of his youth. If he were over 21, we would likely check the L4–5 disc by discogram.
   c. Even if the L4 disc showed early degenerative changes, if the pain reproduction test was nearly painless, the L4 would not be included in the fusion.
2. We used the paraspinal approach,[3] because by saving the midline structures:
   a. Further slip or roll virtually does not occur.
   b. The fusion rate is a little better.
3. Autologous bone was used because we believe the fusion rate is better with autologous bone.
4. We chose not to do a decompression on the painful side for the following reasons:
   a. The patient had a negative EMG and normal neurological exam.

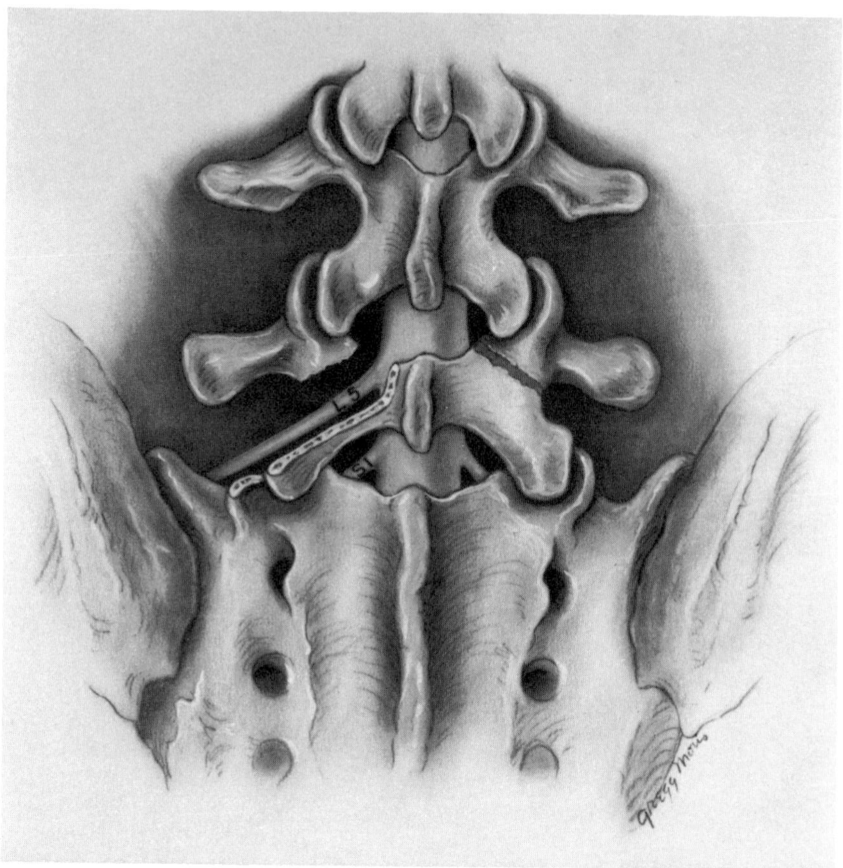

FIGURE 5. Method of channeling to decompress the L5 nerve. *Not done in this case.* (From Wiltse LL, Bateman JG, Hutchinson RH, Nelson WE: The sacrospinalis-splitting approach to the lumbar spine. J Bone Joint Surg 50A:923, 1968, with permission.)

b. His MRI showed equal narrowing of the L5 neurovascular canal on both sides, yet only one side hurt. Just because the lateral canal is narrow does not mean that the nerve is compressed to the point of producing pain.
c. His leg pain was more sclerotomal than dermatomal in distribution and accounted for only 30% of his total pain. Had the leg pain accounted for over 50% of his symptoms, we would have considered doing a unilateral decompression of the L5 spinal nerve only (Fig. 5). Had the leg pain been bilateral, even though severe, we would not decompress, since decompressing both sides severely destabilizes the spine, and one would have to consider the use of pedicle screws.

5. As a routine, we take the bone from the side opposite the leg pain. Thus, we can separate continued sciatic pain from bone graft site pain.
6. We would not implant a bone stimulator or use an external unit post-operatively unless a pseudarthrosis seemed to be developing. We have

not had a pseudarthrosis in a person below age 21 in our L5 to S1 fusions. There would be no contraindication to the spinal bone stimulator, however.

7. We have never used internal fixation in this operation in people of this age.

Operation

A one-level spinal fusion was done through a paraspinal approach, using bone graft from the painless right side (Fig. 6).

Postoperative Care

The patient was operated during summer vacation. He was allowed up in a day or two and went home from the hospital in 5 days. A single standing spot lateral x-ray, centered at the lumbosacral joint, was taken the day he left. No further slip had occurred. No corset or brace was used. He returned to school for the fall semester 6 weeks postoperation. A single standing spot lateral x-ray was again taken 1 month postoperatively checking for possible further slip. We do this routinely, but slip of significant degree has never occurred in this situation in our experience. At 6 months, bending films showed the fusion to be solid (Fig. 7). The patient gradually increased his activity and returned to competitive tennis at 1½ years postoperation and has done well since. Figure 8 is an x-ray taken 5 years postoperatively, showing a solid L5 to S1 fusion.

DISCUSSION

If the leg pain had not gone away in about 6 months postoperation and the fusion had been solid, we would have then decompressed the L5 spinal nerve on the painful side. If the fusion had not been solid at 6 months, we would have waited until it was. After fusion is solid, decompression can be done easily, since there is no danger of producing instability. We would probably decompress both the L5 and S1 nerves on the painful side, but in isthmic spondylolisthesis it is nearly always the L5 nerve that is involved. I have very rarely had to do this late decompression. If the fusion had not been solid at 6 months, I would have put on a bone stimulator.

We have not used corsets or braces in these cases.

If the leg pain is very severe postoperatively, we keep the patient horizontal for 2 to 3 weeks or even up to 6 weeks to let the pain resolve. This has been necessary only three or four times in our experience.

There have been several cases of paraplegia reported in the literature after *in situ* fusion for high-grade spondylolisthesis.[1] It has been our good fortune not to have had this complication, but patients should be watched carefully during the first few days postoperation. At any sign of neurological trouble, a posterior decompression should be done, and probably the posterior superior portion of the body of S1 should be removed. During surgery, the loose element should never be hammered upon. Only a Leksell or high-speed bur should be used to roughen the loose element, and when the Leksell is used, avoid pushing down on the loose element. The loose element is often lying against the posterior superior border of the body of S1, with only a thin, tight band, the cauda equina, in between. Even the high-speed bur carries some danger.

We used the paraspinal approach, because it leaves the midline structures intact and thus helps prevent further slip or roll.

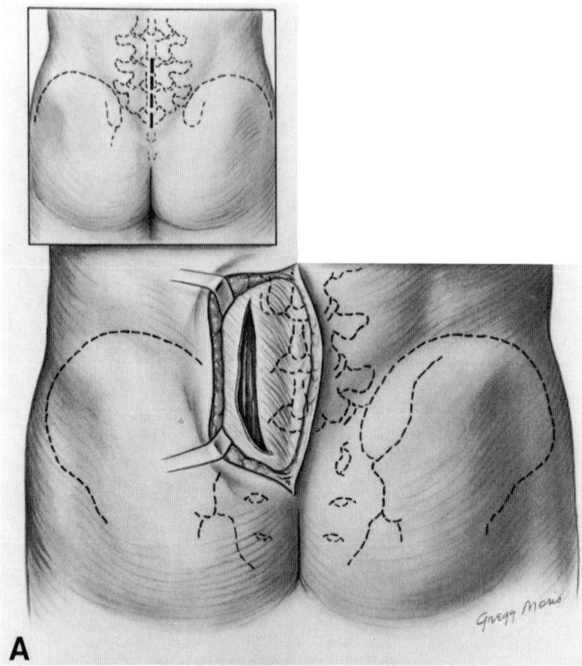

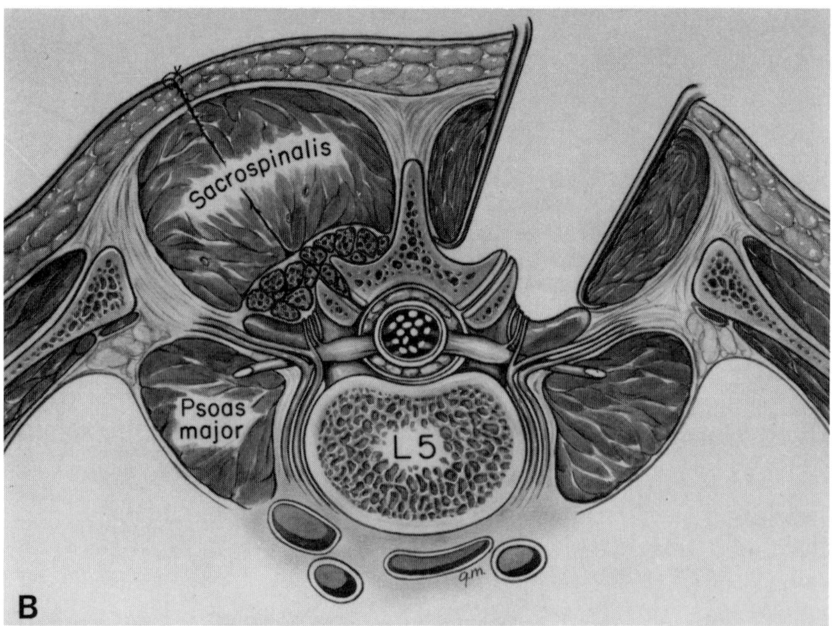

FIGURE 6. *A,* Skin incision for the paraspinal approach that we have used since 1960. Note a midline skin incision is used, but once through the skin, the fascial incisions are made 2 cm lateral to the midline. (From Wiltse LL: The paraspinal sacrospinalis-splitting approach to the lumbar spine. Clin Orthop 91:48, 1973, with permission.) *B,* Cross-sectional drawing of a paraspinal approach. (From Wiltse LL, Bateman JG, Hutchinson RH, Nelson WE: The sacrospinalis-splitting approach to the lumbar spine. J Bone Joint Surg 50A:L923, 1968, with permission.)

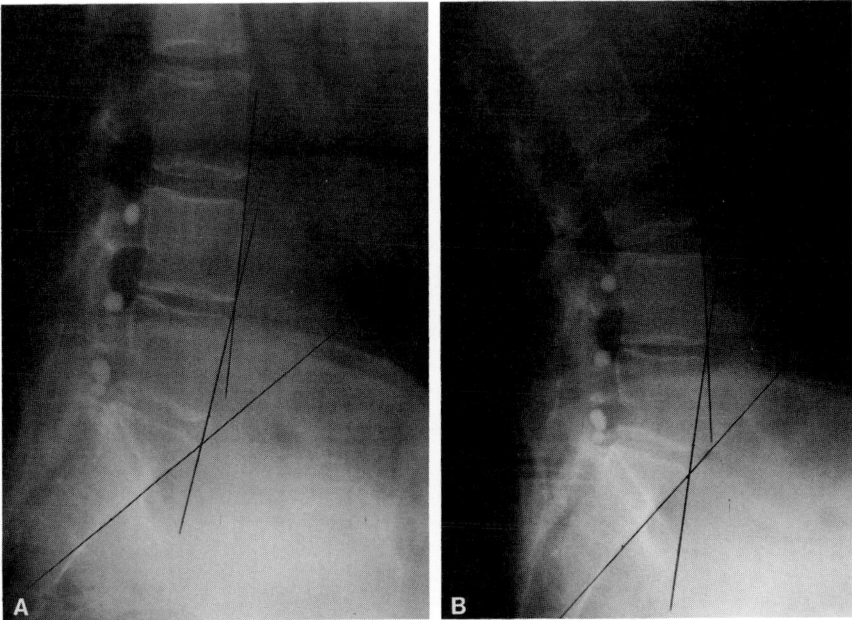

FIGURE 7. *A,* Flexion view. This example of a two-level fusion is shown to demonstrate our method of determining fusion. The case reported here had only a one-level fusion. Lines are drawn along the most definite points on the vertebral bodies. These lines must superimpose within one to two degrees to be considered a solid fusion. *B,* Extension view. We have the patient lie on his side. We find that the flexion and extension views to determine solidity of fusion superimpose better if taken lying down. The patient must not be permitted to roll on flexion and extension. Another advantage of lying-down flexion and extension views is that, if the patient has much pain, it is hard for him to bend while standing, but bending is much less painful if he or she is lying down.

REFERENCES

1. Maurice HD, Morley TR: Cauda equina lesions following fusion in situ and decompressive laminectomy for severe spondylolisthesis. Spine 14:214–216, 1989.
2. Schoenecker P, Cole H, Herring J, et al: Cauda equina syndrome following in situ fusion of severe spondylolisthesis at the lumbosacral junction (in press).
3. Wiltse LL: Paraspinous sacrospinalis-splitting approach to the lumbar spine. Clin Orthop 91:48, 1973.
4. Wiltse LL, Winter RB: Terminology and measurement of spondylolisthesis. J Bone Joint Surg 65A:768–772, 1983.

Editor's Note:

Dr. Wiltse prefers to take his bone graft from the asymptomatic side. Others prefer to take the graft from the symptomatic side, since the patient already has pain in this distribution.

This case is an interesting contrast to Dr. Frymoyer's (p. 313). In the former, fusion was performed from L4 to the sacrum with decompression at the initial surgery. Of note is that in Dr. Wiltse's experience there has been no pseudarthrosis associated with L5-S1 fusion in patients less than 21 years old.

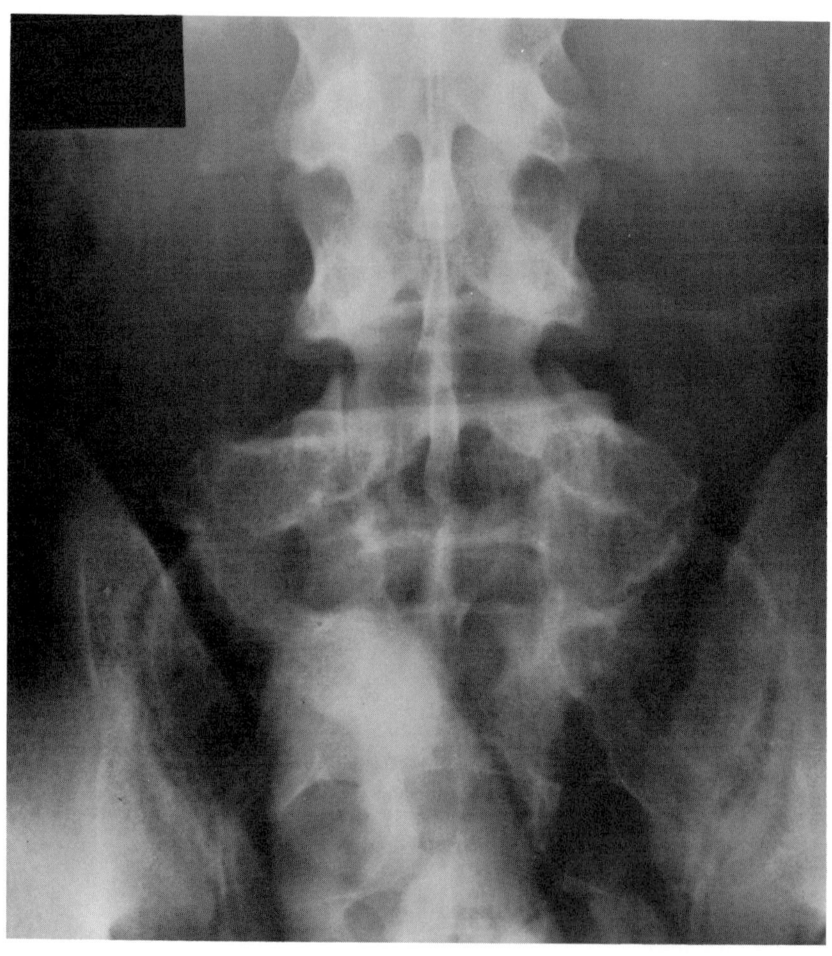

FIGURE 8. AP view showing solid fusion, L5 to S1.

Case Report 6

PAINFUL SPONDYLOLYSIS IN A YOUNG FOOTBALL PLAYER

Lyle J. Micheli, MD and James R. Kasser, MD

D.C. first presented with complaints of activity-related low back pain in November of 1987. At that time he was participating in basketball activities but had also had back pain in association with high school-level football activities the previous fall.

At the time of initial evaluation, he was found to have pain on hyperextension testing. He had no pain on forward-bending and could actually forward-bend to the level of his ankles. He had no tenderness in the back. Straight leg raising was limited to 80 degrees bilaterally by hamstring tightness, but there was no radicular pain or increase in back pain. He had full range of motion otherwise about the hips, knees, and ankles, and was neurologically intact in the lower extremities.

Plain x-rays obtained at the time showed lysis of the pars interarticularis at the L4 level bilaterally (Fig. 1). CT scan obtained at that time also showed evidence of a fracture lesion through the pars interarticularis bilaterally. Radionucleotide bone scan technetium-99 obtained at that time also showed evidence of increased uptake at the pars interarticularis.

The patient was begun on a program of exercises directed to decrease the lumbar lordosis and to increase the abdominal strength as well as pelvic flexibility and range of motion. In addition, he was fitted for an antilordotic thermoplastic brace designed with zero degrees of lordosis. He was asked to maintain fulltime use of the brace for a period of 6 months.

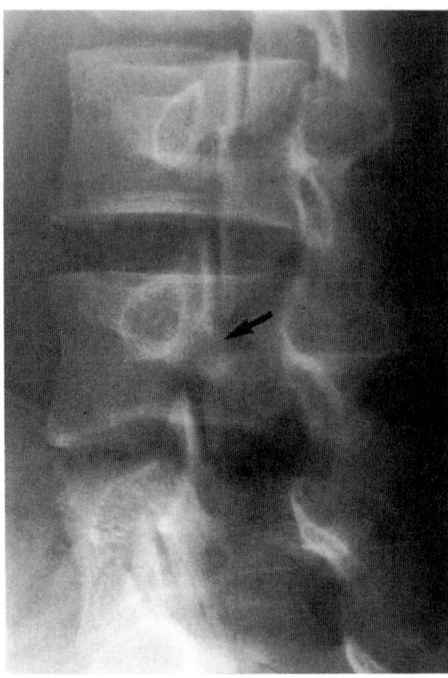

FIGURE 1. Initial oblique radiograph views demonstrate lysis of the left pars interarticularis at L4.

At the time of reevaluation on May 25, 1988, the patient was totally free of pain, had no pain on hyperextension testing in particular, and had improved his flexibility on forward-bending and rotation.

Plain x-rays at that time revealed apparent bony consolidation of the pars lesions at L4 (Figs 2, 3). In addition, repeat CT scan obtained at the time showed

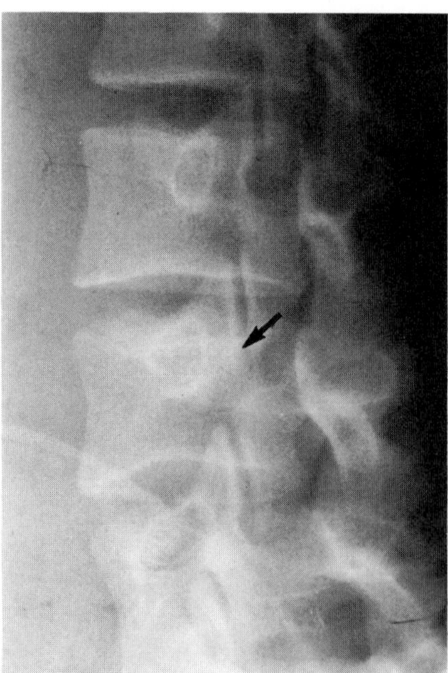

FIGURE 2. Oblique radiograph views of the left pars interarticularis at L4 following 6 months of brace treatment show bony union of the pars defect.

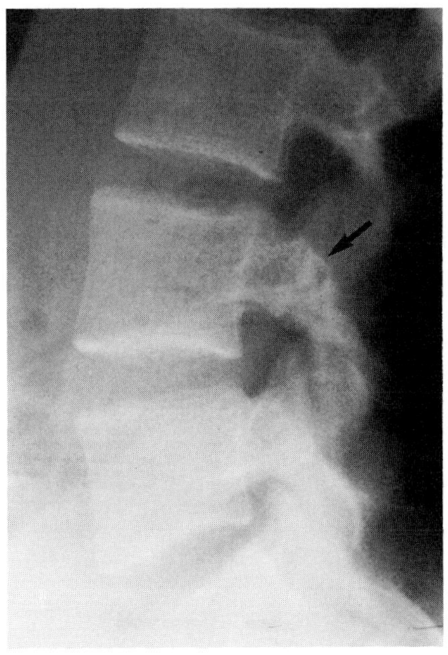

FIGURE 3. Lateral radiographs of the lumbar spine following 6 months of brace treatment show bony union at the site of previous lysis at L4.

evidence of union at the L4 level (Fig. 4). He subsequently resumed full sports activities, including football, and has remained asymptomatic.

DISCUSSION

The evidence is increasing that symptomatic spondylolytic defects of the lower lumbar spine presenting in the sports-active young athlete are most probably acquired lesions.[1,2,9,10] These lesions are, in effect, stress fractures of the pars interarticularis related to repetitive flexion or extension activities of the spine.

It is well known that there is a congenital predisposition in certain groups and certain individuals to the occurrence of lysis of the pars defect. In the study by Steiner and Micheli in 1985, the incidence of spina bifida occulta found in

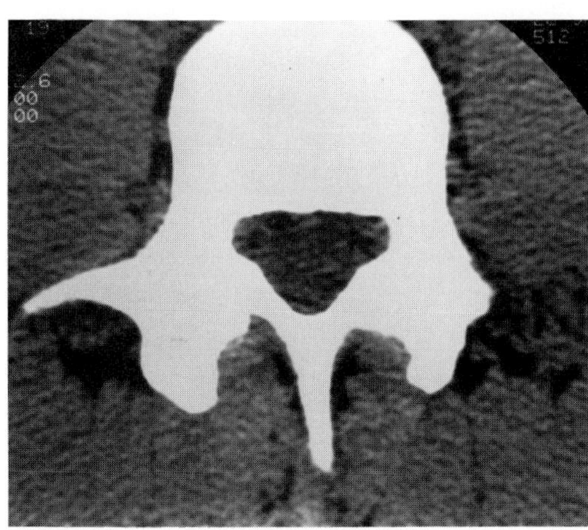

FIGURE 4. CT cut at the level of previous pars defect at L4 demonstrates bony union bilaterally.

association with symptomatic spondylolysis was significantly higher than the previously reported incidence in the general population.[8] This case suggests that immobilization combined with antilordotic exercises for a period of 6 months can be useful in assisting the healing of these lesions and allowing the restoration of full, painless sports activity.[5,7]

These observations of a congenital predisposition to the occurrence of this lesion do not contravene the acquired etiology of these injuries in athletic populations, but rather emphasize the need for careful screening of athletic candidates. The presence of spina bifida occulta in a young athlete with back pain is an important diagnostic observation that should increase the suspicion of pars injury, despite initial negative plain radiographs.[3,4,6]

REFERENCES

1. Beeler JW: Further evidence on the acquired nature of spondylolisthesis. AJR 108:796–798, 1970.
2. Ciullo JV, Jackson DW: Pars interarticularis stress reaction, spondylolysis and spondylolisthesis in gymnastics. Clin Sports Med 4:95–110, 1985.
3. Ferguson RI, McMasters JH, Stanitski CL: Low back pain in college football lineman. J Sports Med 2:63, 1974.
4. Jackson DW, Wiltse LL, Cirincione RL: Spondylolysis in the female gymnast. Clin Orthop 117:68–73, 1976.
5. Letts M, Smallman T, Afanasiev R, Gouw G: Fracture of the pars interarticularis in adolescent athletes: A clinical-biomechanical analysis. J Pediatr Orthop 6:40–46, 1986.
6. Micheli LJ: Back injuries in gymnastics. Clin Sports Med 4:85–93, 1985.
7. Micheli LJ, Hall JE, Miller ME: Use of the modified Boston brace for back injuries in athletes. Am J Sports Med 8:351–356, 1980.
8. Steiner ME, Micheli LJ: Treatment of symptomatic spondylolysis and spondylolisthesis with the modified Boston brace. Spine 10:937 943, 1985.
9. Wiltse LL: The etiology of spondylolisthesis. Clin Orthop 10:48–59, 1957.
10. Wiltse LL, Widell EH, Jackson DW: Fatigue fracture: The basic lesion in isthmic spondylolisthesis. J Bone Joint Surg 57A:17–22, 1975.

Editor's Note

This case presents a good example of conservative management leading to a return to sports and a healed anatomical situation. The use of an anti-lordotic thermoplastic brace combined with an abdominal strengthening program has proven effective. Whether this treatment regimen will be successful in a prospective group of patients with spondylolysis and a corresponding positive bone scan is yet to be determined.

Case Report 7

A 17-YEAR-OLD WHITE FEMALE GYMNAST WITH LOW BACK PAIN

Jose E. Rodriguez, MD and Stephen H. Hochschuler, MD

In August 1987, a 17-year-old white female Olympic-class gymnast presented with a history of low back pain. The patient related the onset to a relatively powerful gymnastic maneuver having occurred in April 1987. She was diagnosed as having a sprain. An anti-inflammatory medication was started and she was told to stay off gymnastics until pain-free. Two days later she resumed regular activities. At that time she was involved in gymnastic competition in Hungary and Romania and complained of intermittent symptoms.

In July 1987, the patient went on vacation with her family and engaged in wind surfing. She noted that her low back discomfort was increasing and consequently came to our attention in August of that year. She complained of severe pain in the low back region. She experienced no radiation of pain to either lower extremity and denied any numbness or tingling, or any trouble with either bowel or bladder function. There was no history of blood in either urine or stool, and she denied any history of weight loss or loss of appetite. The patient was an extremely healthy female with no medical illnesses. There was no history of allergies, and she was not taking any medication at the time of our evaluation.

On initial physical exam the patient was noted to be a well-developed, muscular, athletic female. She was able to ambulate on her toes and heels and had a normal gait. She had an excellent range of motion of her lumbar spine, but during this maneuver she complained of pain in the lumbosacral region in the area of the L4–5 facet joints. Her sitting root tests were negative bilaterally. She had normoactive and symmetric patellar and Achilles deep tendon reflexes associated with a normal sensory exam. The motor strength of the quads, hamstrings, adductors, abductors, tibialis anterior, extensor hallucis longus, and gastrocnemius were 5/5 bilaterally. She had a negative Patrick's test and normal straight leg raising and popliteal compression tests. In the prone position she had local tenderness in the lumbosacral region with a negative femoral stretch test. The x-ray studies done at that time revealed a mild left-sided lumbosacral scoliotic curve of approximately 10 degrees to the left (L3–sacrum). There was a question of a pars defect on the right side at L4. Flexion/extension views revealed hypermobility, but there was no spondylolisthesis evident. The preliminary diagnosis was lumbar syndrome with a question of a pars defect at L4 on the right. The work-up at that time included a CT scan and a bone scan. The patient was continued on nonsteroidal anti-inflammatories and was told to refrain from gymnastic activities.

A bone scan performed in August 1987 revealed mild asymmetrical increased activity on the right side of L4 (Fig. 1). Otherwise, the bone scan was considered unremarkable. A CT scan of the lumbar spine demonstrated a pars interarticularis defect on the right at L4, and thinning and sclerosis of the L4 pars interarticularis on the left. The above was associated with a 2 mm generalized central disc bulge at L4–5 and minimal degenerative changes of the facet joints. There was no bony, foraminal, or canal stenosis present.

The patient was treated conservatively. She was to avoid extension activities, with instructions to go back to gymnastics only when she was completely

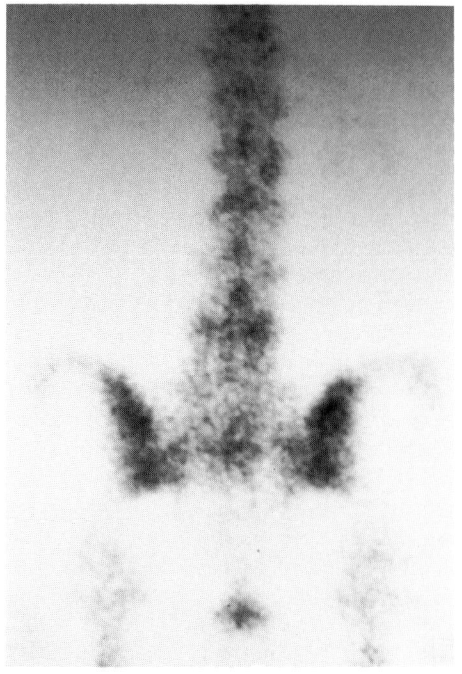

FIGURE 1. Bone scan of lumbar and pelvic area that showed mild increased uptake on the right side of L4.

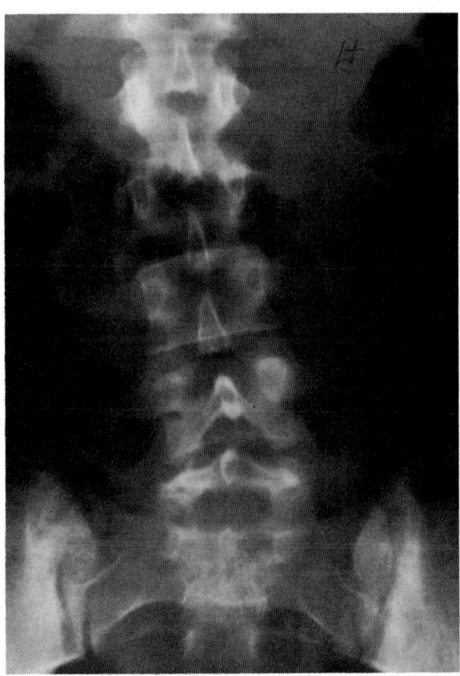

FIGURE 2. AP x-rays of the lumbar spine showing sclerosis of left L4 pedicle, which is associated with a mild curve to the left as well.

asymptomatic. In October she resumed gymnastics. On December 12, 1988, she complained of increased lumbar pain. She was told to stop her gymnastic activities, to rest, and to continue taking the nonsteroidal anti-inflammatory medication. In January 1989 she returned, complaining of lumbar pain more on the left than on the right. Repeat x-rays demonstrated no progression of her spondylolysis, but the left L4 pedicle was hypertrophic and sclerotic (Figs. 2, 3, and 4). The presence of an osteoid osteoma or osteoblastoma was considered.

A CT scan demonstrated the previously discovered spondylolysis at L4 without spondylolisthesis. There was increased bony density at the left L4 pedicle (Fig. 5). This did not appear to be either lytic or blastic. A central nidus was not identified and an osteoid osteoma was thought to be ruled out. the radiologist noted that the pedicular hypertrophy was associated with increased trabeculations probably secondary to biomechanical stresses placed on this pedicle from the contralateral pars defect. The scan showed no lumbar disc herniation and no other abnormalities.

The patient was again treated conservatively. She was advised to decrease sports activities to a minimum until her symptoms resolved. Although her symptoms have resolved, she has elected not to resume active gymnastic competition but does engage in recreational activities.

DISCUSSION

Other chapters in this issue have addressed pars interarticularis defects in the athlete. This occurs frequently in gymnasts. Wiltse reported that a spondylolytic defect often develops as a fatigue fracture secondary to repeated trauma in a predisposed individual.[2] Sherman et al. reported the incidence of unilateral hypertrophy of the pedicle associated with unilateral pars defects in 11 patients.[1]

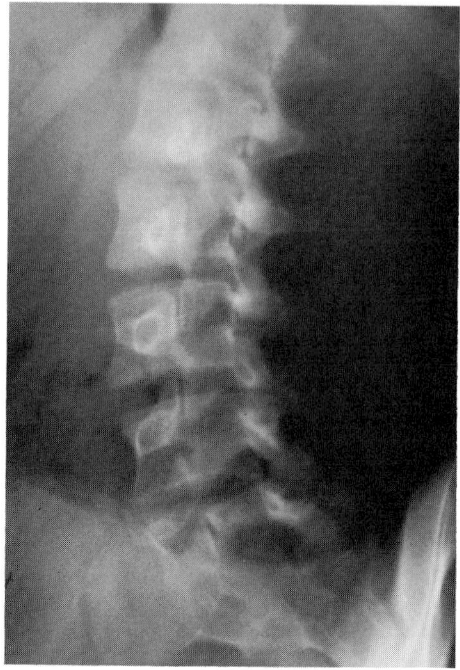

FIGURE 3. Right oblique view showing L4 PA-1 interarticularis defect.

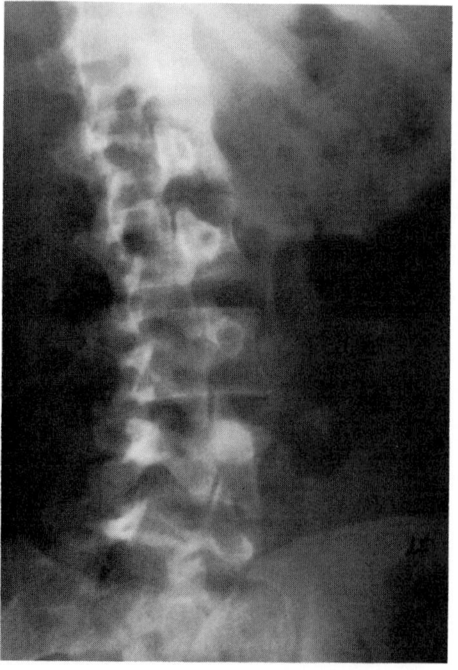

FIGURE 4. Left oblique view showing a sclerotic and hypertrophic pedicle of L4.

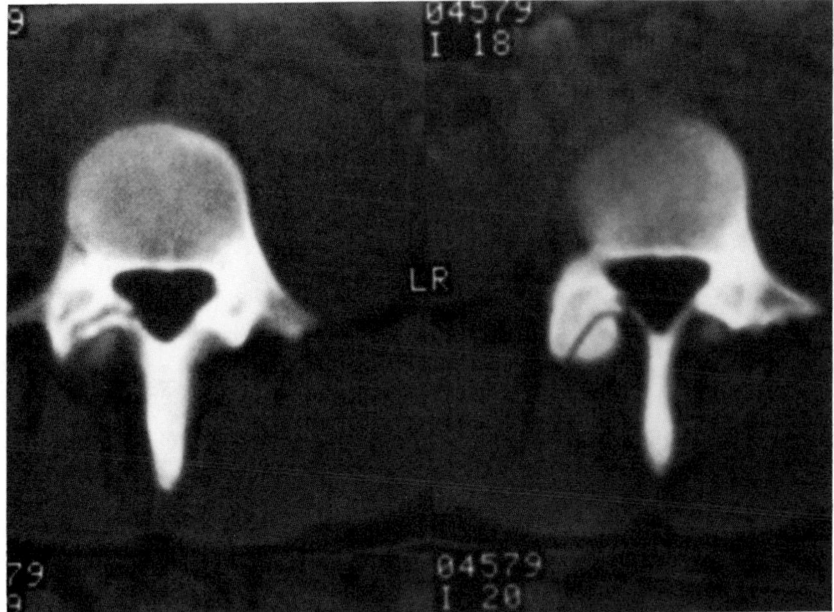

FIGURE 5. CT scan through pedicles of L4 where mild widening of the left as compared to the right is observed.

In that report, it was indicated that the unilateral hypertrophy of the pedicle represented a physiological reaction to stress on an unstable neural arch. The investigators inferred that this physiologic reaction acted as a buttressing effect. If this did not occur, a bilateral defect would develop.

It is important to rule out neoplastic lesions such as osteoid osteoma and osteoblastomas, which are seen sporadically in the spine. Osteoid osteomas can occur with painful scoliosis. The importance of making the proper diagnosis in patients with a sclerotic lesion of the posterior elements of the lumbar spine is obvious. Excision of this lesion without spine fusion has been recommended in cases with osteoid osteoma; however, excision of a pedicle without fusion in the presence of a contralateral pars defect can be expected to cause a painful instability.

CONCLUSION

When a sclerotic lesion of the posterior elements of the lumbar spine is found in the young athlete with lumbar pain, a thorough evaluation is indicated. It is important to obtain a detailed roentgenographic examination. This should include a CT scan, bone scan, and in some situations tomography. The homogeneous density of the sclerotic lesion supports a diagnosis of stress hypertrophy, whereas the presence of a nidus confirms the diagnosis of an osteoid osteoma. If there is destruction of the bone, then an osteoblastoma may be a consideration. The patient's management should be directed towards stabilizing and/or protecting further progression of the defect.

In this particular patient, our approach was to try to control the further progression of the spondylolysis and thus prevent the development of bilateral pars defects. Activities were limited and a brace was prescribed. If a neoplastic lesion is ruled out, surgery should not be considered unless spinal instability, unrelenting pain, or a neurological deficit is demonstrated.

REFERENCES AND SUGGESTED READING

1. Sherman FC, Wilkinson RH, Hall RE: Reactive sclerosis of a pedicle and spondylolysis in the lumbar spine. J Bone Joint Surg 59A:49–54, 1977.
2. Wiltse LL: Spondylolisthesis in children. Clin Orthop 21:156–163, 1961.
3. Boxall D, Bradford DS, Winter RB, Moe JH: Management of severe spondylolisthesis in children and adolescents. J Bone Joint Surg 61A:479–495, 1979.
4. Hensinger RN: Spondylolysis and spondylolisthesis in children. Park Ridge, IL, American Academy of Orthopaedic Surgeons. Instructional Course Lectures, 1983.

Editor's Note

This is a good example of a potential dilemma that can arise when dealing with back pain in athletes.

INDEX

Entries in **boldface type** indicate complete chapters.